I0072204

Biochemical Pharmacology

Edited by **Thomas Haldane**

SYRAWOOD
PUBLISHING HOUSE

New York

Published by Syrawood Publishing House,
750 Third Avenue, 9th Floor,
New York, NY 10017, USA
www.syrawoodpublishinghouse.com

Biochemical Pharmacology
Edited by Thomas Haldane

© 2016 Syrawood Publishing House

International Standard Book Number: 978-1-68286-075-5 (Hardback)

This book contains information obtained from authentic and highly regarded sources. Copyright for all individual chapters remain with the respective authors as indicated. All chapters are published with permission under the Creative Commons Attribution License or equivalent. A wide variety of references are listed. Permission and sources are indicated; for detailed attributions, please refer to the permissions page and list of contributors. Reasonable efforts have been made to publish reliable data and information, but the authors, editors and publisher cannot assume any responsibility for the validity of all materials or the consequences of their use.

The publisher's policy is to use permanent paper from mills that operate a sustainable forestry policy. Furthermore, the publisher ensures that the text paper and cover boards used have met acceptable environmental accreditation standards.

Trademark Notice: Registered trademark of products or corporate names are used only for explanation and identification without intent to infringe.

Printed in the United States of America.

Biochemical Pharmacology

Contents

Preface

The purpose of the book is to provide a glimpse into the dynamics and to present opinions and studies of some of the scientists engaged in the development of new ideas in the field from very different standpoints. This book will prove useful to students and researchers owing to its high content quality.

Biochemical pharmacology is an emerging field which applies the concepts of biochemistry for producing better quality and effective drugs. This book brings forth some ground-breaking research from across the globe which will contribute to further the scope of this field. The theories, models and techniques discussed in this book will prove beneficial to students, chemists, researchers and professionals. It aims to facilitate the growth of this discipline and set ground for new research.

At the end, I would like to appreciate all the efforts made by the authors in completing their chapters professionally. I express my deepest gratitude to all of them for contributing to this book by sharing their valuable works. A special thanks to my family and friends for their constant support in this journey.

Editor

Efficacy of *Dissotis rotundifolia* on *Trypanosoma brucei brucei* infection in rats

Abdullahi Mann[1]*, Evans C. Egwim[2], Barnabas Banji1, Nda-Umar Abdukadir[1], Mohammed Gbate[1], J. T. Ekanem[3]

[1]Department of Science Laboratory Technology, Federal Polytechnic Bida, P. M. B. 55, Bida, Niger State, Nigeria.
[2]Department of Biochemistry, Federal University of Technology Minna, P. M. B. 65, Minna Niger State Nigeria.
[3]Department of Biochemistry, University of Ilorin, P. M. B. 1515, Ilorin, Kwara State Nigeria.

The therapeutic potential of the crude extract of *Dissotis rotundifolia* was   investigated in rats infected with *Trypanosoma b. brucei*. Animals were treated orally or intraperitoneally at 200, 600 and 800 mg/kg body weight. At 800 mg/kg, parasitemia was reduced by 66.7 and 78.4% after oral and intraperitoneal administration respectively. *In vitro* exposure of blood forms to high concentration (800 mg/kg) crude extract test resulted in complete paralysis or killing within 45 s of exposure. It is concluded that *D. rotundifolia* may contain antitrypanosomal constituents.

Key words: Efficacy, trypanosoma, parasitemia, *Dissotis rotundifolia*, antitrypanosomal activity.

INTRODUCTION

African trypanosomiasis has continued to threaten human health and economical development (Kuzoe, 1993; WHO, 2000). African trypanosomes cause human sleeping sickness and livestock trypanosomiasis in sub-Saharan Africa. *Trypanosome*, the causative parasite, is most prevalent in Africa and has been responsible to a great extent for the under development, poverty and suffering in many parts of Africa (Holmes, 2000). The common parasites are *Trypanosoma brucei brucei*, *T. congolense*, *T. brucei gambiense* and *T. brucei rhodesiense*; they are unicellular and transmitted by the bite of tsetse fly as the vector of sleeping sickness in humans and related diseases in animals (Warren, 1988; Kuzoe, 1993).

Up to 80% of the Nigerian land mass is infested by the vector of the parasite, tsetse fly (genus, Glossina). Presently, the disease in cattle has been on the increase due to the menace of the vector, drug resistance and the presence of other haematophagous flies (Holmes, 2000).

In the chemotherapy of African trypanosomiasis, each of the drugs in use has its drawbacks (Kuzoe, 1993; Onyeyili and Egwu, 1995). The search for vaccination against African trypanosomiasis remains elusive and effective treatment is beset with problems of drug resistance and toxicity (Aldhous, 1994; Gutterridge, 1985;

Onyeyili and Egwu, 1995). Therefore, there is still an urgent need for the development of new, cheap, safe, and easy-to-administer drugs for the treatment of African trypanosomiasis for both human and animal and drugs of natural origin may be more effective and safer. Moreover, among the indigenes of trypanosome prevalent areas, there are several claims of medicinal plants with possible therapeutic activities, which have not been proved scientifically (Atawodi et al., 2002; Mann et al., 2003; Oliver-Bever, 1986; Onyeyili and Egwu, 1995). However, a number of African medicinal plants were evaluated for their *in vitro* trypanocidal activity (Abegaz et al., 2002; Asres et al., 2001; Atawodi et al., 2003; Freiburghaus et al., 1997; Hoet et al., 2004a, 2004b; 2007; Igweh and Onabanjo, 1989; Kamanzi et al., 2004; Ogbunugafor et al., 2007; Owolabi et al., 1990; Nok et al., 1993; Wosu and Ibe, 1989; Wurochekke and Nok, 2004). Furthermore, several plant extracts or plant derivatives were investigated *in vivo* for the antitrypanosomal efficacies in mice (Asuzu and Chineme, 1990; Asuzu and Ugwuja, 1989; Youan et al., 1997).

Dissotis rotundifolia is a medicinal plant which is widely used in Nupe ethnomedicine for treatment of trypanosomiasis (Mann et al., 2003). Gills (1992) in his collection of medicinal plants of Nigeria reported that the active constituents of *D. rotundifolia* include: insulin, saponin and tannins. It is against this background that the present investigation is conducted to primarily justify the acclaimed effi-

*Corresponding author. E-mail: abdumann@yahoo.com.

Table 1. Mean Relative weight of experimental mice infected with *Trypanosoma brucei* and treated with crude extracts of *D. rotundifolia*.

Day-post infection	Dose (mg/kg body wt)	Weight of mice (g)			
		A	B	C	D
0	200	182±2.9a	180±2.4d	173±2.6f	162±2.9h
1	200	182±2.9a	179±2.4c	173±2.6f	162±3.0h
2	600	180±1.8a	178±2.3c	171±2.5f	163±2.9h
3	600	179±2.3b	174±2.5c	168±2.6g	163±3.0h
4	800	187±1.6a	192±2.0e	166±2.7g	164±3.0h
5	800	189±1.5a	196±2.0e	162±3.2g	165±2.9

Mean = SD followed by different letters in a column are significantly different at $p < 0.05$.

cacy of *D. rotundifolia* used in curing human trypanosomal infections among the Nupe tribe in Northern Nigeria.

MATERIAL AND METHODS

Uninfected adult whistar rats were obtained from the National Institute of Trypanosomiasis Research (NITR) Jos, Nigeria, while *T. b. brucei* was obtained from the Department of Biochemistry, University of Ilorin, Kwara State, Nigeria. *D. rotundifolia* were collected from the bushes around Bida, Niger state, Nigeria and were identified at the herbarium section of the biology unit of the Federal Polytechnic Bida, Niger State, Nigeria. All the reagents used were of the BDH grades

Extraction procedure

D. rotundifolia leaves were cut into smaller pieces and dried under the laboratory conditions for 2 weeks and pulverized to powder using a hand blender. The leaf powder was extracted with ethanol by cold maceration for 48 h to obtain the ethanol extract. The extract was concentrated in a rotary evaporator under reduced pressure.

Animal handling and infection

The adult whistar rats of both sexes were allowed to acclimatize for two weeks in the animal house of the Biochemistry unit of the Department of Science Laboratory Technology of the Federal Polytechnic, Bida, Niger State, Nigeria. After acclimatizing, the rats were randomly distributed into four groups. Food and water was given without restriction. Rats in groups A, B and C were infected intraperitoneally with 0.2 ml of blood collected from an infected donor rat. Group D was not infected and served as positive control (non-infected, non-treated).

Treatment and evaluation

The crude extract of *D. rotundifolia* was reconstituted in physiological saline to treat the animals. Groups A and B was dosed with increasing concentration of extract: 200, 600 and 800 mg /kg body weight. For group A and B, treatments were conducted in triplicate per concentration that is using three rats per dosage of the extract (nine rats per group). Rats in group A received oral administration while group B received intraperitoneal administration. Rats in group C (oral) received an equivalent volume of normal saline only and

served at negative control (infected, non- treated). The rats were treated 3 times daily while blood parasitemia collected through the tail blood were counted under the light microscope and body weight were determined on daily basis.

Statistical analysis

Statistical analysis was carried out using analysis of variance (ANOVA) at ($p < 0.05$) confidence level. There is significant increase in weight of the animals in groups A and B after 3 days.

Percentage inhibition of parasitemia was calculated using following formula $Y = 100(X_1 - X_0)/ X_1$, where Y = Percentage inhibition of parasitemia, X_1 = highest blood parasitemia, X_0 = lowest blood parasitemia after commencement of treatment. The % inhibition of parasitemia values were compared using ANOVA at ($p < 0.05$) confidence level.

In vitro test

Blood samples from tails of infected rats were collected in different EDTA bottles. 1 ml of infected blood was sampled on a glass slide and exposed to 0.1 ml of the different crude extract concentrations. This was then replicated per concentration. The slides were observed under the light microscope at 15 s interval and the number of motile parasites was recorded.

RESULTS AND DISCUSSION

Table 1 shows the weight of the rats up to day–5–post infection. Rats in group D (non-infected and non-treated) showed consistent gain in weight, groups A and B showed weight loss up to day 3 and picked up there after.

Group C showed consistent loss in weight. Death among group C was recorded from day 4 and continued till the end of the experiment while no death was recorded in groups A, B and D. This result suggests that the crude extract of *D. rotundifolia* may contain antitrypanosomal constituents.

Table 2 shows parasitemia count in blood of treated infected rat at 200 and 600 mg/kg, no reduction in blood parasitemia was observed.

However, at 800 mg/kg body weight, blood parasitemia was reduced from 12.6×10^4 to 4.2×10^4 after oral dosing and from 9.7×10^4 to 2.1×10^4 after intraperitoneal dosing

Table 2. Blood parasitemia from mice infected with T. *brucei* and treated with crude extract of *D. rotundifoli*a at day post infection.

Day-post infection	Dose mg/kg	Parasitemia in blood			
		A	B	C	D
1	-	Nil	Nil	Nil	Nil
2	200	2.50×10^4	3.0×10^4	2.2×10^4	Nil
3	600	4.20×10^4	4.0×10^4	4.0×10^4	Nil
4	600	9.02×10^4	7.3×10^4	6.0×10^4	Nil
5	800	12.60×10^4	9.7×10^4	10.0×10^4	Nil
6	800	6.30×10^4	5.2×10^4	12.0×10^4	Nil
7	800	4.20×10^4	2.1×10^4	Death	
% inhibition		66.7	78.4	0	-

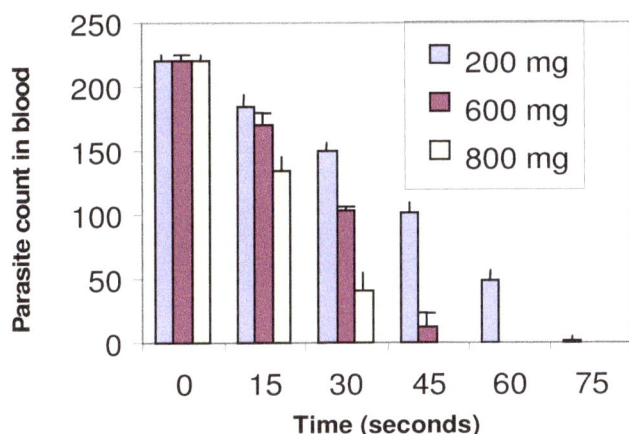

Figure 1. Exposure of blood parasite to crude extract of *D. rotundifolia*.

compared the parasitemia in group C which continued to increase. The present result confirms that the crude extract of *D. rotundifolia* contains active compounds against *T. brucei*. Oral and intraperitoneal administration showed 66.7 and 78.4% inhibition of parasitemia respectively, which can be considered as a positive result. According to Cartier (1973) who reported that 50% deparasitation is an indication of significant activity. The intraperitoneal route is more effective which can be expected because the active constituents may reach the blood stream faster and to a larger extent. The lower activity after oral administration may be due to enzymatic inactivation of active compounds in the gut or reduced absorption from the gut or a combination of both. The crude extract of *D. rotundifolia* could not eliminate blood parasitemia completely even at high concentration of 80 mg/100 g- body weight up to day 7 at which the animals in control group C were all dead.

The present observation suggests a possible treatment failure as observed by Legros et al. (1999). Legros et al. (1999) have shown that treatment failure is possible in cases of massive parasitemia at the time of the thera- peutic intervention. It is possible that the early treatments with lower concentrations of the crude extract may have

favoured treatment failure. It may be that blood parasite- mia could be completely eliminated if the treatment is initiated at high dose of crude extract of *D. rotundifolia* which is illustrated by the *in vitro* results (Figure 1).

The *in vitro* test showed that the crude extract at high concentration (800 mg/kg) was able to paralyze or kill the parasite completely within 45 s.

Further investigations should include purification of the crude extract in order to identify and isolate the active ingredient(s) before recommending the crude extract for treatment and management of trypanosomal infection.

REFERENCES

Abegaz BM, Bezabih M, Msuta T, Brun R, Menche D, Muhlbacher J, Bringmann G (2002). Gaboroquinones A and B and 4'-O-demethylknipholone-4'-O-beta-D-glucopyranoside, phenylanthraquinones from the roots of *Bulbine frutescens*. J. Nat. Prod. 65(8):1117-1121.

Aldhous P (1994). Fighting parasites on a shoe string, Science 264:1857-1859.

Asres K, Bucar F, Knauder E,Yardley V, Kendrick H, Croft SL (2001). *In vitro* antiprotozoal activity of extract and compounds from the stem bark of *Combretum molle*. Phytother. Res. 15(7):613-617.

Atawodi SE, Ameh DA, Ibrahim S, Andrew JN, Nzelibe HC, Onyike E, Anigo KM, Abu EA, James DB, Njoku GC, Sallau AB (2002). Indigenous knowledge system for treatment of trypanosomiasis in Kaduna state of Nigeria. J. Ethnopharmacol. 79:279 – 282.

Atawodi SE, Bulus T, Ibrahim S, Ameh DA, Nok AJ, Mamman M, Galadima M (2003). In vitro trypanocidal effect of methanolic extract of some Nigerian savannah plants. Afr. J. Biotech. 2(9):317-321.

Asuzu IU, Chineme CN (1990). Effects of Morinda lucida leaf extracts on Trypanosoma brucei brucei infection in mice. J. Ethnopharmacol. 30:307- 313.

Asuzu IU, Ugwuja MO (1989). A preliminary study of the biological activities of the bark extract of Piliostigma thonningii (Schum) in mice. Phytother. Res. 35:209-211.

Carver R (1973). Chemotherapy of Helminthiasis. Pergamon Press vol .1 .

Freiburghaus F, Jonker SA, Nkuna MHN, Mwasunbi LB, Brun R (1997). *In vitro* trypanocidal activity of some rare Tanzanian medicinal plants. Acta Trop. 67: 181-185.

Gills LS (1992). Ethnomedical uses of Plants in Nigeria. University of Nigerian press, Edo state Nigeria. p.103

Guttering WE (1985). Existing chemotherapy and its limitations. Br. Med. Bull. 41:162-168.

Hoet S, Opperdoes FR, Brun R, Quetin-Leclercq J (2004a). Natural products active against African trypanosomes: a step towards new drugs. Nat. Prod. Rep. 21(3):353-364.

Hoet S, Stévigny C, Block S, Opperdoes FR, Colson P, Baldeyrou

B, Lansiaux A, Bailly C, Quetin-Leclercq J (2004b). Alkaloids from *Cassytha filiformis* and Related Aporphines: Antitrypanosomal Activity, Cytotoxicity, and Interaction with DNA and Topoisomerases. Planta Med. 70 (5):407-513.

Hoet S, Pieters L, Muccioli GG, Habib-Jiwan J-L, Opperdoes FR, Quetin-Leclercq J (2007). Antitrypanosomal Activity of Triterpenoids and Sterols from the Leaves of *Strychnos spinosa* and Related Compounds. J. Nat. Prod. 70(8):1360 -1363.

Holmes P (2000). Programme against African Trypanosomiasis. Journal of Tsetse and Trypanosomiasis Information Quarterly. 23:1

Igweh AC, Onabanjo AO (1989). Chemotherapautic effects of *Annona senegalensis* in *Trypanosoma brucei brucei*. Ann. Trop. Med. Parasitol. 83:527-534.

Kamanzi AK, Schmid C, Brun R, Kone MW, Traore D (2004). Antitrypanosomal and antiplasmodial activity of medicinal plants from Cote d'Ivoire. J. Ethnopharmacol. 90(2-3):221-227.

Kuzoe FAS (1993). Current situation of African trypanomiasis. Acta Tropica 54:153- 162.

Le Grand A (1989). Anti-infectious Phytotherapy of the tree savannah, Senegal (West Africa) III: A review of the phytochemical substances and antimicrobial activity of 43 species. J. Ethnopharmacol. 25: 315-338.

Legros D, Evans S, Maino F, Enyarel JCK, Mbulanuberi D (1999). Risk factors for treatment failure after melarsoprol for *Trypamosoma brucei gambianse* Trypanosomiasis in Uganda. Journal of transactions of the Royal Society of tropic Medicine and Hygiene. 93(4):439 – 442.

Mann A, Gbate M, Nda Umar A (2003). Medicinal and Economic Plants of Nupeland. Jube-Evans Books and Publications, Bida, Niger State, Nigeria, p. 276.

Ogbunugafor HA, Okochi VI, Okpuzor J, Adedayo T, Esue S (2007). *Mitragyna ciliata* and its trypanocidal activity. Afri. J. Biotech. 6(20):2310-2313.

Oliver-Bever B (1986). Medicinal plants in tropical West Africa. Cambridge University press, Cambridge, MA.

Onyeyili RA, Egwu GO (1995). Chemotherapy of Africa trypanomiasis: A historical review. Protozool. Abstr. 5:229-243.

Owolabi OA, Makanga B, Thomas EW, Molyneux DH, Oliver RW (1990). Trypanocidal potentials of Africa woody plants. *In vitro* trials of *Khaya grandifolioli* seed extracts. J. Ethnopharmacol. 30:227-231.

Nok AJ, Esievo KAN, Lingdet I, Arowosafe S, Onyenekwe PC, Gimba CE, Kagbu JA (1993). *In vitro* activity of leaf extracts against *Trypanosoma brucei brucei*. J. Clin. Biochem. Nutr. 15:113-118.

Warren KS (1988). The global impact of parasitic diseases. In: The Biology of parasitism (Eds. England PT, Sher A.) Alan R. Liss, New York, pp 3-12.

World Health Organization (WHO) (2000). Sleeping sickness treatment and drug resistance. Journal of Tsetse and Trypanosmiasis Information Quarterly; 23:4.

Wosu LO, Ibe CC (1989). Use of extracts of *Picrilima nitida* in the treatment of experimental trypanosomiasis: A preliminary study. J. Ethnopharmacol. 25:263-268.

Wurochekke AU, Nok AJ (2004). *In vitro* anti trypanosomal activity of some medicinal plants used in the treatment of trypanosomosis in Northern Nigeria. Afr. J. Biotech. 3(9):481-483.

Youan BBC, Coulibaly S, Miezan TB, Doua F, Bamba M (1997). *In vivo* evaluation of sixteen plant extracts on mice inoculated with *Trypanosoma brucei Gambiense*. Bull. World Health Org. 75:343-348.

A Biflavonoid and a Carotenoid from *Rhus leptodictya*: Isolation, Characterization and Antibacterial Properties

Songca SP[1]*, Sebothoma C[2], Samuel BB[3] and Eloff JN[3]

[1]Faculty of Science, Engineering and Technology, P.O. Box 19712, Tecoma, 5247, East London, South Africa.
[2]Department of Chemistry and Biochemistry, Faculty of Science, University of Limpopo, Private Bag X 235, Medunsa, 0204, South Africa.
[3]Department of Paraclinical Science, Faculty of Veterinary Science, University of Pretoria, Onderstepoort, 0110, Pretoria, South Africa.

Acetone extracts of the leaves of *Rhus Leptodictya* were studied for antibacterial activity using bioautography and micro titre plate assay techniques against four nosocomial bacterial pathogens - *Escherichia coli*, *Pseudomonas aeruginosa*, *Staphylococcus aureus*, and *Enterococcus faecalis*. A bioassay guided fractionation showed that the activity was concentrated in the carbon tetrachloride fraction. A bioautography fingerprint showed that three major compounds were responsible for the antibacterial activity. Two of these compounds were isolated by a combination of solvent - solvent fractionation and chromatographic techniques. They were characterised by ^{1}HNMR, ^{13}CNMR and 2D-NMR as 2,3-dihydro-amentoflavone, a biflavonoid and lutein, a carotenoid. This is the first report on the isolation of bioactive compounds from *Rhus leptodictya*. The four test organisms were sensitive to the two bioactive compounds. We found that Gram-positive organisms were more sensitive to 2,3-dihydro-amentoflavone with MIC values of 0.03 and 0.02 mg/ml to *E. faecalis* and *S. aureus*, respectively; while Gram-negative organisms were more sensitive to Lutein with MIC values of 0.06 and 0.09 to *P. aeruginosa* and *E. coli*, respectively. The cytotoxicity was determined using a methyl thiazole tetrazolium (MTT) based colorimetric assay against Vero monkey kidney cells. The MTT assay indicated that the LC_{50} of 2,3-dihydroxy-amentoflavone to Vero cells was 9.4 µg/ml while the LC_{50} of lutein was 9.8 µg/ml. Therefore, while the two compounds were very active against test organisms of nosocomial origin, they were also quite toxic.

Key words: *Rhus leptodictya*, bioautography, 2,3-dihydro-amentoflavone, lutein, anacardiaceae.

INTRODUCTION

The emergence of antibiotic resistance by bacteria has made the development of new microbial compounds for resistant organisms critically important (Martini and Eloff, 1998). Plant-derived medicines have been part of traditional health care in most parts of the world for thousands of years and there is increasing interest in plants as a source of agents to fight microbial diseases (Palombo et al., 2001). Medicinal and poisonous plants have always played an important role in African society.

More than 80% of the population in developing countries depends on plants for their medicinal needs. Traditions of collecting, processing and applying plants and plant-based medication have been handed down from generation to generation (Fyhrquist et al., 2001). Plants have provided and will continue to provide not only directly usable drugs, but also a great variety of chemical compounds that can be used as starting points for the synthesis of new drugs with improved pharmacological properties (Ballabh, 2008); hence the need to continuously study plants for their bioactive components and the toxic effects thereof.

Rhus leptodictya is a member of the economically im-

*Corresponding author. Email: spsongca@wsu.ac.za.

portant mango family, which has about 200 species worldwide. It has about 75 to 80 trees and shrubs in southern Africa, which makes it one of the largest tree families in the region. The common names for *R. leptodictya*are mountain karee, rock karee (English); bergkaree, klipkaree (Afrikaans); inHlangushane (siSwati); Mohlwehlwe (Northern Sotho). The Manyika people use powdered roots *of R. leptodictya*for acute pain in the chest and abdominal areas. The Xhosa people use roots for gall sickness in cattle. Branch lotion and smoke from burning is used for eye complaints by Swati people (Hutchings et al., 1996). Pillay (2008) previously reported anticancer potential of this plant. Apart from the local applications for various infections, there has been no previous scientific report of the antimicrobial activities of this plant; also there is no previous report of the isolation of any compound from this plant; hence the need for the current study. We report here for the first time the antimicrobial assessment and the isolation of antibacterial compounds from *R. leptodictya*.

The leaves of *R. leptodictya* had previously been screened for anticancer activity at the Council for Scientific and Industrial Research (CSIR) in Pretoriaamong several other plants species (Fouche et al., 2008). Most of the plants showedmoderate anticancer activity with total growth inhibition (TGI) being observed at concentrations of between 6.25 and15 µg/ml. The TGI for the leaves of *R. leptodictya* against renal TK10, breast MCF7 and melanoma UACC62 cell lines were were 8.72, 55.42 and 9.83 µg/ml, respectively. The study focused on anticancer activity and there were no isolated compounds reported.

MATERIALS AND METHODS

Thin layerchromatographic plates(TLC; Kieselgel60 F254) were purchased fromMerck. The following solvents and chemicalswere obtained from Sigma-Aldrich as analytical reagents: berberine chloride, benzene, ethanol, ammoniumhydroxide, ethylacetate, methanol, chloroform, formicacid, acetone, vanillin,sulphuricacid, the *p*-iodonitrotetrazolium violetreagent and the gentamicin standard. The orbital shaker used was an MRC with twelve positions for 250 to 500 ml Erlenmeyer flasks, purchased from Labotec. The Büchner funnel was a Corning and the filter paper was a Whatman No. 1. The rotary evaporator was a Buchi R-114 fitted with a diagonally sloping water-cooled condenser. The autoclave was an Optima B class from Prestige Medical. The microplate reader was a Versamax. The water was triple distilled and passed through a deionising column before use. The test bacterial strains were obtained from the National Health Laboratory Services (NHLS). Minimal Essential Medium (MEM) and Foetal Calf Serum (FCS) were obtained from Highveld Biological, South Africa.

The plant material

The leaves and twigs of *R. leptodictya* were collected from the botanical garden at the University of Pretoria in May 2008. The plant was identified by the Botanist, Ms Laurens Middleton of the Department of Botany. A voucher specimen was deposited at the herbarium of Phytomedicine Programme Department of Paraclinical Science, University of Pretoria Onderstepoort, South Africa. The

plant was powdered and stored in glass storage containers maintained at ambient temperature in the dark in the Phytomedicine laboratory until used.

Extraction procedure

The powdered leaves and twigs (500 g) *of R. leptodictya* were extracted with 5 L of extraction solvent with shaking for 5 h on a Labotec shaking machine to facilitate the extraction process. The supernatant was filtered through Whatman No. 1 filter paper using a Buchner funnel and was evaporated at 40°C using a Buchi rotavapor R-114 Labotec. The extract was finally dried under a stream of cold air to dryness. After drying the weight of the extract was determined (26 g yield: 5.2%). Concentrations of 10 mg/ml were prepared in acetone for biological assays.

Thin layer chromatographic analysis of extracts

The extracts were analyzed using thin layer chromatography(TLC), Merck,Kieselgel60 F254 with the following solvent systems : benzene : ethanol: ammonium hydroxide (BEA)(36:4:0.4), ethylacetate : methanol : water (EMW) (40:5.4:4)and chloroform: ethylacetate:formicacid (CEF)(20:16:4).The TLC separated components were visualized as coloured spots on the plates after spraying the plates with the vanillin-sulphuric acid spray reagent (0.1 g vanillin, 28 ml methanol,1 ml sulphuric acid), followed by gently heatingthe plates to 110°C until the colour of the spots were fully developed (approximately one minute).

Bioautography assay

Four thin layer chromatography (TLC) plates were loaded with 100 µg of the extract, and dried in a stream of air before they were developed in mobile phases of varying polarities (BEA, CEF and EMW) until the solvent front reached the top of the TLC plate. The plates were dried in a stream of air. In the mean time 10 ml of a dense fresh bacterial suspension was transferred to two centrifuge tubes and centrifuged at 3500 r.p.m. for 20 min to concentrate the bacteria. The supernatant was discarded and the pellet was resuspended in 2 to 4 ml of fresh Muller Hinton (MH) broth. This was mixed on the vortex shaker and approximately 4 ml medium was then added to give the concentrated bacterial culture of each test organism. The dried plates were sprayed with the concentrated bacterial cultures of *E. coli, P. aeruginosa, S. aureus,* and *E. faecalis* until completely moist with the aid of spraying gun, and enhanced using a humidified chamber for 24 h to allow the microorganisms to grow on the plates. The plates were then sprayed with 2 mg/ml of p-iodonitrotetrazolium violet (INT) (Sigma) and incubated for 30 min. The emergence of purple-red colour resulting from the reduction of INT into the respective formazan was a positive indicator of cell viability. Clear zones were indicative of antibacterial growth activity of the extracts.

Minimal inhibitory concentration assay of the plant extracts

Minimal inhibitory concentration (MIC) is accepted as the lowest concentration of extract that inhibits growth of test organisms. The method of Eloff (1998b) was used. The assay was initiated by pouring sterile water aliquots (100 µl) into wells of microtitre plates. Exactly 100 µl of 10 mg/ml extract prepared in acetone was added in row A and mixed using a micropipette. From row A, 100µl was aspirated and added into row B and mixed with sterile water aliquots (100 µl). The procedure was repeated until all the wells were filled. An additional 100 µl in row H was discarded. Two columns were used as control, one as sterility control (no cultures were added) and the other for growth control (the extracts were replaced with 100 μl of acetone). Concentrated suspensions of microorganisms (100 μl) were added to each well except the sterility controls. The microtitre plates were sealed in a plastic bag with a plastic film sealer (Brother) before they were incubated at 37°C in a humidified incubator for 18 h. After incubation 40 μl of 0.2 mg/ml INT was added to each well and the plates were incubated for a further 2 h before observation. The development of red/purple colour, resulting from the formation of the red/purple formazan, was indicative of growth (positive indicator of cell viability). MIC values were regarded as the lowest concentrations of the extracts that inhibit the growth of the test organisms (the well of first disappearance of the red formazan colour). Gentamicin was used as reference. The experiments were performed in triplicate.

Methyl thiazole tetrozolium-based colorimetric assay (MTT)

The two isolated compounds were tested for cytotoxicity against Vero African monkey kidney cells (Vero cells) using the method described by Mosmann (1983). Berberine chloride (Sigma) was used as positive control in this method. The intensity of colour is directly proportional to the number of surviving cells. The MTT is described in detail including the cell preparations, calibration curve and the actual cyctotoxicity testing.Tests were carried out in quadruplicate and each experiment was repeated three times.

Cell preparations

A suitable passage of cells of a subconfluent culture were harvested and centrifuged at 200 g for 5 min, and the cell pellet resuspended in growth medium to a density of 2.4×10^3 cells/ml. Minimal Essential Medium (MEM) (Highveld Biological, South Africa) supplemented with 0.1% Gentamicin (Sigma) and 10% Foetal Calf Serum (FCS) (Highveld Biological, South Africa) was used as growth medium. Cells were incubated at 37°C in a 5% CO_2 atmosphere in this growth medium under sterile conditions for 48 h. The cells were subsequently dispersed. The growth medium was then removed by centrifugation and the cells were re-suspen-ded in fresh growth medium. Cells prepared in this way were ready for use in the preparation of the calibration curve and for the cytotoxicity tests.

Calibration curve

To calibrate the method, a series of cell densities ranging from 0 to 600 cells/ml were prepared and placed in the wells of microtitre plates with 96 wells. The plateswere incubated for 48 h . A 5 mg/ml solution of INT in PBS was added to the wells and the plates were incubated for 5 h, after which no further colour development was observed. Acidic DMSO was added to dissolve the blue crystals, and to make up to a final volume of 25 ml. The absorbance was measured on a UV/Vis spectrophotometer, using a test wavelength of 570 nm, a reference wavelength of 630 nm, and calibration settings of 0.00 to 1.00. The absorbance was plotted against cell density to give a linear calibration curve.

Cytotoxicity tests

Cell suspension (200 μl) was added into each well of columns 2 to 11 of a sterile 96-well microtitre plate. Growth medium (200 μl) was added into wells of columns 1 and 12. The plates were incubated for 24 h at 37°C in a 5% CO_2 incubator, until no further colour development was observed. The medium was then removed from wells using a thin tube attached to a hypodermic needle and immediately

replaced with 200 μl of test compound or berberine chloride (Sigma) (positive control) at various known concentrations. The concentration gradient of test compound and berberine chloride was obtained by quadruplicate serial dilutions prepared in growth medium. The microtitre plates containing treated and untreated cells were incubated at 37C in a 5% CO_2 incubator for 24 h. MTT (30 μl) (Sigma) (stock solution of 5 mg/ml in phosphate-buffered saline [PBS]) was added to each well and the plates incubated for a further 4 h at 37C. The medium in each well was carefully removed without disturbing the MTT crystals in the wells. The MTT formazan crystals were dissolved by adding 50 μl of DMSO to each well, followed by gentle shaking of the MTT solution. The amount of MTT reduction was measured immediately by detecting absorbance at 570 nm using a microplate reader (Versamax). The wells in column 1, containing only medium and MTT but no cells, were used to blank the reader. The LC50 values were calculated as the concentration of test compound or plant extract resulting in a 50% reduction of absorbance compared to untreated cells.

Isolation of antibacterial compounds

The dried acetone extract (26 g) was subjected to the solvent - solvent fractionation method described by Suffness and Dourous (1999) and adapted by Eloff (1998a). The bioautography fingerprint showed that two spots in the carbon tetrachloride fraction were responsible for its activity. The carbon tetrachloride extract (6 g), which had the most antibacterial compounds, was subjected to fraction collection based column chromatography on silica gel 60 (Merck). Fifty-seven fractions were collected in 100 ml test tubes. Based on TLC fingerprint, the fractions were combined to 5 fractions. Compound D1 was obtained from fraction 4 (412 mg) by precipitating with hexane. Compound D2 was obtained from Fraction 5 (669 mg) by running a second column on silica gel with a narrow gradient of Chloroform: Methanol (98:2 to 90:10). The activi-ties of these compounds on four nosocomial bacterial pathogens and their cytotoxic effects were tested using the standard proce-dures as described above.

RESULTS AND DISCUSSION

The Bioautogram in Figure 2 showed that the active compounds were mainly in the carbon tetrachloride extract. This extract showed three major active spots. Column chromatographic separation of the carbon tetrachloride fraction led to the isolation of two bioactive compounds. Compound D1 was isolated as yellowish-reddish amorphous solid. Inspection of the carbon NMR spectra showed the presence of 40 carbon resonances, with signals in the upfield and downfield region. The spectra of the isolated compound showed a characteristic pattern for carotenoids (C40 derivatives). The ^{13}C chemical shift data was compared with the ^{13}C data of previously isolated carotenoids. That the ^{13}C data for isolated compounds compared perfectly with data from the previously isolated carotenoid-lutein is shown in Table 1 (Arigoni et al., 1999). The correlation of the ^{13}CNMR data in Table 1 was considered to present conclusive identification of the compound as lutein.

The mass spectrum of compound D2 (Figure 1) shows a molecular ion at m/z 539[M - 1], which is consistent with molecular formulae of $C_{30}H_{20}O_{10}$. The fragmentation pattern is consistent with the characteristic pattern of a

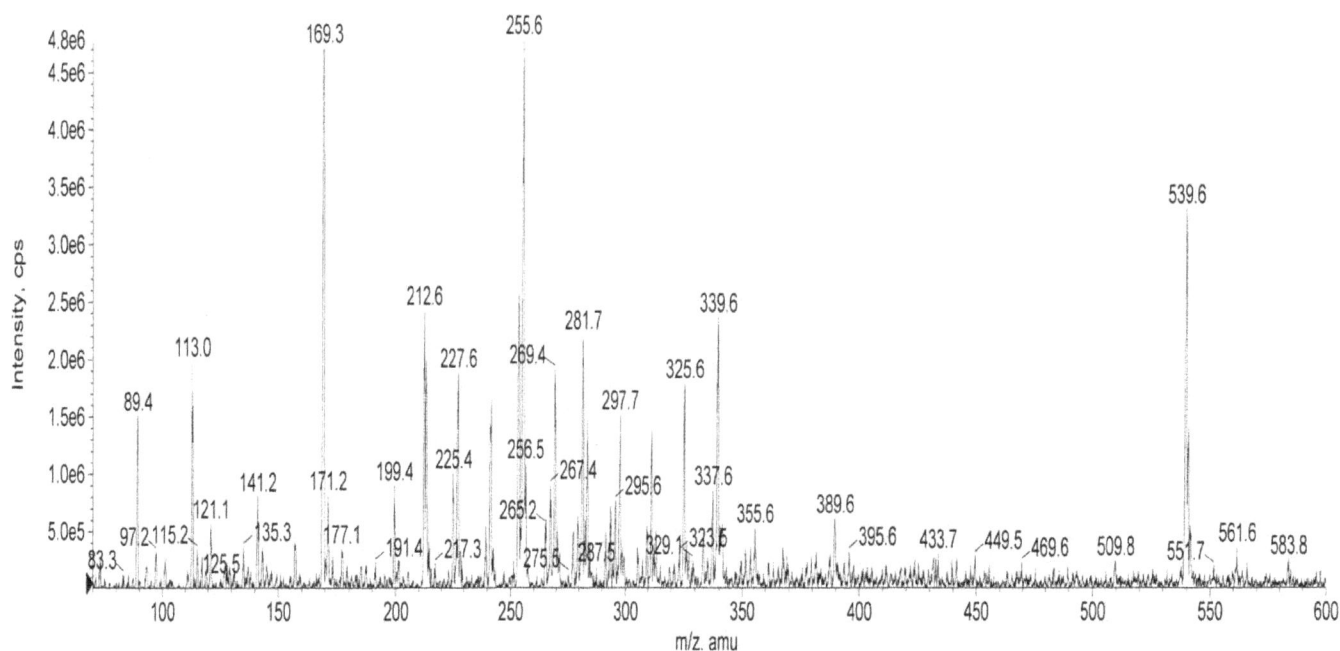

Figure 1. MS spectrum of Compound D2 .

Table 1. ^{13}C data for isolated compound compared perfectly with known data for lutein.

Carbon	Lutein	BSRL-1	Carbon	Lutein	BSRL-1	Carbon	Lutein	BSRL-1
1	37.09	37.11	7'	128.79	128.71	14	132.56	132.58
1'	34.01	34.16	8	138.47	138.49	14'	132.56	132.58
2	48.30	48.35	8'	137.68	137.56	15	130.09	130.09
2'	44.60	44.64	9	135.68	135.68	15'	130.04	130.04
3	65.04	65.09	9'	135.06	135.06	16	30.26	30.26
3'	65.89	65.94	10	131.28	131.31	16'	24.19	24.19
4	42.46	42.49	10'	130.77	130.81	17	28.72	28.68
4'	124.39	124.45	11	124.90	124.93	17'	29.50	29.46
5	126.13	126.17	11'	124.77	124.81	18	21.62	21.63
5'	137.98	137.98	12	137.53	137.56	18'	22.86	22.88
6	137.68	137.56	12'	137.53	137.56	19	12.75	12.76
6'	54.87	54.95	13	136.40	136.40	19'	13.10	13.10
7	125.53	125.59	13'	136.48	136.46	20.20'	12.81	12.81

biflavonoid, which consists of a flavanone and a flavone. The NMR spectra of compound D2 indicated two flavone units linked through the C-3 of a flavone ring to the C-8 of the second flavone. This class of compounds consists of three ring systems A, B, and C.Ring B which has a hydroxy substitution at C-4 often gives a typical 4 peak pattern of two doublets (AA'BB' system) with a characteristic coupling constant; this pattern was clearly shown in C-3, C-5, C-2 and C-6 with resonance from 6.86 to 7.68 ppm and a coupling constant of 9 Hz at ring IIB (Figure 3). The data obtained correlate with data obtained on previous isolation of biflavonoid; 2,3-dihydro amentoflavone com-

pound (Chen et al., 2005) (Figure 4).

Antibacterial studies

From the bioautography and MIC studies as shown in Figure 1 and Table 2, the four microorganisms are susceptible to the two compounds. The most susceptible organism to D1 is *P.* aeruginosa with MIC Value of 0.06 mg/ml, while compound D2 shows better activity against Gram-positive organisms with MIC value of 0.02 mg/ml. The activity of the isolated compounds compares well

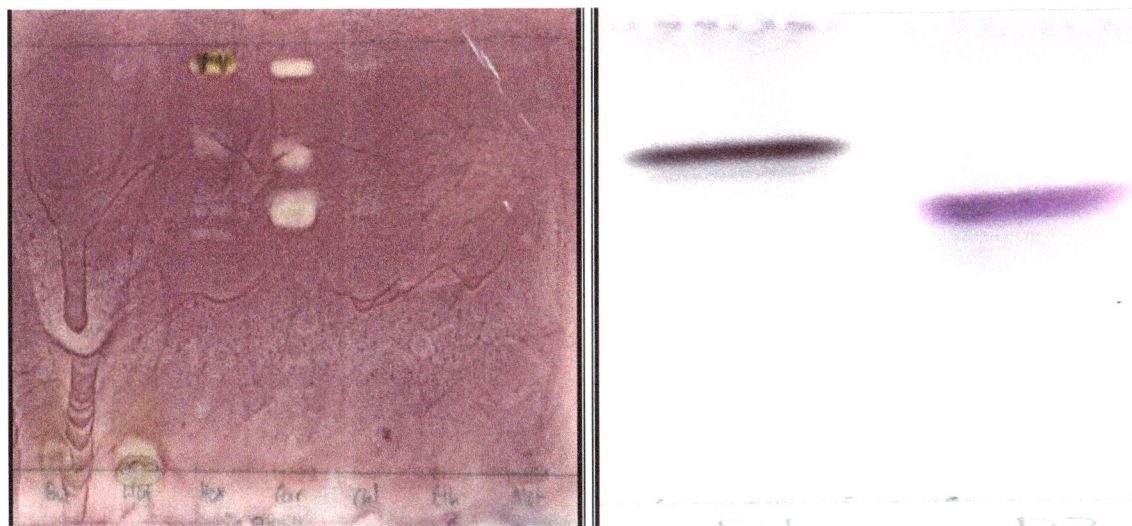

Figure 2. (a) Bioautogram of different extracts of *Rhus leptodictya*. Colorless areas denote inhibition of bacterial growth. (b) TLC chromatogram of the isolated compounds (D1 and D2).

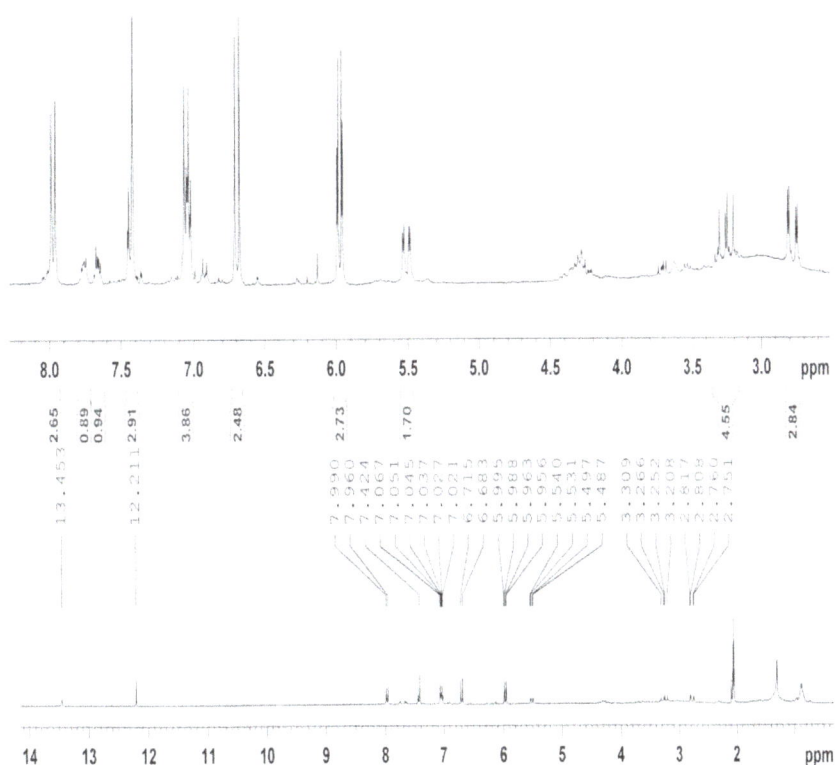

Figure 3. 1HNMR spectrum of compound D2.

with the reference compound (Gentamicin) as shown in Table 1. This could possibly account for the local application of this plant extract forvarious infections

Toxicity studies

The compounds indicated high level of cell toxicity against the cell line with LC50 of 9.4 µg/ml for 2,3-amentoflavone and 9.8 µg/ml forlutein. While the carotenoids are known from literature to show some measure of toxicity (Leal et al., 1998); 2,3-dihydro amentoflavone can be subjected to some structure activity studies to obtain an optimum compound with minimum toxicity while maintaining its good bioactivity.

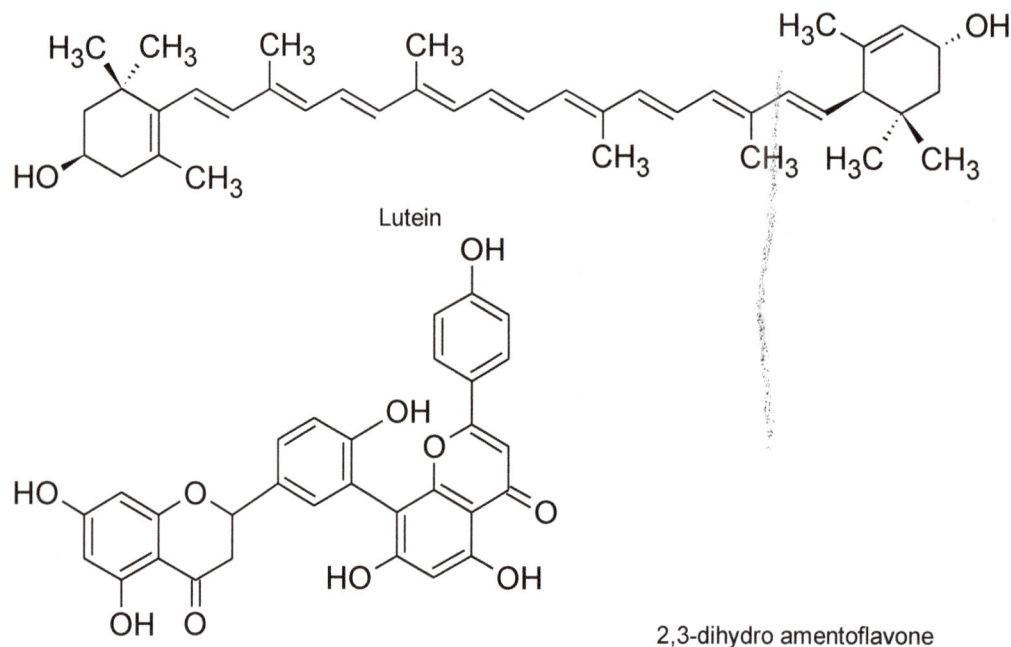

Lutein

2,3-dihydro amentoflavone

Figure 4. Compound D1: lutein, a carotenoid and D2: 2,3-dihydro amentoflavone, a biflavonoid.

Table 2. MIC values of the isolated compounds and Gentamicin control against bacterial species.

Isolated compounds	Lutein(D1) (mg/ml)	2,3-dihydro amentoflavone (D2 (mg/ml)	Gentamicin control (mg/ml)
S. aureus (+)	0.16	0.02	0.02
E. faecalis (+)	0.16	0.03	0.02
P. aeruginosa (-)	0.06	0.02	0.02
E. coli (-)	0.09	0.19	0.03

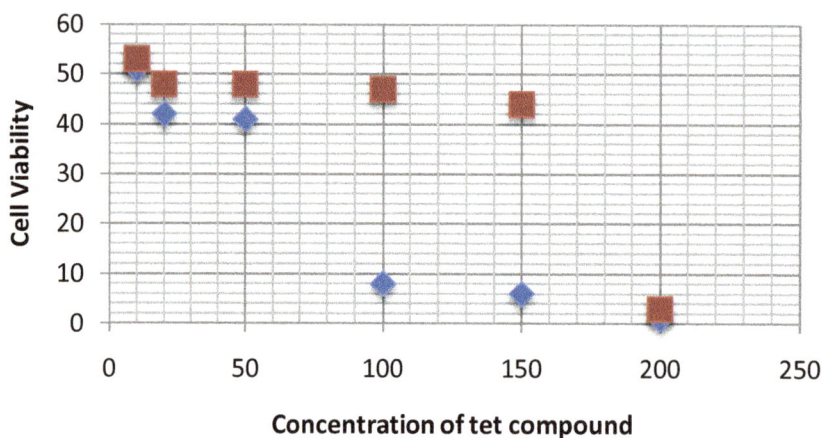

Figure 5. Dose response curve for compound D1 and D2.

The cytotoxicity dose response curve for the two compounds is shown in Figure 5.

Conclusions

Current studies report for the first time the isolation of antibacterialcompounds from the leaves of Rhus leptodictya. Of the three compounds observed in the zones of inhibition in the bioautographic fingerprint, two antibacterial compounds were isolated and identified as lutein and 2,3-dihydro amentoflavone. Four microorganisms are susceptible to the two compounds. The Gram-negative organisms were more sensitive to lutein; while Gram-positive organisms had higher sensitivity to 2,3-dihydro amentoflavone. The activity of the isolated compounds compares well with the activity of the reference compound, Gentamicin used in this study.The compounds indicated high cell toxicity against Vero monkey kidney cell lines with LC50 of 9.4 µg/ml and 9.8 µg/ml for 2,3-amentoflavoneand luteinrespectively. While the carotenoid, luteinis known from literature for its cytotoxicity, 2,3-dihydro amentoflavone can be subjected to some structure activity studies to obtain an optimum compound with minimum toxicity while maintaining its good bioactivity. The study validated the use of this plant extract in the treatment of eye, abdominal and chest ailments of infectious origin. These compounds could be lead compounds for the development of other antibacterial pharmaceuticals.

ACKNOWLEDGEMENT

We acknowledge the University of Limpopo, National Research Foundation (NRF) and PlantBio trust for financial support. Prof Abegaz of the University of Botswana for assistance with acquisition of 2D NMR spectra.

REFERENCES

Arigoni D, Esenreich W, Latzel C, Sagners S, Radykewicz T, Zenk MH, Bacher A (1999). Dimethylallyl pyrophosphate is not the committed preusor of isopentenyl pyrophosphate during terpenoid biosynthesis from 1-deoyxylose in higer plants. Biochemistry 96: 1309-1314.

Ballabh B, Chaurasia OP, Amed Z, Signh SB (2008). Traditional medicinal plants of cold desert Ladakh-Used against kidney and urinary disorders. J. Food Chem. 118: 331-339.

Chen J, Duh C, Chen JF (2005). New cytotoxic biflavonoids from Selaginella discatula. Planta Med. 71:659-665.

Eloff JN(1998a). Which extractant should be used for the screening and isolation of antimicrobial components from plants? Planta Med. 64:711-713.

Eloff JN (1998b). A sensitive and quick method to determine the minimum inhibitory concentration of plant extracts for bacteria. J. Ethnopharmacol. 60:1-8.

Fyhrquist P, Mwasumbi L, Haeggström CA, VuorelaH, Hiltunen R, Vuorela P(2001). Ethnobotanical and antimicrobial investigation on some species of Terminalia and Combretum (Combretaceae). J. Ethnopharmacol. 79:169-177.

Hutchings A, ScottA, Lewis A, Cunningham AB (1996). Zulu Medicinal Plants: An Inventory. University of Natal Press, Pietermaritzburg.

Leal M, Gonzalez E, Ruiz F, Shimada A (1998). Effects of carotenoids on cytotoxicity of T-2toxin chicken hepatocytes in vitro. Toxicol. In Vitro 12:133-139.

Martini N, Eloff JN(1998). The preliminary isolation of several antibacterial compounds from Combretum erythrophyllum (Combretaceae). J. Ethnopharmacol. 62: 255-2643.

Mosmann T(1983). Rapid colorimetric assay for cellular growth and survival: application to proliferation and cytotoxicity. J. Immunol. Methods. 65: 55-63.

Palombo EA, Semple SJ (2001). Antibacterial activity of traditional Australian medicinal plants. J. Ethnopharmacol. 77: 151-157.

Fouche G, Cragg GM, Pillay P, Kolesnikova N, Maharaj VJ, Senabe J (2008). In vitro anticancer screening of South African plants. J. Ethnopharmacol.119(3): 455-461.

3

Screening of antioxidant activity, total phenolics and GC-MS study of *Vitex negundo*

P. Praveen Kumar[1]*, S. Kumaravel[1] and C. Lalitha[2]

[1]Food Testing Laboratory, Indian Institute of Crop Processing Technology, Pudukkottai Road, Thanjavur-613 005. Tamil Nadu, India.
[2]Department of Biochemistry, Dhanalkshmi Srinivasan Arts and Science College for Women, Perambalur-621212, Tamil Nadu, India.

The present study was carried out for identification of the phytochemicals present in the *Vitex negundo* leaves and also evaluate the total phenols, total flavonoids and antioxidant activity of the leaf extract. Total phenols was carried out by Folin Ciocalteu method and the phenolic content was 27.72 mg/100 of gallic acid equivalent (GE). Antioxidant activity was evaluated by DPPH method and the leaves of *V. negundo* showed 23.21 mg/100 of Ascorbic acid Equivalent Antioxidant Capacity (AEAC). The GC-MS study also carried out and it showed the presence of phytochemicals like 4H-Pyran-4-one, 2,3-dihydro-3,5-dihydroxy-6-methyl-(RT:6.17), Phytol (RT:19.67) and Vitamin E (RT:25.11).

Key words: Total Phenols, total flavonoids, antioxidant activity, DPPH, GC-MS.

INTRODUCTION

Vitex negundo belongs to the family verbenaceae is a large aromatic shrub or a small tree of about 3M in height (Kirtikar and Basu, 1976). *V. negundo* leaves may have both central and peripheral analgesic action and also possesses antiinflammatory activity by acting through inhibition of prostaglandin biosynthesis (Telang et al., 1999). The mature fresh leaves of *V. negundo* have oral anti-inflammatory, analgesic and antihistamine properties (Dharmasiri et al., 2003).

Oxygen derived free radicals and their products are known to play an important role in the pathogenesis of chronic inflammatory disorders (Blake et al., 1981). *V. negundo* contains many polyphenolic compounds, terpenoids, glycosidic iridoids and alkaloids. Since polyphenolic compounds have high antioxidant potential, the antioxidant potency of *V. negundo* was investigated by employing various established *in vitro* systems (Om Prakash et al., 2007). The present study was carried out to study the flavonoids, phenols and antioxidant activity of *V. negundo* and the chemical constituents were studied by GC-MS.

MATERIALS AND METHODS

Collection and processing of plant material

The leaves of the plant *V. negundo* collected from Thanjavur District in the month of January, 2009 and authenticated by Dr. John Britto, Rapinat Herbarium, St. Joseph's College, Tiruchirappalli. The leaves were cleansed and shade dried for a week and grounded into uniform powder. 1 g of plant material was added to 20 ml of aqueous methanol (20%, v/v) for 18 h at room temperature. The extracts were filtered and used for the estimation of total phenols and antioxidant activity.

Total phenols

0.5 ml of freshly prepared sample was taken and diluted with 8 ml of distilled water. 0.5 ml of Folin Ciocalteu Reagent (1 N) was added and kept at 40˚C for 10 min. 1 ml of Sodium Carbonate (20%) was added and kept in dark for one hour. The color was read at 650 nm using Shimadzu UV-1650 Spectrophotmeter (Malick et al., 1980). The same procedure was repeated for all standard gallic acid solutions and standard curve obtained. The sample concentration was calculated as Gallic acid equivalent (GE).

Total flavonoids

0.5 ml of aqueous extract of sample is diluted with 3.5 ml of distilled water at zero time and 0.3 ml of 5% Sodium Nitrate was added to

*Corresponding author. E-mail: pravee.21msc@gmail.com.

*Vitex negundo-*231

IICPT TANJORE. 13-MAR-2009 + 13:40:17

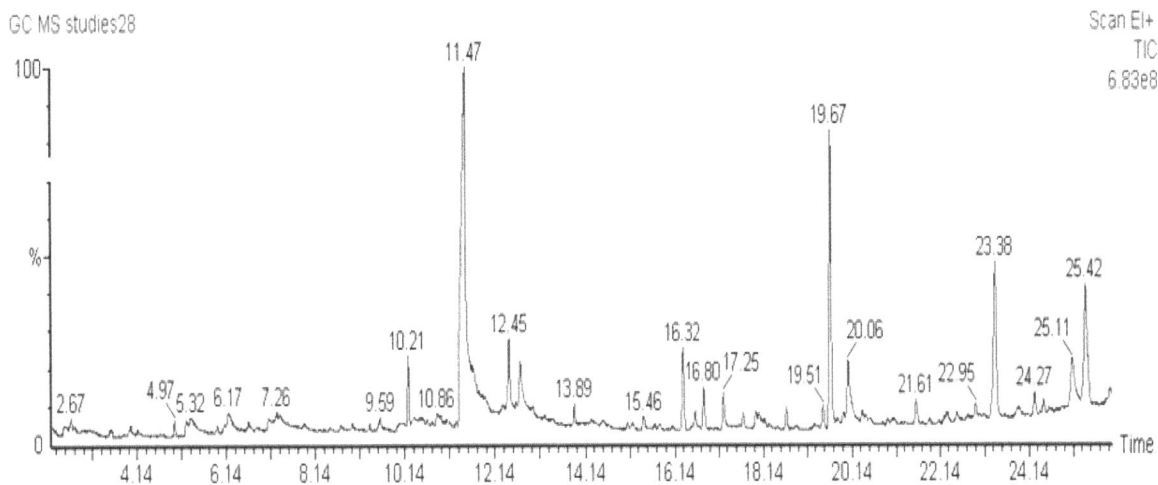

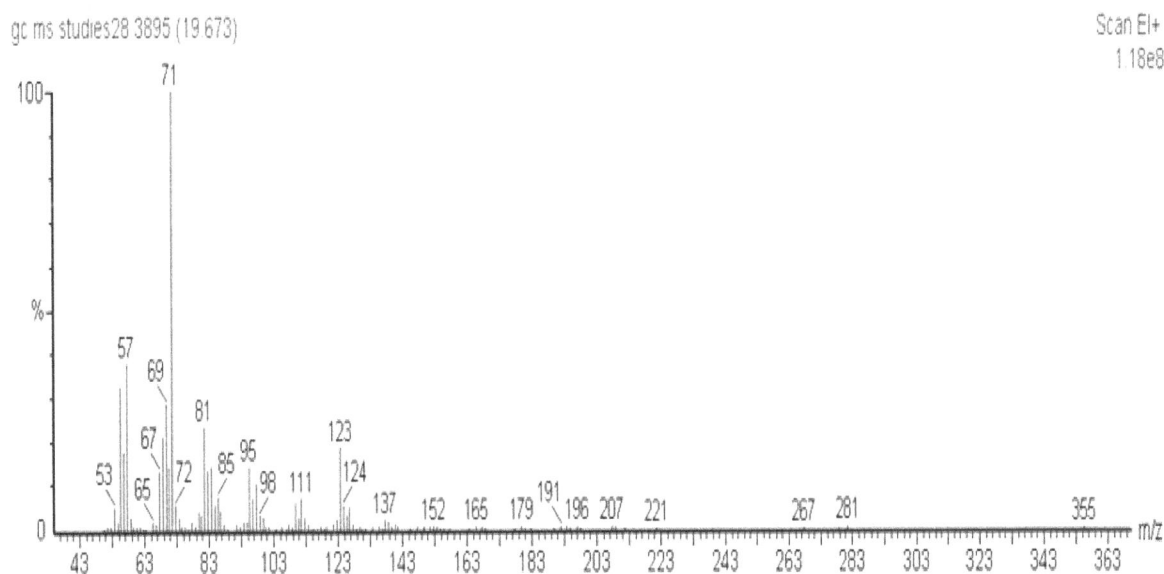

Figure 1. Chromatogram of *V. negundo* leaves by GC-MS.

*Vitex negundo-*231

IICPT TANJORE. 13-MAR-2009 + 13:40:17

Figure 2. Mass spectrum of Benzoic acid, 3-hydroxy-

the tubes. After 5 min, 0.3 ml of Aluminium Chloride (10%) was added to all the tubes. At the 6th minute, 2 ml of Sodium Hydroxide (1 M) was added to the mixture. Immediately, the contents of the reaction mixture were diluted with 2.4 ml of distilled water and mixed thoroughly. Abosorbance of the mixture was determined at 510 nm versus a prepared blank immediately. Gallic acid was used as the standard compound for quantification of total flavonoids as mg/100 g (Zhisen et al., 1999).

Antioxidant activity

DPPH method

0.1 ml of the freshly prepared sample was taken in test tubes. 6 ml of DPPH solution (0.1 mM) was added and the tubes kept in dark for one hour. The color was read at 517 nm. The difference in the O.D of DPPH solution and DPPH solution + sample was calculated.

Table 1. Total phenols, flavonoids and antioxidant activity in the leaves of *V. negundo*.

S/No.	Parameter analysed	Values obtained
1	Total phenols (mg/100 g) GE[*]	27.72 ± 0.3
2	Total flavonoids (mg/100 g) GE[*]	196.04 ± 0.8
3.	Antioxidant activity (mg/100 g) AEAC[**]	23.21 ± 0.96

The values are mean value of three replicates. [*] - Gallic acid equivalent, [**] - Ascorbic acid equivalent antioxidant capacity.

The decrease in OD with sample addition is used for calculation of the antioxidant activity. Ascorbic acid standards were prepared in different concentrations and antioxidant was determined as ascorbic acid equivalent antioxidant capacity (AEAC) mg/100 g of sample (Koleva et al., 2002).

GC –MS analysis

Preparation of extract

Leaves of *V. negundo* were shade dried. 20 g of the powdered leaves were soaked in 95% ethanol for 12 h. The extracts were then filtered through Whatmann filter paper No.41 along with 2 gm sodium sulfate to remove the sediments and traces of water in the filtrate. Before filtering, the filter paper along with sodium sulphate was wetted with 95% ethanol. The filtrate was then concentrated by bubbling nitrogen gas into the solution. The extract contained both polar and non-polar phytocomponents of the plant material used. 2 µl of these solutions was employed for GC/MS analysis (Merlin et al., 2009).

GC analysis

GC-MS analysis was carried out on a GC clarus 500 Perkin Elmer system comprising a AOC-20i autosampler and gas chromatograph interfaced to a mass spectrometer (GC-MS) instrument employing the following conditions: column Elite-1 fused silica capillary column (30 × 0.25 mm ID ×1EM df, composed of 100% Dimethyl poly siloxane), operating in electron impact mode at 70 eV; helium (99.999%) was used as carrier gas at a constant flow of 1ml/min and an injection volume of 0.5 EI was employed (split ratio of10:1) injector temperature 250°C; ion-source temperature 280°C. The oven temperature was programmed from 110°C (isothermal for 2 min), with an increase of 10°C/min, to 200°C, then 5°C/min to 280°C, ending with a 9 min isothermal at 280°C. Mass spectra were taken at 70 eV; a scan interval of 0.5 s and fragments from 40 to 550 Da.

Identification of components

Interpretation on mass spectrum GC-MS was conducted using the database of National Institute Standard and Technology (NIST) having more than 62,000 patterns. The spectrum of the unknown component was compared with the spectrum of the known components stored in the NIST library. The name, molecular weight and structure of the components of the test materials were ascertained.

RESULTS AND DISCUSSION

Total phenolics and flavonoid content in the leaves of *V. negundo*

It has been recognized that flavonoids show antioxidant activity and their effects on human nutrition and health are considerable. The mechanisms of action of flavonoids are through scavenging or chelating process (Kessler et al., 2003). Phenolic compounds are a class of antioxidant agents which act as free radical terminators (Om Prakash et al., 2007). The flavonoid contents of the extracts in terms of gallic acid equivalent (Table 1). Total phenolic content of the methanolic extract of *V. negundo* leaves is 27.72 mg/100 g of GE. The highest value of phenolic content indicates that the plant has high antioxidant activity.

GC-MS Study

The GC-MS study of *V. negundo* leaves has shown many phytochemicals which contributes to the medicinal activity of the plant (Tables 2 and 3). The major components which present in the leaves of the plant *V. negundo* was Benzoic acid 3-hydroxy (RT:11.47) (Figure 2), Ledol (RT:12.45), 9,12,15-Octadecatrienoic acid, (Z,Z,Z)-(RT:23.38) and Vitamin E. The other components like 4H-Pyran-4-one, 2,3-dihydro-3,5-dihydroxy-6-methyl- (RT: 6.17), Caryophyllene (RT: 10.21) and n-Hexadecanoic acid also present in the leaves of *V. negundo* (Figure 1).

Conclusion

The study clearly indicates that the leaf extract was rich in antioxidants, phenolics and flavonoids. The GC-MS study also showed many Phytochemicals Hexanoic acid, ethyl ester, 4H-Pyran-4-one, 2,3-dihydro-3,5-dihydroxy-6-methyl-, Hexadecanoic acid, ethyl ester, Caryophyllene, Benzoic acid, 3-hydroxy-, Ledol, Aromadendrene oxide-(1), n-Hexadecaonoic acid, Phytol, 9,12,15-Octadecatrienoic acid, (Z,Z,Z)- and Vitamin E which contributes the activities like antimicrobial, antioxidant anticancer, Hypercholesterolemic, Antiulcerogenic and

Table 2. Phytocomponents identified in the methanolic extract of the leaves of *V. negundo* by GC-MS.

RT	Name of the compound	Peak area (%)
2.67	d-Mannose	0.24
3.53	Butane, 1,1-diethoxy-3-methyl	0.06
3.98	Hexanoic acid, ethyl ester	0.22
4.97	Propane, 1,1,3-triethoxy-	0.12
5.32	2,3-Dihydrothiophene 1,1-dioxide	0.67
6.17	4H-Pyran-4-one, 2,3-dihydro-3,5-dihydroxy-6-methyl-	0.55
7.26	2,4-Pentadien-1-ol, 3-propyl-, (2Z)-	0.29
7.34	D-Glucose, 6-O-α-D-galactopyranosyl-	0.78
8.46	Ascaridole epoxide	0.03
8.71	4,9-Decadienoic acid, 2-nitro-, ethyl ester	0.07
9.35	Hexadecanoic acid, ethyl ester	0.05
9.59	10, 13-Octadecadiynoic acid, methyl ester	0.23
10.01	4-Decynoic acid, methyl ester	0.18
10.21	Caryophyllene	0.56
11.47	Benzoic acid, 3-hydroxy-	13.51
12.45	Ledol	1.19
13.89	Azulene, 1,4-dimethyl-7-(1-methylethyl)-	0.27
15.46	Ethanol, 2-(9-octadecenyloxy)-, (Z)-	0.18
16.10	Ethyl iso-allocholate	0.06
16.32	(7α-Isopropenyl-4,5-dimethyloctahydroinden-4-yl)methanol	0.91
16.80	Aromadendrene oxide-(1)	0.75
17.25	n-Hexadecaonoic acid	0.44
17.70	2-Methyl-4-(2,6,6-trimethylcyclohex-1-enyl)but-2-en-1-ol	0.15
18.17	6,9,12,15-Docosatetraenoic acid, methyl ester	0.12
19.67	Phytol	3.18
19.95	Ethanol, 2-(9,12-octadecadienyloxy)-, (Z,Z)-	0.12
20.06	9,12,15-Octadecatrienoic acid, (Z,Z,Z)-	1.08
23.38	12-Bromo-13-hydroxy-2,5,9,13-tetramethyltetradeca-4,8-dienoic acid, methyl ester	2.52
25.11	Vitamin E	0.62

Table 3. Activity of phyto-components identified in *V. negundo* leaf extract by GC-MS.

RT	Name of the compound	Compound nature	Activity
6.17	4H-Pyran-4-one, 2,3-dihydro-3,5-dihydroxy-6-methyl-	Flavonoid fraction	Antimicrobial, antiinflammatory
7.34	D-Glucose, 6-O-α-D-galactopyranosyl-	Sugar moiety	Preservative
9.35	Hexadecanoic acid, ethyl ester	Palmitic acid ester	Antioxidant, hypocholesterolemic nematicide, pesticide, anti androgenic flavor, hemolytic, 5-Alpha reductase inhibitor
10.21	Caryophyllene	Sesquiterpene	Anti-tumor, analgesic, antibacterial, antiinflammatory, sedative, fungicide
11.47	Benzoic acid, 3-hydroxy-	Benzoic acid compound	Antimicrobial

Table 3. Contd.

12.45	Ledol	Sesquiterpene alcohol	Antimicrobial, antiinflammatory
16.10	Ethyl iso-allocholate	Steriod	
16.80	Aromadendrene oxide-(1)	Sesquiterpene oxide	Anti-tumor, analgesic, antibacterial, antiinflammatory, sedative, fungicide
17.25	n-Hexadecaonoic acid	Palmitic acid	Antioxidant, hypocholesterolemic nematicide, pesticide, anti androgenic flavor, hemolytic, 5-Alpha reductase inhibitor
18.17	6,9,12,15-Docosatetraenoic acid, methyl ester	Unsaturated fatty acid	Anti cholesterol compound
19.67	Phytol	Diterpene	Antimicrobial, anticancer, antiinflammatory, diuretic
20.06	9,12,15-Octadecatrienoic acid, (Z,Z,Z)-	Linolenic acid	Antiinflammatory, hypocholesterolemic cancer preventive, hepatoprotective, nematicide, insectifuge, antihistaminic antieczemic, antiacne, 5-Alpha reductase inhibitor, antiandrogenic, antiarthritic, anticoronary, insectifuge
25.11	Vitamin E	Vitamin E	Antiageing, analgesic, antidiabatic antiinflammatory, antioxidant, antidermatitic, antileukemic, antitumor, anticancer, hepatoprotective, ypocholesterolemic, antiulcerogenic, vasodilator, antispasmodic, antibronchitic, anticoronary

**Source: Dr.Duke's phytochemical and ethnobotanical databases [Online database].

other activities.

ACKNOWLEDGEMENT

The authors thank very much Dr. K. Alagusundaram, Director, Indian Institute of Crop Processing Technology, Thanjavur for providing all the facilities and support used to carry out the work.

REFERENCES

Blake DR, Hall DA, Treby D, Halliwell B, Gutteridge JMC (1981). Protection against superoxide and hydrogen peroxide in synovial fluid from rheumatoid patients. Clin. Sci. 61: 483-486.

Dharmasiri MG, Jayakody JRAC, Gallhena G, Liyanage SSP, Ratnasooriya WD (2003). Anti-inflammatory and analgesic activities of mature fresh leaves of Vitex negundo. J. Ethnopharmacol., 2003.

Kessler M, Ubeaud G, Jung L (2003). Anti- and pro-oxidant activity of rutin and quercetin derivatives. J. Pharm. Pharmacol. 55: 131-142.

Kirtikar KR, Basu BD (1976). Indian medicinal plant, Orient Longman. 5: 387.

Koleva II, Van Beek TA, Linssen JPH, de Groot A, Evstatieva LN (2002). Screening of plant extracts for antioxidant activity: a comparative study on three testing methods. Phytochem. Anal. 13: 8-17.

Malick CP, Singh MB (1980). In: Plant Enzymology and Histo Enzymology, Kalyani Publishers, New Delhi, p. 286.

Merlin NJ, Parthasarathy V, Manavalan R, Kumaravel S (2009). Chemical Investigation of Aerial Parts of Gmelina asiatica Linn by GC-MS. Pharmacognosy Res.1(3): 152-156.

Om Prakash Tiwari, Yamini B, Tripathi (2007). Antioxidant properties of different fractions of Vitex negundo Linn, Food Chem. 100(3): 1170-1176.

Telang RS, Chatterjee S, Varshneya C (1999). Studies on Analgesic and Anti-inflammatory activities of Vitex negundo Linn. Indian J. Pharmacol. 31: 363-366.

Zhisen J, Meng Cheng T, Jianming W (1999). Food Chemistry 64: 555-559.

4

Anti-malarial activity of cocoa powder in mice

Jayeola, C. O.[1]*, Oluwadun, A.[2], Olubamiwa, O.[1], Effedua, H. I.[2] and Kale, O. E[3]

[1]Crop Processing and Utilization Division, Cocoa Research Institute of Nigeria, P. M. B., 5244, Ibadan, Oyo State, Nigeria.
[2]Department of Medical Microbiology and Parasitology, Obafemi Awolowo College of Health Science, Olabisi Onabanjo University Sagamu, Ogun State, Nigeria.
[3]Department of Pharmacology, Obafemi Awolowo College of Health Science, Olabisi Onabanjo University Sagamu, Ogun State, Nigeria.

At present, malaria is one of the most important parasitic diseases in the world killing more than one million people annually. It is an important public health problem because many of the drugs that are being prescribed for the treatment of malaria have become ineffective to the disease. This study was therefore carried out to determine the anti-malaria activity of cocoa powder through the use of mouse model. Natural cocoa powder was used to compound mice feed and this was both pre-fed and post-fed to mouse that had been infected with *Plasmodium berghei*. The results indicated that cocoa powder had both therapeutic and prophylactic effects against *P. berghei*. The mean percentage plasmodial reduction expressed in mice post-fed with cocoa and those treated with chloroquine were 60.82 ± 8.47% and 60.09 ± 7.84% respectively. This is an indication that both agents exhibited plasmodial reduction almost at equal frequency. Though, percentage *plasmodium* reduction was more in mice pre-fed with cocoa than those post-fed with cocoa, but the difference was not significant (P > 0.05). The observation of higher percentage of plasmodial reduction in mice pre-fed with cocoa suggested it may possess an immune-booster effect which action is anti-malarial. There was a decline in weight of mice demonstrating that cocoa might contain some weight trimming ingredients.

Key words: *Plasmodium berghei,* chloroquine, therapeutic immune booster.

INTRODUCTION

Malaria is a potentially, fatal tropical parasitic disease that is spread through the bite of an infected female mosquito. Malaria parasites are members of the genus *Plasmodium* (Phylum Apicomy plexa). It is wide spread in tropical and subtropical regions including parts of the Americas, Asia and Africa. Malaria in humans is caused by one of four protozoan species of the genus *Plasmodium*: *Plasmodium falciparum*, *Plasmodium vivax*, *Plasmodium ovale*, or *Plasmodium malariae* and *Plasmodium knowlesi*, a parasite of Old World monkeys also infects man. Investigations are ongoing to determine the extent of its transmission to humans (Mveller et al., 2007). Malaria is passed on by the female anopheles mosquito biting a person who has malaria parasites in their blood. Malaria can also be passed on by blood transfusions and the use of infected needles. Malaria causes an average loss of 1.3% of annual economic growth in countries with intense transmission. Severe malaria is almost exclusively caused by *P. falciparium* infection. The infected person may have feverish attacks, influenza-like symptoms, tiredness, diarrhea or a whole range of other symptoms (Trampuz et al., 2003). In most severe cases of the disease, fatality rates can exceed 20%, even with intensive care and treatment (Kain et al., 1998). In endemic areas, treatment is often less satisfactory and the overall fatality rate for all cases of malaria can be as high as one in ten (Mochenhaupt et al., 2004). Over the longer term, developmental impairments have been documented in children who have suffered episodes of severe malaria (Carter, 2005). It is responsible for the death of an estimated 10,000 pregnant women and up to 200,000 infants each year in Africa alone (Trampuz et al., 2003).

It is well-known that cocoa contains a wide range of polyphenols, especially procyanidins with a high degree of polymerization. Procyanidin is a class of polyphenolic

---
*Corresponding author. E-mail: yinktay@yahoo.com.

polymer composed of flavan-3-ol (catechin) and epicathechin as monomers, moreover small amounts of flavonoids and phenolic acids have been found in various cocoa-derived products. Flavonoids are polyphenolic compounds that are ubiquitous in nature and are categorized, according to chemical structure, into flavornols, flavones, flavanones, isoflavones, catechins, anthocyanidins and chalcones. Over 4,000 flavonoids have been identified, many of which occur in fruits, vegetables and beverages (tea, coffee, beer, wine and fruit drinks) (Ortega et al., 2008). Cocoa was reported to have high polyphenols content, which comprises 12 to 18% of the whole beans dry weight (Richelle et al., 2001). A study reported that in raw cocoa beans, 60% of total phenolics were flavonol monomers (epicatechin and catechin) and procyanidin oligomers (Dreosti et al., 2000). (–)-Epicatechin content in freshly prepared beans ranged from 21.89 to 43.27 mg/g dry defatted samples. Cocoa is rich in other polyphenols such as (+)-catechin, (–)-epicatechin, and oligomers of these monomeric base units, namely procyanidins, and anthocyanidins (Hammerstone et al., 1999). Kelm et al. (2006) later indicated that unfermented cocoa beans contain monomers up to tetradecamers. Cocoa contains flavanol which has potential beneficial effects on human health such as antiviral, anti-allergic, anti-platelet, anti-inflammatory, anti-tumor and anti-oxidant activities. Numerous studies have reported a relationship between the consumption of cocoa derivatives especially dark chocolate with beneficial health effects on cardiovascular diseases as a result of the antioxidant activity of procyanidins (Keen et al., 2005, Cooper et al., 2008). The flavonoids have aroused considerable interest recently because of their potential benefits on human health. Murakami (2003) have shown that diglycosides of flavanols (a specific type of flavonoids) retard life cycle of malaria parasites, whereas monoglycosides completely inhibited proliferation of trophozoite stage of parasites. The health benefits of consuming cocoa based products have recently been recognized, indeed reports have suggested that cocoa may protect against cancer (Masharinec, 2009), cardiovascular disease (Galleano et al., 2009; Corti et al., 2009) and various other medical conditions (Visioli et al., 2009). Such qualities of cocoa have largely been attributed to the catechins, which are polyphenols of the flavanol group, which function as antioxidants and which cocoa contains in significant amounts (Vinson et al., 2006). This study was therefore geared towards confirming the previously reported good attributes of cocoa in human health through the use of mouse models to determine its anti-malaria activity.

MATERIALS

Parasite

P. berghei was obtained from Malaria Research and Reference Repository Centre (MR4) 10801 University Boulevard, Manassas, Virginia United States of America (Batch Number S0594596) was used. It was collected from the Institute of Medical Research and Training (IMRAT), College of Medicine, University of Ibadan, Nigeria and maintained by mouse-to-mouse passage.

Mice

Male and female Naïve BALB/C mice of 8 to 12 weeks old (14 to 22 g) were used for this study. They were purchased from commercial animal breeding house in Ibadan Oyo State, Nigeria.

Cocoa

Natural cocoa powder (non-alkalized) as packaged by Cocoa Research Institute of Nigeria (CRIN), Idi-Ayunre, Ibadan, Oyo State, Nigeria, was used for this experiment.

Chloroquine

Chloroquine injection produced by Pfizer Nig. Ltd was purchased at Ogun State University Teaching Hospital Pharmaceutical Centre at Shagamu, Ogun State, Nigeria.

Modified cocoa feed

The experimental feed was specially formulated on request to be made of the normal rat diet with inclusion of 2% natural cocoa powder. The modified feed consisted of maize starch, sucrose, soybean oil, fibre (cellulose powder), mineral premix, choline bitartrate, tert-butyl-hydroquinone (Katsuhiko et al., 2009) and 2% cocoa powder. This was made into rat feed pellet by Pfizer feed mill, Iwo Road, Ibadan.

Experimental animals

Mice were housed in cages and maintained under standard condition (12 h light/dark cycle 25± 3°C, 45 to 65% humidity). The animals had access to modified standard mouse feed and water ad libidum. All the animals were acclimatized to laboratory condition for 3 days before commencement of the experiment as described by Karunakar et al. (2009). Experimental mice were randomly put grouped into six groups randomly containing 5 animals each, according to their weight and sex. Each group comprises of both male and female mice.

Group A - normal (rat) feed
Group B - compounded cocoa feed
Group C - normal (rat) feed + infection with P. berghei
Group D - normal (rat) feed + infection with P. berghei + treatment with chloroquine
Group E - normal (rat) feed + infection with P. berghei + post feeding with cocoa feed
Group F - pre-fed with cocoa feed (one week before) + infection with P. berghei + post feeding with cocoa feed
Group G - normal (rat feed) + infection with P. berghei + cocoa feed + chloroquine.

Inoculation of mice

Infected blood containing P. berghei was obtained from donor mouse with 20 to 40% parasitemia. Blood for innocular was obtained by cardiac bleeding using 3% sodium citrate as an

Table 1. Parasitaemia (cells/µl) in cocoa and chloroquine treated mice.

Groups	$\overline{X} \pm$ SEM	F	P-value
Untreated (control)	23,937.50 ± 1499.77	27.20	< 0.05
Treated with chloroquine	3,412.50 ±1499.77		
Post-fed with cocoa	2,989.59 ± 361.80		
Pre-fed with cocoa	3,166.67 ± 2333.34		
Treatment with cocoa and chloroquine	2,375.00 ±125.00		

Table 2. Variation in parasitaemia (cells/µl) in cocoa and chloroquine treated mice.

Groups	$\overline{\overline{X}} \pm$ SEM (%)	t	P-value
Untreated (control)	+258.33 ± 56.49	0.96	< 0.05
Treated with chloroquine	-60.09 ± 7.84		
Post-fed with cocoa	-60.82 ± 8.47		
Pre-fed with cocoa	-73.81 ± 6.86		
Treatment with cocoa and chloroquine	-52.38 ± 11.60		

anticoagulant. Experimental mice received one innoculum of 0.2 ml of *P. berghei* which was applied intraperitoneallly (IP).

Determination of parasitemia

For the detection of malaria infection, thin and thick blood smears were prepared from all experimental mice before the start of experiment. Less than 1 mm section of the distal end of the tail was cut and approximately 3 µl of blood was sported unto a microscope slide. Slides were air dried, and smears were stained with a 10% Giemsa solution and were observed in a light microscope with X 1000 objective (oil immersion). The percentage parasitemia and parasite density were taken at each follow-up day that is day 0, 3, 5, 7, 11 and 14. The mean weights were taken, parasite counts were expressed as parasite density per microlitre (µl) of blood, (Cheesebrough, 2005). Also, percentage change in parasite density was determined as stated below:

$$\text{Percentage (\%) change in parasite density} = \frac{\text{Initial MP density before treatment - Density of MP after treatment}}{\text{Initial MP density before treat}} \times \frac{100}{}$$

Note: MP = Malaria parasite

Weight gain/loss

Weights of the experimental mice were taken before the commencement of the experiment (that is, day 0) and on days 3, 5, 7, 11, and 14 days. Mean weights were taken and percentage weight loss or gain was determined through comparison of the mean weight before and after infection with *P. berghei*.

Statistical analysis

Data analysis was carried out with (SPSS version 15). Comparison of weights and parasite density in mice was done by using Analysis of Variance (ANOVA) and Student's t-test. Level of significance was determined at 95%.

RESULTS AND DISCUSSION

The results of the experiment on plasmodium infection on mice and the effect of cocoa powder ingestion as compared with chloroquine treatment as demonstrated in this study. In Table 1, the result of parasitaemia (cells/µl) in cocoa and chloroquine treated mice were indicated, the highest parasitaemia (plasmodial density) of 23,937.50 ± 2,782.25 cells/µl of blood was recorded in the untreated mice (P< 0.05) while others showed decrease in their plasmodial densities. On comparison of percentage change in parasite density as indicated in Table 2, the untreated mice recorded a mean percentage increase of +258.33 ± 56.49% while mean percentage decrease was recorded by various groups of treated mice such as those injected with chloroquine (-60.82 ± 8.47%), post-fed with cocoa (-60.82 ± 8.47%), pre-fed with cocoa (-73.81 ± 6.86%) and those treated with chloroquine and cocoa (-52.38 ± 11.60%). Observation of significantly lower parasite density in blood of mice group treated with chloroquine and cocoa (P< 0.05) showed that both agents have anti-plasmodial activities. This experiment was in agreement with the research findings of de Monbrinson et al. (2006) who observed that flavonoid derivatives such as dehydrosilybin and 8-(1,1)-DMA-kaempferide, which were extracted from cocoa, exerted significant anti-malarial activity against five strains of *P. falciparum*. The author also recommended that flavonoid derivatives could be used as adjunct to already available anti-malarial drugs to delay the spread of resistance in *P. falciparum*. The mean percentage plasmodial reduction

Table 3. Weight variations in cocoa treated mice.

Period of treatment (weeks)	Values $\overline{X} \pm$ SEM	F	P-value
Before treatment (0)	17.60 ± 1.27	1.41	< 0.05
1st week of treatment (1)	16.65± 1.63		
2nd week of treatment (2)	15.60 ± 0.10		

Table 4. Total parasite density in male and female mice.

	Total parasite density (cells/µl of blood)		
Sex	$\overline{X} \pm$ SEM (%)	t	P-value
Male	45666.867 ± 10443.83	0.061	< 0.05
Female	44900.200 ± 7154.43		

expressed in mice post-fed with cocoa (60.82 ± 8.47%) and those treated with chloroquine (60.09 ± 7.84%) indicated that both agents exhibit plasmodial reduction almost at equal level. In this study, therapeutic and prophylactic effects of cocoa against *P. berghei* were compared in mice. Though, higher percentage of plasmodium reduction was observed in mice pre-fed with cocoa (73.81 ± 6.86%) than those post-fed (60.82 ± 8.47%), but the difference was not significant (t = 0.96, P> 0.05).

Insignificant difference in the percentage plasmodial reduction between mice pre-fed with cocoa and those post-fed with cocoa (P> 0.05) is an indication that both method of anti-malaria treatment are equally effective. However, the observation of higher percentage of plasmodial reduction in mice pre-fed with cocoa suggests that cocoa may contain immune-booster whose action is anti-malarial. The effect of cocoa consumption on mice weight was determined in Table 3, a systematic decline was observed in the weight of mice with mean weight of 17.60 ± 1.27 g before administration of cocoa, 16.65 ± 1.63 g after first week of treatment and 15.60 ± 0.00 g after second week of treatment. The difference was however, found to be insignificant (F = 1.41, P> 0.05).

The systematic decline in weight of mice after being fed with cocoa for a period of two weeks demonstrated that cocoa may contain some weight trimming ingredients. The insignificant observation may be attributable to the short duration of this study. The result of total parasite density in male and female mice as observed in Table 4 showed comparison between the total parasite density of male and female mice. The result of this analysis indicated that there was no significant difference in the level of parasitaemia observed in mice from both gender (t = 0.61, P> 0.05).

Conclusion

From this study it can be concluded that cocoa powder

exhibited *in vivo* anti-malaria activity. It further confirmed that cocoa powder possesses both therapeutic and prophylactic effects against *P. berghei*. This means that regular consumption of cocoa will reduce the occurrence of malaria attack. However, extensive research work is required for the study of its anti-malaria agents and their possible, precise mechanism of action.

RECOMMENDATION

From the outcome of this study, we hereby recommend that cocoa consumption should be promoted in areas where malaria is endemic. This will surely reduce incessant cases of drug-resistance and as well prevent the devastating effect of malaria on human. Since cocoa powder is a food drink, it is not likely for malaria causing parasite (*Plasmodium spp.*) to become resistance to cocoa powder. The immune booster effect of cocoa powder is an area to look into in the nearest future.

ACKNOWLEDGEMENT

We are grateful to the Executive Director of Cocoa Research Institute of Nigeria Prof. G. Iremiren for the permission given to publish this paper. We also appreciate Mrs Oyelami for her secretarial assistant during the course of this project.

REFERENCES

Carter JA, Ross AJ, Neville BG, Obiero E, Katana K, Mungala-Odera V, Less JA, Newton CR (2005). Developmental impairments following severe falciparum malaria in children. Trop. Med. Int. health, 10(1): 3-10.

Cheesebrough M (2005) Counting parasite numbers. In District Laboratory Practice in Tropical Countries. Second Ed. Cambridge University Presss, The Edinburgh Building, Cambridge CB2 2RU, U.K., p. 251.

Cooper K, Donovan,J, Waterhouse A, Willisamson, G (2008). Cocoa health: A decade of Research. Br. J. Nutr., 99-111.

Corti R, Flammer AJ, Hollenberg NK, Luscher TF (2009). Cocoa and cardiovascular health. Circulation, 119: 1433-41.

de Monbrison F, Maitrejean M, Latour C, Bungnazet F, Peyron F, Barron F, Picot S (2006). In vitro antimalaria activity of flavonoid derivatives dehydrosilybin and 8-(1,1)-DMA-kaempferide Acta Trop., 97(1):102-107.

Dreosti IE (2000). Antioxidant polyphenols in tea, cocoa, and wine. Nutrition, 16: 692-694.

Galleano M, Oteiza PI, Frag CG. (2009). Cocoa chocolate and cardiovascular disease. J. Cardiovasc. Pharmacol., pp; 54(6):483-490.

Hammerstone JF, Rucker RB, Ritter KA, Schmitz HH (1999). HPLC method for the quantification of procyanidins in cocoa and chocolate samples and correlation to total antioxidant capacity. J. Agric. Food Chem., 47: 4184-4188.

Kain K, Harrington M, Tennysan S, Keptone J (1998). Impaired malaria prospective analysis of problems in diagnosis and management. Clin. Infect. Dis., 27(1): 142-9.

Karunakar H, Thakken SP, Aron BJ, Shastry CS, Chandrashekha KS (2009). Anticonvulsant activity of Carissa carandas lin. Root extract in experimental mice. Trop. J. Pharmaceutical Res., 8(2):117-125.

Katchuhiko Y, Aki K , Miki O (2009). Iron bioavailability of cocoa powder as determined by Hb regeneration efficiency method. British J. Nutr., 102: 215-220.

Keen, C, Holt R, Oteiza P, Fraga, C, Schmitz, H (2005). Cocoa antioxidants and cardiovascular health. An. J. clin. Nutr., 8: 2985-3035.

Kelm MA, Johnson JC, Robbins RJ, Hammerstone JF, Schmitz HH (2006). High-performance liquid chromatography separation and purification of cacao (Theobroma cacao L.) procyanidins according to degree of polymerization using a diol stationary phase. J. Agric. Food Chem., 54: 1571-1576.

Masharinec G (2009). Cancer protective properties of cocoa: a review of the epidemiologic evidence. Nutr Cancer, 61: 573-9.

Mockenhaupt F, Ehrhardt J, Bosomtwe S, Laryea S, Anemama S, Otchwemah R, Cramer J, Dietz E, Gellert S, Bienzle U (2004). Manifestation and outcome of severe malaria in children in Northern Ghana. Am. J. Trop. Med. Hygiene, 71(2): 167-172.

Murakami N (2003). Exploration for new functions of polyphenol food additives and investigation on structures and safety of their metabolites. The Japan Food Chemical Research Foundation Research Reports No. 9 Abstract. http"/www.ffcr.or.jp/zaidan/FFCRHOME.nsf/a.

Mweller I, Zimmermen PA, Reeder, JC (2007) Plasmodium malariae and plasmodium ovale-the bashful malaria parasites. Trends in parasitol., 23(6): 278-83.

Richelle, M, Tavazzi I, Offord E (2001). Comparison of antioxidant activity of commonly consumed polyphenolic beverages (coffee, cocoa, and tea) prepared per cup serving. J. Agric. Food Chem., 49: 3438-3442.

Trampuz A, Jeeb M, Muziovic I, Prabhu R (2003). Clinical review. Severe malaria Crit care, 7(4): 315-23.

Vinson JA, Proch J, Bose P, Muchler S, Taffera P, Shuta D, Samman N, Agbor GA (2006). Chocolate is a powerful ex vivo and in vivo antioxidant, an antiatherosclerotic agent in an animal model, and a significant contributor to antioxidants in the European and American Diets. J Agric Food Chem., 54: 8071-6.

Visioli F, Bernaert H, Corti R, Ferri C, Heptinstall S, Molinar E, Poli A, Serafini M, Smit HJ, Vinson JA, Violi F, Paoletti R (2009). Chocolate, lifestyle and health. Crit. Rev. Food Sci. Nutr., 49: 299-312.

5

Screening of antioxidant activity, total phenolics and gas chromatography-mass spectrophotometer (GC-MS) study of ethanolic extract of *Aporosa lindleyana* Baill

S. Ramakrishnan[1]* and R. Venkataraman[2]

[1]Department of Biotechnology, Sri Paramakalyani College, Alwarkurichi – 627 412, Tirunelveli District, Tamil Nadu, India.
[2]Post graduate and Research Department of Chemistry, Sri Paramakalyani College, Alwarkurichi – 627 412, Tirunelveli District, Tamil Nadu, India.

The present study was carried out for the identification of phytochemicals present in the roots of *Aporosa lindleyana* and also to evaluate the total phenol, total flavonoids and antioxidant activity. Total phenol was carried out by Folin Ciocalteu method and the phenolic content was 31.20 mg/100 g of gallic acid equivalent (GE) and the flavonoid content was 203.10±0.9. Antioxidant activity was evaluated by 2,2-diphenyl-1-picrylhydrazyl (DPPH) method and the roots of *A. lindleyana* showed 19.91 mg/100 g of ascorbic acid equivalent antioxidant capacity (AEAC). The gas chromatography-mass spectrophotometer (GC-MS) study was also carried out and it showed the presence of phytochemicals like 1,2-benzenedicarboxylic acid, diphenyl ester (RT: 11.97), pthalic acid, bis (7 methylocytyl) ester (RT: 20.86) and squalene (RT: 24.70).

Key words: *Aporosa lindleyana*, antioxidant, flavonoids, gas chromatography-mass spectrophotometer (GC-MS), 2,2-diphenyl-1-picrylhydrazyl (DPPH).

INTRODUCTION

Aporosa lindleyana belongs to the family of Euphorbiaceae, is a much branched, evergreen, glabrous tree, grown in India and Sri Lanka. It possesses antioxidant activity (Badami et al., 2005) and hepatoprotective effect (Ramakrishnan et al., 2010) and also having antihyperglycemic effect (Jayakar and Suresh, 2003). So far, very few research works were carried out in this plant. *A. lindleyana* Baill have much medicinal properties such as diuretic, antiviral and a good analgesic. Its leaves are used to treat diabetics. Its bark and roots were used to treat headache, fever and jaundice. Decoctions of roots are used to treat insanity, seminal loss and excessive thirst.

The preliminary phytochemical studies reveal the presence of phytosterol, alkaloids and flavonoids.

Polyphenolic compounds have high antioxidant potential, the antioxidant activity of *A. lindleyana* was investigated by employing various *in vitro* tests. The present study was carried out to investigate the antioxidant activity, flavonoids and total phenolic content of *A. lindleyana*. In addition, chemical constituents of *A. lindleyana* was analyzed by gas chromatography-mass spectrophotometer (GC-MS).

MATERIALS AND METHODS

Collection and processing of plant material

The roots of *A. lindleyana* was collected from Keeriparai, Kanyakumari District, Tamilnadu during the month of January 2009. The specimen was identified by Dr. V. Chelladurai, Taxonomist, Department of Ayurvedic Sciences, Tirunelveli District. The roots were cleansed and shade dried for a weak and grounded into uniform powder. 1 g of plant material was added to 20 ml of aqueous ethanol (20% v/v) for 18 h at room temperature. The

---
*Corresponding author. E-mail: sramkrish1978@gmail.com.

Table 1. Total phenols, flavonoids and antioxidant activity in the roots of *A. lindleyana.*

S/N	Parameter analysed	Value obtained
1	Total Phenols (mg/100 g) GE*	31.20±0.2
2	Total flavonoids (mg/100 g) GE*	203.10±0.9
3	Antioxidant activity ((mg/100 g) AEAC**	19.91±0.5

The values are mean value of three replicates, *Gallic acid equivalent, **Ascorbic acid equivalent antioxidant capacity.

extracts was filtered and used for the estimation of total phenols and antioxidant activity.

Total phenols

0.5 ml of freshly prepared sample was taken and diluted with 8 ml of distilled water. 0.5 ml of Folin Ciocalteu reagent (1 N) was added and kept at 40°C for 10 min. 1.0 ml of sodium carbonate (20%) was added and kept in dark for one hour. The color was read at 650 nm using shimadzu UV-1650 spectrophotometer (Malick et al., 1980). The same procedure was repeated for all standard gallic acid solution and standard curve obtained. The sample concentration was calculated as gallic acid equivalent (GE).

Total flavonoids

0.5 ml of ethanolic extract of sample is diluted with 3.5 ml of distilled water at zero time and 0.3 ml of 5% sodium nitrate was added to the tubes. After 5 min, 0.3 ml of aluminium chloride (10%) was added to all the tubes. At the 6th min, 2 ml of sodium hydroxide (1 M) was added to the mixture. Immediately, the contents of the reaction mixture were diluted with 2.4 ml of distilled water and mixed thoroughly, after which absorbance of the mixture was then determined at 510 nm versus a prepared blank. Gallic acid was used as the standard compound for quantification of total flavonoids as mg/100 g (Zhisen et al., 1999).

Antioxidant activity

0.1 ml of the freshly prepared sample was taken in the test tubes. 6.0 ml of 2,2-diphenyl-1-picrylhydrazyl (DPPH) solution (0.1 mM) was added and the tubes kept in dark for one hour. The color was read at 517 nm. The difference in the optical density (O.D) of DPPH solution and DPPH solution + sample was calculated. The decrease in O.D with sample addition is used for the calculation of the antioxidant activity. Ascorbic acid standards were prepared in different concentration and antioxidant activity was determined as ascorbic acid equivalent antioxidant capacity (AEAC) mg/100 g of sample (Koleva et al., 2002).

GC-MS analysis

Preparation of extract

The ratio of *A. lindleyana* was shade dried and 20 g of the powdered roots was soaked in 95% ethanol for 12 h. The extract was filtered through Whatmann filter paper No. 41 along with 2 g sodium sulfate to remove the sediments and traces of water in the filtrate. Before filtering, the filter paper along with sodium sulphate was wetted with 95% ethanol. The filtrate was then concentrated by bubbling nitrogen gas into the solution. The extract contained both polar and nonpolar phytocomponents of the plant material used. 2 µl of this solution was employed for GC-MS analysis (Merlin et al., 2009).

GC analysis

GC-MS analysis was carried out on a GC clarus 500 perkin Elmer system comprising a AOC-20i autosampler and gas chromatography interfaced to a mass spectrophotometer (GC-MS) instrument employing the following condition. Column Elite – 1 fused silica capillary column (30 × 0.25 mm ID × IEM df, composed of 100% trimethyl poly siloxane) operating in electron impact mode at 70 eV; helium (99.999%) was used as carrier gas at a constant flow of 1 ml/min and an injection volume of 0.5 EI was employed (split ratio of 1:1) injector temperature (280°C). The oven temperature was programmed from 110°C (isothermal for 2 min), with an increase of 10 C/min to 200°C, then 5 C/min to 280°C, ending with a 9 min isothermal at 280°C. Mass spectrum was taken at 70 eV; a scan interval of 0.5 s fragments from 40 to 550 Da.

Identification of components

Interpretation on mass spectrum GC-MS was conducted using the database of National Institute of Standard and Technology (NIST) having more than 62,000 patterns. The spectrum of the unknown component was compared with the spectrum of the known components stored in the NIST library. The name, molecular weight and structure of the components of the test materials were ascertained.

RESULTS AND DISCUSSION

Total phenol and flavonoid content

Plant polyphenols, a diverse group of phenolic compounds (flavonols, anthocyanins, phenolic acids, etc.) possess an ideal structural chemistry for free radical scavenging activity. Antioxidative properties of polyphenols arise from their high reactivity as hydrogen or electron donors from the ability of the polyphenol derived radical to stabilize and delocalize the unpaired electron (chain-breaking function) and from their potential to chelate metal ions (termination of the Fenton reaction) (Rice-Evans et al., 1996).

The flavonoid contents of the extracts were expressed in terms of gallic acid equivalent (Table 1). Total phenolic content of the ethanolic extract of *A. lindleyana* root was

Table 2. Phytochemicals and their activity identified in the ethanolic extract of the roots of *A. lindleyana* by GC-MS.

S/N	RT	Name of the compound	Molecular formula	MW	Peak area (%)	Nature of compound	**Activity
1	9.00	1,3-Dioxolane-2-heptanenitrile, à-methyl-ë-oxo-2-phenyl-	$C_{17}H_{21}NO_3$	287	1.16	Aromatic nitrile compound	Antimicrobial
2	11.97	1,2-Benzenedicarboxylic acid, diheptyl ester	$C_{22}H_{34}O_4$	362	3.10	Plasticizer compound	Antimicrobial, antifouling
3	13.08	1,2-Benzenedicarboxylic acid, butyl cyclohexyl ester	$C_{18}H_{24}O_4$	304	1.15	Plasticizer compound	Antimicrobial, antifouling
4	20.86	Phthalic acid, bis(7-methyloctyl) ester	$C_{26}H_{42}O_4$	418	10.46	Plasticizer compound	Antimicrobial, antifouling
5	21.38	4-Methoxymethoxy-hex-1-ene	$C_8H_{16}O_2$	144	4.79	Alkene compound	No activity reported
6	24.70	Squalene	$C_{30}H_{50}$	410	32.34	Triterpene	Anticancer, antimicrobial, antioxidant, chemo preventive pesticide, anti- tumor sunscreen
7	28.77	Silane, 1,4-phenylenebis[trimethyl-	$C_{12}H_{22}Si_2$	222	16.25	Aromatic silica compound	No activity reported
8	32.40	2,4,6-Cycloheptatrien-1-one, 3,5-bis-trimethylsilyl-	$C_{13}H_{22}OSi_2$	250	30.76	Ketone compound	No activity reported

**Source: Dr. Duke's: Phytochemical and ethnobotanical databases.

31.20 mg/100 g of GE. The highest value of phenolic content indicates that the plant has high antioxidant activity.

The antioxidant properties of flavonoids are due to several different mechanisms, such as scavenging of free radicals, chelation of metal ions, such as iron and copper, and inhibition of enzymes responsible for free radical generation (Benavente-Garcia, 1997). Depending on their structure, flavonoids are able to scavenge practically all known reactive oxygen species (ROS). Total flavonoid content of ethanolic extract of *A. lindleyana* roots was 203.10 mg/100 g of GE.

GC-MS study

The GC-MS study of roots of *A. lindleyana* has shown many phytochemicals which contributes to the medicinal activity of the plant (Table 2 and Figure 1). The major component present in the roots of *A. lindleyana* was 1,3 –Dioxolane – 2 – hepanenitrile a'-methyl-e-oxo-2-phenyl (RT:9.00), 1,2-Benzene dicarboxylic acid, diphenyl ester (RT: 11.97), 1,2 – Benzene dicarboxylic acid butyl cyclohexyl ester (RT:13.08)– (Figure 2) and phthalic acid (RT:20.86) , 4- Methoxymethoxy hex-1-ene, Squalene (RT: 24.70) - (Figure 3), Silane 1,4, phenylene bis(trimethyl), 2,4,6 cycloheptatrien -1-ene-3,5 bis-trimethyl silyl found in the roots of *A. lindleyana*.

Squalene plays a major role in the protection and enhancement of human skin. Like glutathione (GSH), Squalene is one of the few antioxidants manufactured within the body, both of which detoxify, help balance our protective metabolisms and protect us from other threats. Squalene also has anticancer and blood cholesterol lowering effects (Nakagawa et al., 1985).

In our study, Squalene, an antioxidant found in the ethanolic extract, may give antioxidant properties of the *A. lindleyana*.

Conclusion

Our present study showed that the root extract was rich in antioxidants, phenolics and flavonoids. The GC-MS study also proved many phytochemicals such as Squalene, Pthalic acid and 1,2 benzene dicarboxylic acid, butyl cyclohexyl ester etc., which contributes to the activities like antioxidant, antimicrobial and antifouling activity.

ACKNOWLEDGEMENT

We are immensely thankful to Indian Institute of Crop Processing Technology, Thanjavur and The Management, The Principal of Sri Paramakalyani College, Alwarkurichi for providing all the facilities and constant encouragement during these period of work.

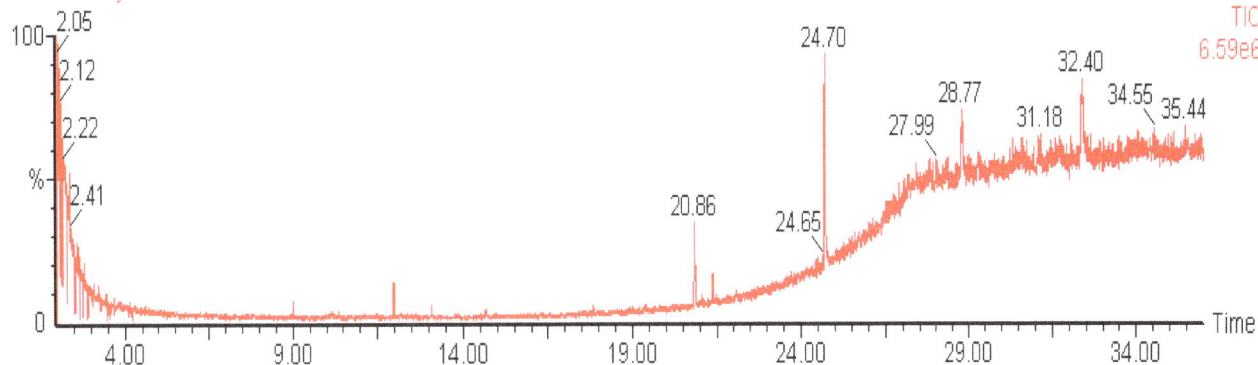

SAMPLE - 653

GC-MS Analysis154

IICPT, Thanjavur, 22-FEB-2011 + 15:44:52

Scan EI+
TIC
6.59e6

Figure 1. Chromatogram of *A. lindleyana* roots by GC-MS.

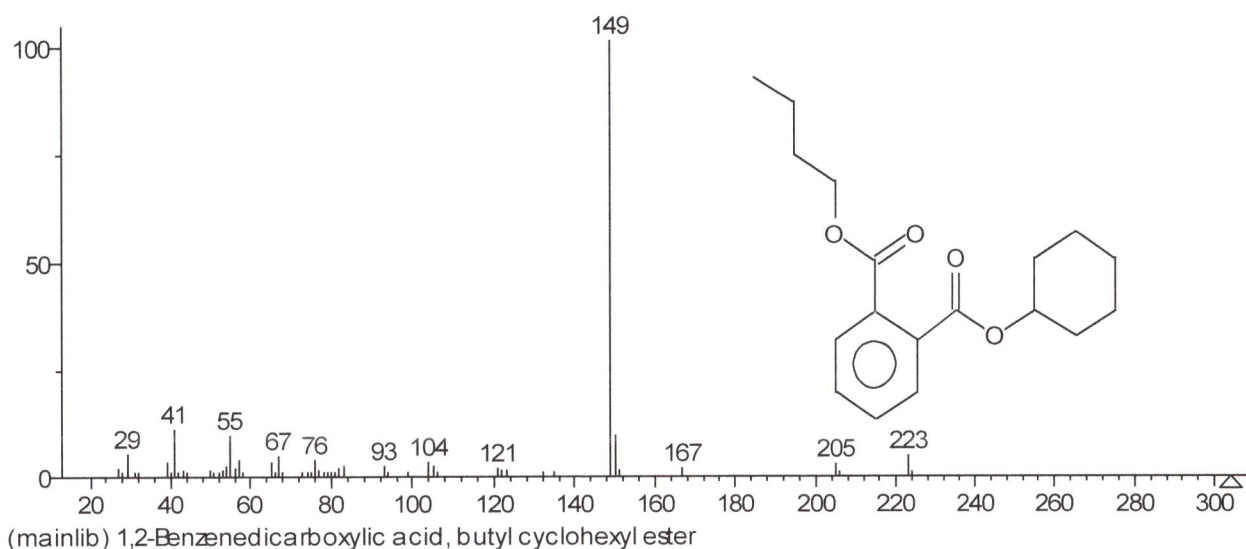

(mainlib) 1,2-Benzenedicarboxylic acid, butyl cyclohexyl ester

Name: 1,2-Benzenedicarboxylic acid, butyl cyclohexyl ester

Formula: $C_{18}H_{24}O_4$

MW: 304 CAS#: 84-64-0 NIST#: 75987 ID#: 87207 DB: mainlib

Other DBs: None

Contributor: RADIAN CORP

10 largest peaks:

    149 999 | 41 104 | 150 92 | 55 89 | 29 50 |
    223 44 | 67 44 | 57 37 | 76 37 | 65 30 |

Synonyms:

1.Phthalic acid, butyl cyclohexyl ester
2.Butyl cyclohexyl phthalate
3.Cyclohexyl butyl phthalate
4.Elastex 50B
5.1-Butyl 2-cyclohexyl phthalate #

Figure 2. Mass spectrum of 1,2-Benzenedicarboxylic acid, butyl cyclohexyl ester.

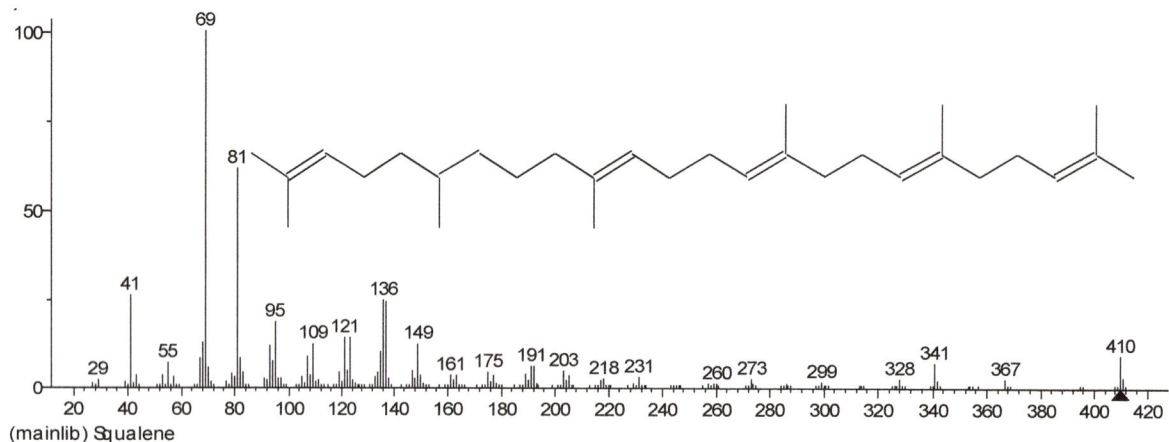

Name: Squalene
Formula: C$_{30}$H$_{50}$
MW: 410 CAS#: 7683-64-9 NIST#: 227620 ID#: 27655 DB: mainlib
Other DBs: None
Contributor: Japan AIST/NIMC Database- Spectrum MS-NW-8230
10 largest peaks:
  69 999 | 81 612 | 41 257 | 136 243 | 137 240 |
  95 184 | 121 139 | 123 137 | 68 124 | 149 119 |
Synonyms:
1.2,6,10,14,18,22-Tetracosahexaene, 2,6,10,15,19,23-hexamethyl-
2.Skvalen
3.Spinacene
4.Supraene
5.(6E,10E,14E,18E)-2,6,10,15,19,23-Hexamethyl-2,6,10,14,18,22-tetracosahexaene

Figure 3. Mass spectrum of squalene.

REFERENCES

Badami S, Om Prakash, Dongra SH, Suresh B (2005b). *Invitro* antioxidant properties of *Solanum pseudocapsicum* leaf extracts. Indian J. Pharmacol., 37: 251-252.

Badami S, Rai SR, Suresh B (2005a). Antioxidant activity of *Aporosa lindleyana* root. J. Ethnopharmacol., 101: 180-184.

Benavente-Garcia (1997). Uses and properties of Citrus flavonoids. J. Agri. Food Chem., 45: 4505-4515.

Jayakar B, Suresh B (2003). Antihyperglycemic and hypoglycemic effect of Aporosa lindleyana in normal and alloxan induced diabetic rats. J. Ethnopharmacol., 84(2-3): 247-249.

Koleva II, Van Beek TA, Linssen JPH, Groot AD, Evstatieva LN (2002). Screening of plant extracts for antioxidant activity: a comparative study on three testing methods. Phytochem. Anal., 13: 8-17.

Malick CP, Singh MB (1980). In: Plant Enzymology and Histoenzymology, Kalyani Publishers, New Delhi, p. 286.

Merlin NJ, Parthasarathy V, Manavalan R, Kumaravel S (2009). Chemical investigation of Aerial parts of Gmelina asiatica Linn. by GC-MS. Pharmacognosy Res., 1(3): 152-156.

Nakagawa M, Yamaguchi T, Fukawa H, Ogata J, Komiyama S, Akiyama S, Kuwano M (1985). Potentiation by squalene of the cytotoxicity of anticancer agents against cultured mammalian cells and murine tumor. Jpn. J. Cancer Res., 76(4): 315-320.

Rice-Evans CA, Miller NJ, Paganga G (1996). Structure–antioxidant activity relationship of flavonoids and phenolic acids. Free Radic. Biol. Med., 20: 933-956.

Zhisen J, Mengcheng T, Jianming W (1999). The determination of flavonoid contents in mulberry and their scavenging effects on superoxide radicals. Food Chem., 64: 555-559.

6

Purification of human serum paraoxonase: A simple and rapid method

A. J. Mahadesh Prasad*, K. Kemparaju, Elizabeth A. Frank and Cletus J. M. D'Souza

Department of Biochemistry Manasagangotri, University of Mysore, Mysore-570006, India.

Paraoxonase/arylesterases (EC.3.1.8.2) is an enzyme found tightly associated with high density lipoprotein particle in serum. Because of its unique enzyme activity, antioxidant property and its role as an anti atherosclerotic molecule, various methods are used for its purification from human serum. Methods involved in its purification are elaborate and complicated. Also the yield and final activity are highly variable. Here, we report a 2 step method of purification involving affinity chromatography on cibacron blue sepharose followed by gel filtration on sephadex G50.The final preparation was 27.7 fold purified compared with the serum and gave a single band in SDS-PAGE by silver staining.

Key words: Cibacron blue sepharose, paraoxonase, phenyl acetate, SDS-PAGE, silver staining.

INTRODUCTION

Paraoxonase (E.C. 3.1.8.2), (PON) is an enzyme ubiquitously distributed in nature (La Du et al., 1992). In animals it is mainly found in blood in association with high density lipoprotein (HDL) particle, by a strong hydrophobic association through the N-terminal hydrophobic peptide (Kuo and La Du, 1995). Consequently methods of purification have employed isolation of HDL, dissociation of HDL-PON and subsequent purification of PON.

PON was first purified by Main (1968). This method involved a series of ethanol precipitation and ammonium sulphate fractionation steps. The purified enzyme had a molecular weight ranging from 35 - 50 KDa.

The other methods of purification involved precipitation of HDL using heavy metal salts (Burstein et al., 1970) or by density gradient centrifugation to separate HDL fraction. More recent methods employ gel filtration of HDL on sepharose or affinity purification of HDL by affinity material like cibacron blue sepharose or heparin-agarose (Chapman et al., 1971) .These methods also use other additional steps of purification.

We report a 2 step method using affinity purification on cibacron blue sepharose followed by gel filtration on sephadex G-50.

MATERIALS AND METHODS

Materials

Glycine, tris buffer, ammonium per sulphate, acrylamide, bis

acrylamide, coomassi brilliant blue, TEMED, SDS and ethylene diaminetetraaceticacid (EDTA) were purchased from SRL chemicals (Mumbai, India). Cibacron blue 3GA and deoxycholate were purchased from Sigma Aldrich company USA. Acetic acid was purchased from Ranbaxy chemicals (New Delhi). All other chemicals, acids, bases, solvents and salts used for the purification were of analytical grade. Dialysis bags used during dialysis was purchased from Thermo scientific life science research products, Rockford, USA.

Human blood was collected from normal healthy volunteers according to guidelines mentioned by the institutional ethical committee for biomedical research.

Methods

Purification of human serum PON on affinity chromatography

Human serum paraoxonase was purified by nonspecific affinity chromatography on cibacron blue 3GA. Cibacron blue sepharose (30 ml) was washed and suspended in column buffer which contained 10 mM tris-HCl, 1 mM $CaCl_2$ and the pH was adjusted to 8.2 (Kuo and La Du, 1995). The ratio of gel to serum was maintained 4:5 (v/v). Serum (45 ml) was mixed with an equal volume of column buffer and the mixture was loaded on cibacron blue gel column, (40 × 2 cm). The eluate was recycled through the column twice. The eluate was then collected in one fraction. The column was then washed with 30 ml of 4 M NaCl solution. The 4 M NaCl salt solution greatly reduces albumin or other soluble proteins from binding to cibacron blue gel and thus most of the soluble proteins and other lipoproteins are washed out of column. The salt fraction was collected in a separate tube to check whether it contained the esterase activity (Rodrigo et al., 1997).

The column was then eluted with 30 ml of 0.1% deoxycholate and fractions were collected (1 ml). Optical density of the eluted fractions was measured at 280 nm. PON activity in the eluted fractions was monitored by assaying the aryl esterase activity. The fractions containing PON were pooled separately. The pooled frac-

*Corresponding author. E-mail: prasadjavarappa@hotmail.com.

tions were concentrated and further purified by gel filtration on sephadex G-50 column.

Gel filtration on G- 50

The pooled deoxycholate fraction (containing the aryl esterase enzyme activity) was loaded on sephadex G-50 column (50 × 2 cm) pre-equilibrated with 0.5 M NaCl solution. The column was also eluted with 0.5 M NaCl. 20 fractions (1 ml) were collected and the optical density was measured at 280 nm (Cordle et al., 1985).

Dialysis

The diluted protein fractions from G-50 with esterase activity were pooled (about 10 ml) and kept for dialysis in a dialysis bag with 8 KDa cut-off. Dialysis was carried out overnight against double distilled water with 2 changes. This process facilitates removal of deoxycholate which was used during the elution of HDL fraction from affinity column and the salt from gel filtration column. Long time association of deoxycholate with paraoxonase affects its activity as well as its half life.

Protein estimation by Lowry's method

Protein estimation was carried out according to Lowry's method (Lowry, 1951) to estimate serum protein as well as protein in purified fractions.

Assay of enzyme activity

Synthesis of phenyl acetate

10 ml of distilled phenol was taken in a round bottom flask and 20 ml acetyl chloride was added and refluxed at 70°C for 1 h. The contents of the flask were cooled and 200 ml of ice cold water was added. Free acid was neutralized by adding calculated amount of NaOH. The oily layer was separated by dissolving it in petroleum ether. Petroleum ether layer was evaporated to yield Phenyl acetate (Gan et al., 1991).

Aryl estrase activity

PON 1 activity towards phenyl acetate was measured spectrophotometrically at 270 nm in an automated shimadzu UV-1601, UV visible spectrophotometer. Buffer substrate was prepared by adding 50 mM Tris-HCl buffer pH 8.0 containing 2 mM Calcium. Phenyl acetate in Isopropyl alcohol was added such that the Phenyl acetate concentration was 2 mM and the isopropyl alcohol concentration was less than one percent. To 2.99 ml of buffered substrate 10 μl of the sample from different fractions was added and the optical density was measured at 270 nm continuously at intervals of 30 sec for 3 min. PON 1 activity was calculated from the linear part of the curve by calculating the change in OD per min. One unit of activity was defined as that amount of enzyme which produced 1 micromole of phenol per min. The molar extinction coefficient of phenol was 1310 M^{-1} cm^{-1} (Gan et al., 1991).

Inactivation of PON

Heat inactivation

PON activity in serum samples was also confirmed by the heat inactivation of PON. Selected serum, HDL or purified protein samples were heated at 80°C for 15 min prior to determining their PON activity as described above. There was no precipitation of protein by this treatment and the activity was essentially zero

Electrophoresis

SDS –page

Polyacrylamide gel electrophoresis (10% cross linking) was carried out for purified human serum paraoxonase as described by Davis (1964) using an alkaline buffer. (Tris-glycine buffer pH 8.8) The electrophoresis was performed at constant voltage for 2 - 4 h. The gels were stained using coomassi brilliant blue dye.

Silver staining

Silver staining was carried out essentially by the method of Switzer et al. (1980). Protein detection by silver staining depends on the binding of silver ions to the amino acid side chains, the sulphydryl and carboxyl groups of proteins followed by reduction to free metallic silver. As a result, the image of protein distribution within the gel is based on the difference in oxidation-reduction potential between the gel's area occupied by proteins and the free adjacent sites. It is sensitive enough to detect nanogram level of contaminating proteins if any.

Regeneration of cibacron blue gel

This is the most important and necessary step employed in the purification of PON from human serum sample. Initially the cibacron blue gel was washed with 3 M NaCl to remove any protein which was bound to cibacron blue gel. The gel was then washed with excess of water to remove chloride ions. This facilitated rapid purification and higher yield. The gels could be regenerated to maximum of 4 times.

RESULTS

The total protein concentration in the partially purified paraoxonase (Deoxycholate fraction) was 0.7 g/l with a specific activity of 1.4 mU/mg and total protein concentration of purified paraoxonase was 0.023 g/l with a specific activity of 4.6 mU/mg.

The elution profile of PON activity from cibacron blue affinity column is shown in Figure 1. Protein was eluted in 5 protein peaks while the enzyme activity was eluted in only 2 peaks namely peak 2 and 3. The protein elution and enzyme elution did not overlap. The elution of PON activity from sapahadex G-50 column is shown in Figure 2. The protein and enzyme activity elution overlapped. However a single symmetrical peak was not obtained.

The electrophoretic pattern of the purified protein is shown in Figure 3A and B, a single band was obtained both in coomassi blue staining as well as silver staining. The scheme of purification of PON is summarized in Table 1. The final product was 27.7 fold purified compared with pooled serum.

DISCUSSION

Since PON and HDL are tightly associated, during purifi-

Deoxy cholate Fraction

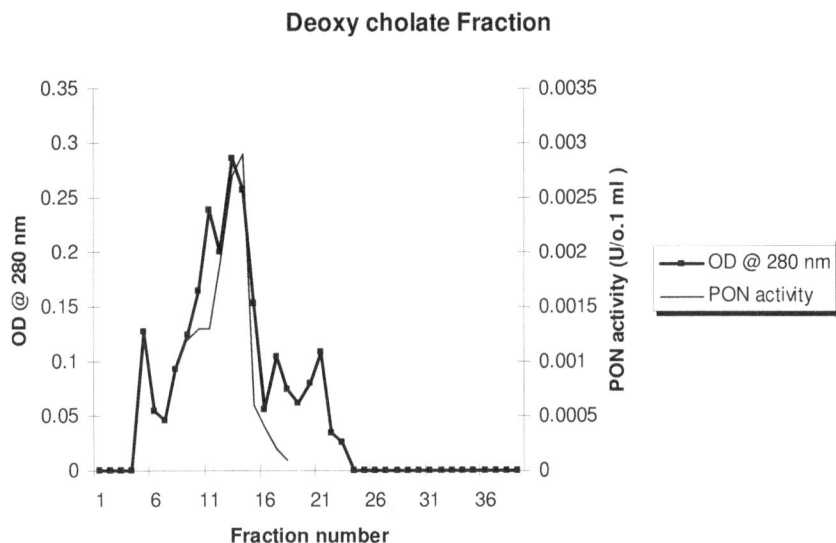

Figure 1. Elution of PON activity from cibacron blue sepharose column by deoxy cholate cibacron blue sepharose (30 ml) was packed in a column (40 × 2 cm). Pooled human serum was diluted with load buffer and passed through the column. Column was washed with 4 M NaCl followed by elution with 0.1% deoxycholate solution. Protein in the eluted fraction was monitored at 280 nm. The activity was monitored by measuring aryl esterase activity.

G-50 Fraction

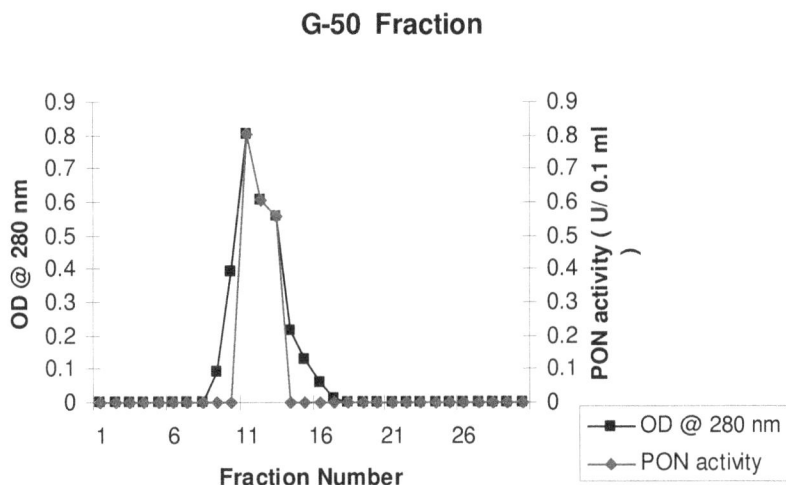

Figure 2. Elution profile of PON activity from sephadex G-50 column. Fraction having PON activity from cibacron blue column was pooled, concentrated and dialyzed against water. It was loaded on a column of sephadex G-50 (50 × 2 cm) preequilibrated and eluted with 0.5 M NaCl. Protein in the fractions (1 ml) was monitored at 280 nm and the activity was monitored by measuring the aryl esterase activity.

purification of PON, it is generally associated with APO-A1 and separating the 2 has been very difficult. APO-A1 is a major protein component of high density lipoprotein (HDL) with molecular weight of 29 KDa. APO-AI promotes cholesterol efflux from tissues to the liver for excretion and also play a major role in preventing accumulation of cholesterol loaded macrophage with in the

arterial wall as a foam cells. APO-AI is also a cofactor for LCAT factors that up regulate PON1 gene also up regulate Apo A1 gene (Hirz and Scanu, 1970). Apo A1 up regulation is associated with increase in HDL. (Hesler et al., 1988) PON 1 is also shown to strongly associate with apo A1 (Mackness, 1998) in HDL. This may be responsible for keeping PON completely associated with

Table 1. Scheme for purification of PON activity.

Fraction	Amount of Protein	Specific activity (mU/mg)
Serum	8.750 g/l	0.166
oxycholate fraction (Dialyzed)	0.7 g/l	1.4
G- 50 fraction	0.023 g/l	4.6

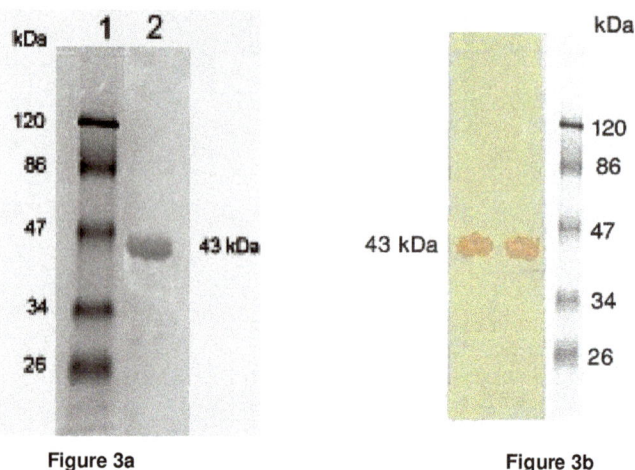

Figure 3a

Figure 3b

Figure 3. Electrophoresis –SDS PAGE
(a) Coomassi staining (10%).
(b) Silver staining.

HDL in the serum (Jenne et al., 1991). Separation of APO AI and PON may result in the loss of PON activity. In this study the total recovery of enzyme activity was only 7.3% of the initial activity. It is possible that the entire PON enzyme may not be associated with HDL. It is also possible that there may be pool of modified HDL which does not bind to the affinity matrix. During purification the loss of activity of PON may also be because of the loss of its natural lipid environment. It is also possible that the PON may not be as active in the dissociated form as it in the native form. This is consistent with the report that purified PON loses its activity rapidly (Aviram et al., 1998). However our data show that the specific activity at the cibacron blue step is about 8 fold higher than that of the serum and in the sephadex gel filtration step it is further improved 3 fold.

Since aryl esterase was used to monitor the elution of PON, the enzyme assayed as PON may not be entirely PON, but may have represented other esterases also. For example, serum cholinesterase also shows arylesterase activity but their contribution to the total activity would be less than 5%. However, this esterase would not be active in high salt solution where only PON is active. We have also shown that the non specific esterase hydrolyzes phenyl acetate at high pH and the activity of non specific esterase at pH 8 is negligible. Hence the phenyl acetate hydrolyzing PON activity alone may be seen in the deoxycholate fraction.

It is interesting that a single band was obtained even when the sephadex G-50 fraction did not show a symmetrical peak. It is possible that some of the PON may still attach to lipid non-covalently in the gel filtration step, since PON is known to bind to lipid it may still be associated in the fractionation. However in SDS – page the lipid would be dissociated giving only single band.

It is interesting to note that the PON activity recovered from the purification steps is low. Since Indians have a high prevalence for cardiovascular diseases (Goyal and Yusuf, 2006; Singh et al., 2007). it is tempting to speculate that the active HDL which would be cardio protective is low among Indians while the non functional HDL even though high, may not contain PON or may contain some inactive form of PON.

Conclusion

We report a simple and rapid method of purification of PON from human serum in sufficient quantity in very short time and also we show the regeneration of the affinity gel for reuse.

ACKNOWLEDGEMENT

EAF thanks DST for research grant (SR/WOS-A/LS-209/2004).

REFERENCES

Abhinav G, Salim Y (2006). The burden of cardiovascular disease in the Indian subcontinent. Indian. J. Med. Res .124: 235-244.

Aviram, RM, Bisgaier CL, Newton RS, Primo-parmo SL, La Du BN (1998). Paraoxonase inhibits high-density lipoprotein oxidation and preserves its functions. A possible peroxidative role for paraoxonase. J. Clin. Invest. 101: 1581-1590.

Burstein HR, Scholnick R, Morfin (1970). Rapid method for the isolation of lipoproteins from human serum by precipitation with polyanions . J. Lip. Res. 11: 583-595.

Chapman S, Goldstein D, Lagrange PM, Laplaud (1981). A density gradient ultracentrifugal procedure for the isolation of the major lipoprotein classes from human serum. J. Lip. Res. 22: 339-358.

Cordle RA, Clegg SJ, Yeaman (1985). Purification and characterization of bovine lipoproteins: resolution of high density and low density lipoproteins using heparin-Sepharose chromatography. J. Lip. Res. 26: 721-725.

Gan A, Smolen HW, Eckerson BN, La Du (1991). Purification of human serum paraoxonase/arylesterase. Evidence for one esterase catalyzing both activities. American Society for Pharmacology and Experimental Therapeutics. 19 (1): 100-106.

Hesler CB, Tall AR, Swenson TL, Weech PK, Marcel YL, Milne RW(1988). Monoclonal antibodies to the Mr 74,000 cholesteryl ester transfer protein neutralize all of the cholesteryl ester and triglyceride transfer activities in human plasma. J. Biol. Chem. Apr. 15;263(11): 5020–5023.

.Hirz R, Scanu AM (1970). Reassembly *in vitro* of a serum high-density lipoprotein. Biochim Biophys Acta. May 26;207(2): 364–367.

Jenne B, Lowin MC, Peitsch A, Bottcher G, Schmitz TJ (1991). Clusterin (complement lysis inhibitor) forms a high density lipoprotein complex with apolipoprotein A-I in human plasma. J. Biol. Chem. 266: 11030–11036.

Kuo, La Du BN (1995) .Comparison of purified human and rabbit serum paraoxonases. Drug Metab. Disposition 23: 935-944.

La Du BN, Kalow W (1992).Human serum paraoxonase/arylesterase. Pharmacogenetics of Drug Metabolism .Pergamon Press, New Yark. pp. 51-94.

GIL LF, HERNANDEZ AF, MARINA A, VAZQUEZ J, PLA A (1997). Purification and characterization of paraoxon hydrolase from rat liver. Biochem. J. 321: 595–601.

Lowry OH, Rosebrough NJ, Farr AL, Randall RJ (1951). Protein measurement with Folin phenol reagent. J. Biol. Chem. 193: 265–275.

Switzer RC, Merril CR, Shifrin S. (1979). A highly sensitive silver stain for detecting proteins and peptides in polyacrylamide gels. Anal. Biochem. 98(1), 231-7.

Main AR (1968) The purification of enzyme hydrolyzing diethyl- p-nitrophenyl phosphate (paraoxon) in sheep serum. Biochem. J. 74: 10, 20.

Singh S, Venketesh S, Verma JS, Verma M, Lellamma CO, Goel RC (2007). Paraoxonase (PON1) activity in North West Indian Punjabis with coronary artery disease & type 2 diabetes mellitus. Indian. J .Med. Res .125: 783-787.

7

Anti-inflammatory and anti-ulcerogenic activity of the ethanol extract of ginger (*Zingiber officinale*)

Chioma A. Anosike, Onyechi Obidoa, Lawrence U. S. Ezeanyika and Meshach M. Nwuba

Department of Biochemistry, University of Nigeria, Nsukka. Enugu State, Nigeria.

The acute toxicity test carried out on the ginger extract gave the LD_{50} value as 1000 mg/kg. The anti-inflammatory and anti-ulcerogenic effects of the ethanol extract of ginger (*Zingiber officinale*) in adult Wistar rats were studied using values below the lethal dose. Inflammation was induced by injecting 0.1 ml undiluted fresh egg albumin (philogistic agent) into the subplantar surface of the right hind paw of the rats. Ethanol extract of ginger with doses of 100, 200 and 400 mg/kg and indomethacin 100 mg/kg were administered intraperitoneally to separate groups of the rats. Control group received 1 ml of normal saline (vehicle). All the doses of the extract (100, 200 and 400 mg/kg) significantly ($p < 0.05$) reduced the fresh egg albumin induced rat paw oedema, though not in a dose dependent manner. The oedema reductions were more than that obtained for indomethacin, the standard anti-inflammatory drug used. The ginger extract also showed good protective effect against indomethacin – induced gastric ulcer in the rats. Administration of the extract doses (100, 200 and 400 mg/kg) evinced a significant ($p < 0.05$) reduction in the indomethacin – induced gastric erosion in all the experimental groups when compared to control. The percent ulcer inhibition by the extract doses was comparable with that of ranitidine (100 mg/kg), the reference drug. These results show that ginger possess good potential as an anti-oedema and anti-ulcer agent.

Key words: Ginger extract, inflammation, oedema reduction, gastric ulcer, indomethacin, ulcer inhibition.

INTRODUCTION

In recent times, focus on plant research has increased all over the world and a large body of evidence has been collected to show immense potential of medicinal plants used in various traditional systems (Dahanuka et al., 2002). *Zingiber officinale* (ginger) which belongs to the family Zingiberaceae is a slender perennial plant that reaches the height of 2 feet and has greenish yellow flowers resembling orchids. The rhizome of ginger has an aromatic pungent taste. Its exact country of origin is uncertain, but it was thought to be originally native of tropical South East Asia before it spread to Africa. It is now grown abundantly in Northern Nigeria.

Ginger has extensive medicinal history. It is used as spice in food and beverages and in traditional medicine as carminative, antipyretic and in the treatment of pain, rheumatism and bronchitis (Afzal et al., 2001). Its extracts have been extensively studied for a broad range of biolo-

gical activities including antibacterial (Mahady et al., 2003; Azu et al., 2007), analgesic and anti-inflammatory (Raji et al., 2002; Grzanna et al., 2005), anti-angiogenesis and antitumor (Surn et al., 1999; Kim et al., 2005). It is also used for the treatment of gastrointestinal disorders including gastric ulcerogenesis (Agrawal et al., 2000; Mohsen et al., 2006). It performs the above role by eliminating the bacteria *Helicobacter pylori* whose secretions of ammonia in the stomach are responsible for many ulcers, especially of the duodene and for other stomach problems like gastritis. The plant also neutralizes the excess gastric acid in the stomach which causes other forms of ulcers. Ginger has also been reported to be an effective anti-emetic, used in the treatment of both motion sickness and the nausea and vomiting associated with pregnancy (Backon, 1991; Ernest and Pittler, 2000). It reduces the stickiness of blood platelets, hence may help reduce the risk of artherosclerosis and heart attacks (Verma et al., 2004). On the basis of these common uses of *Z. officinale* in ethnomedicine, this work was therefore aimed at assessing the effect of the ethanol extract of ginger on induced inflammation and ulcer.

*Corresponding author. E-mail: chiomanos@yahoo.com.

MATERIALS AND METHODS

Animals

Swiss Albino mice (22 – 28 g) and adult Wistar rats (120 – 200 g) of both sexes obtained from the animal house of the Faculty of Biological Sciences, University of Nigeria, Nsukka were used for the studies. They were acclimatised for seven days before the experiment and maintained *ad libitum* on water and growers mash (Pfizer Feeds, Aba) bought from Nsukka market. The research was conducted in accordance with the ethical rules on animal experimentation approved by the ethical committees of the Faculty of Biological Sciences, University of Nigeria, Nsukka.

Chemicals

All chemicals used in this study were of analytical grade. They were products of May and Baker, England and Merck, Darmstadt, Germany.

Plant materials

The ginger plant material (*Z. officinale*) was purchased from the Nsukka local market and identified by Mr. Ugwuozor of Botany department, University of Nigeria, Nsukka. Voucher specimen was deposited in the herbarium unit of the department of Botany, University of Nigeria, Nsukka. The plant was peeled, chopped into tiny bits, air-dried for 2 weeks and ground with a mechanical grinder. The ground plant (500 g) was macerated in absolute ethanol for 24 h, filtered with a white cloth and the filtrate concentrated using a rotary evaporator at an optimum temperature of 40 -50°C. The dried yield of the extract was 5 g.

Phytochemical analysis

Preliminary phytochemical tests were carried out on the ethanol extract of ginger using the methods of Harborne (1984) and Trease and Evans (1989). Tests for the presence or absence of phytochemical compounds using the above methods involve the addition of an appropriate chemical agent to the extract of the plant in a test tube. The mixture was shaken vigorously or gently as the case may be. The presence or absence of phytochemicals such as saponnins, flavonoids, alkaloids, tanninis, trepenoids, steroids etc was observed.

Test for carbohydrate (Molisch's test)

A known weight of 0.1 g of the ginger extract was boiled with 2 ml of water and filtered. To the filtrate, few drops of naphtol solution in ethanol (Molisch's reagent) were added. Concentrated sulphuric acid was then gently poured down the side of the test tube to form a lower layer.

Test for alkaloids (General tests)

Sulphuric acid (20 ml of 5%) in 50% ethanol was added to about 2 g of the ginger extract sample and heated on a boiling water bath for 10 min, cooled and filtered. Filtrate (2 ml) was tested with a few drops of: Mayer's reagent (Potassium mercuric iodide solution), Dragendorff's reagent (Bismuth potassium iodide solution), Wagner's reagent (Iodide in potassium iodide solution) and Picric acid solution (1%). The remaining filtrate was placed in 100 ml separating funnel and made alkaline with dilute ammonia solution. The aqueous alkaline solution was separated and extracted with

two 5 ml portions of dilute sulphuric acid. The sample was tested with a few drops of Mayer's, Wagner's and Dragendorff's reagent.

Test for glycosides (Fehling's test)

A quantity of 5 ml of a mixture of equal parts of Fehling's solution I and II were added to 5 ml of the ginger extract sample and then heated on a water bath for 5 min.

Test for Saponnins (Fehling's method)

Water (20 ml) was added to 0.25 g of the ginger extract in 100 ml beaker and boiled gently on a hot water bath for 2 min. The mixture was filtered hot and allowed to cool and the filtrate used for the following test: Fehling's Test: To 5 ml of the filtrate was added 5 ml of Fehling's solution (equal parts of I and II) and the content heated. A reddish precipitate indicated the presence of saponnins. It was then heated further with sulphuric acid.

Test for tannins (Ferric chloride method)

Ginger extract (1 g) was boiled with 50 ml of water, filtered and used for the Ferric Chloride test: To 3 ml of the filtrate, few drops of ferric chloride were added.

Test for flavonoids (Ammonium test method)

Ethylacetate (10 ml) was added to 0.2 g of the ginger extract sample and heated on a water bath for 3 min. The mixture was cooled, filtered and the filtrate used for the Ammonium test: About 4 ml of the filtrate was shaken with 1 ml of dilute ammonia solution. The layers were allowed to separate.

Test for resins (Precipitation test)

The ginger extract (0.2 g) was extracted with 15 ml of 95% ethanol. The alcoholic extract was then poured into 20 ml of distilled water in a beaker.

Test for proteins (Million's test)

Two drops of million's reagent were added to the filtrate in a test tube.

Test for oils

The ginger extract (0.1 g) material was pressed between a filter paper and the paper was put under serious observation.

Test for steroids and terpenoids

Ethanol (9 ml) was added to 1 g of the ginger extract sample and refluxed for a few minutes and filtered. The filtrate was concentrated to 2.5 ml on a boiling water bath and 5 ml of hot water was added. The mixture was allowed to stand for 1 h and the waxy matter filtered off. The filtrate was extracted with 2.5 ml of chloroform using separating funnel. To 0.5 ml of the chloroform extract in a test tube was carefully added 1 ml of concentrated sulphuric acid to form a lower layer.

Acute toxicity study

The acute toxicity test was carried out by a modified method of Lorke (1983) to define the range of lethal dose and safe dose for the extract. Swiss albino mice were starved of food but allowed access to water prior to the study and were then grouped (three mice per group). They were treated intraperitoneally with different doses of the extract (50, 100, 400, 600, 1000 and 1500 mg/kg). The animals were then observed for 24 h for nervousness, dullness, incoordination or death.

Anti-inflammatory test

The anti-inflammatory test was carried out using a philogistic agent - induced rat hind paw oedema as a model for acute inflammation (Winter et al., 1962). The philogistic agent employed in this study was fresh egg albumin (Akah and Nwambie, 1994). Twenty five (25) adult wistar rats of either sex (120 – 200 g) were divided into five experimental groups of five rats each. They were fasted and deprived of water for 18 h before the experiment. Deprivation of water was to ensure uniform hydration and to minimize variability in oedematous response (Winter et al., 1963).

Various extract doses (100, 200 and 400 mg/kg) suspended in normal saline were administered intraperitoneally into groups I, II and III of the rats. Control group received equivalent amount of normal saline and the reference group was administered 100 mg/kg indomethacin. One hour post treatment, inflammation of the hind paw was induced by injecting 0.1 ml of undiluted fresh egg albumin (philogistic agent) into the subplantar surface of the right hind paw. This treatment was found to cause swelling of the paw which retained about the same degree of oedema for 3 h. The right hind paw volumes of the rats were taken on the principle of volume displacement using LETICA Digital Plethysmometer (LE 7500) immediately before the experiment (zero time) and at 1 h intervals after the injection of egg albumin for a period of 5 h. Average oedema at every interval was assessed in terms of difference in volume displacement after injecting the philogistic agent and zero time volume displacement of the injected paw ($V_t - V_0$). Percent inhibition of oedema was also calculated for each dose (Akah and Njike, 1990) using the relation (Perez, 1996);

$$\text{\% inhibition of oedema} = 1 - \left(\frac{a-x}{b-y}\right) \times 100$$

Where;
a = Mean paw volume of treated rats after egg albumin injection.
x = Mean paw volume of treated rats before egg albumin injection.
b = Mean paw volume of control rats after egg albumin injection.
y = Mean paw volume of control rats before egg albumin injection.

Indomethacin induced ulcer

This assay was carried out using the method of Urushidani et al. (1979). Twenty five adult rats randomly divided into 5 groups of 5 rats each were deprived of food for 18 h and treated per orally with normal saline and varying doses of the ginger extract. The extract and drugs used were freshly prepared as a suspension in normal saline and administered per orally (p.o) to the animals in 5 ml/kg doses. Group 1 (normal control) was administered normal saline (5 ml/kg). Groups II, III and IV were treated with 100, 200 and 400 mg/kg of the ginger extract respectively. Group V (reference group) was administered 100 mg/kg of ranitidine (standard anti ulcer drug).

Thirty minutes later, 50 mg/kg of indomethacin was administered (p.o) to the rats. After 8 h, each animal in the groups was sacrificed

Table 1. Result of phytochemical analysis of the ginger extract.

Plant constituent	Bioavailability
Alkaloid	++
Glycosides	-
Steroids	+++
Terpenoids	+++
Flavonoids	++++
Tannins	-
Acidic compounds	-
Fats and oil	+
Resins	+++
Carbohydrate	+++
Saponnins	-

Key:
- = Not present.
+ = Present in low concentration.
++ = Present in moderately high concentration.
+++ = Present in very high concentration.
++++ = Abundantly present.

by chloroform anaesthesia and the stomach removed and opened along the greater curvature, pinned flat on a board, examined and scored for ulcer. Erosions formed on the glandular portions of the stomach were counted and the ulcer index calculated as described by Main and Whittle (1975).

The ulcer was counted and scored as 0 = no ulcer; 1 = superficial ulcer; 2 = deep ulcer and 3 = perforations. The sum of all the lesions/ulcer in all the animals for each group (Total ulcer score) was used to calculate the ulcer index. Percent ulcer inhibition was calculated relative to control.

Statistical analysis

This was done using SPSS version 14.0 (SPSS Inc. Chicago, IL.USA). All values are expressed as mean ± SD. Data were analysed by one-way ANOVA and difference between means was assessed by a two-tailed Student's T-test. $P < 0.05$ was considered statistically significant.

RESULTS

Phytochemical analysis of the ethanol extract of ginger (Table 1) showed the presence of phytochemicals such as alkaloids, resins, steroids, flavonoids and terpenoids. Other constituents like saponnins, tannins, glycosides and acidic compounds were absent.

The LD_{50} of the crude ethanol extract was calculated to be 1000 mg/kg. All the doses used in this study were therefore carefully chosen to exclude the lethal range. Data from Table 2 show the mean paw volumes for the various groups at different time intervals. On the control rats, fresh egg albumin induced paw oedema which was sustained for 3 h after which it started reducing significantly. The mean paw volumes of groups administered 200 and 400 mg/kg of ginger significantly reduced ($p < 0.05$) from the first hour after oedema induction and that

Table 2. Effect of ethanol extract of ginger on egg albumin induced rat paw oedema.

Groups	Δ paw volume (oedema) ml and % inhibition of oedema				
	1 h	2 h	3 h	4 h	5 h
Control	0.76 ± 0.05	0.68 ± 0.16	0.56 ± 0.23	0.44 ± 0.19	0.3 ± 0.12
100 mg/kg	0.64 ± 0.11	0.4 ± 0.19*	0.3 ± 0.14*	0.17 ± 0.1*	0.11 ± 0.05*
	(15.79)	(41.18)	(46.43)	(63.04)	(63.33)
200 mg/kg	0.6 ± 0.14*	0.46 ± 0.09*	0.3 ± 0.07*	0.22 ± 0.04*	0.1 ± 0*
	(21.05)	(32.35)	(46.43)	(52.17)	(66.67)
400 mg/kg	0.46 ± 0.09*	0.31 ± 0.11*	0.2 ± 0.07*	0.13 ± 0.06*	0.07 ± 0.03*
	(39.47)	(54.41)	(64.29)	(71.74)	(76.67)
100 mg/kg Indomethacin	0.7 ± 0.07	0.5 ± 0.12	0.36 ± 0.09*	0.27 ± 0.08*	0.16 ± 0.05*
	(7.89)	(26.47)	(35.71)	(41.3)	(46.67)

*Reduction in oedema significant at $p < 0.05$ compared to control. Values of oedema shown are mean ± SD (n = 5).
Values in parenthesis are percent inhibition of oedema calculated relative to control.

Table 3. Effect of ginger extract on indomethacin induced gastric ulcer in rats.

Treatment	Dose (mg/kg)	Total ulcer scores	Magnification X 1/10	Ulcer index	% Ulcer inhibition
Control (normal saline)	5 ml/kg	204	20.4	4.08 ± 1.61	-
Extract	100	58	5.8	1.16 ± 0.66*	71.56
Extract	200	105	10.5	2.1 ± 1.23*	48.53
Extract	400	98	9.8	1.9 ± 0.63 *	53.4
Ranitidine	100	44	4.4	0.88 ± 0.33*	78.4

Values shown are mean ± SD. (n = 5). *Significantly different from control at $p < 0.05$.

of group administered 100 mg/kg significantly reduced from the second hour. The paw oedema reduction increased with time but not in a dose dependent manner. The percent inhibition of oedema for the group treated with 100 mg/kg of ginger was 15, 41, 46, 63 and 63% for the 1st, 2nd, 3rd, 4th and 5th hour respectively. That of groups treated with 200 and 400 mg/kg were 21, 32, 46, 52, 66, 39, 54, 64, 71 and 76% respectively.

The oedema reduction for the ginger treated groups was more than that observed for the standard anti-inflammatory drug, indomethacin, which had 7, 26, 35, 41 and 46% inhibition of oedema for the 1st, 2nd, 3rd, 4th and 5th hour respectively. The mean oedema and percent inhibition of oedema in the ginger extract treated rats are shown in Table 2. Data from Table 3 show that indomethacin induced gastric ulcer in all experimental groups. Groups treated with ginger had a significant reduction (p < 0.05) in the gastric erosions formed, when compared to control as is shown from the reduced ulcer indices. The reduction in the ulcer was also not dose dependent. Ginger extract dose of 100 mg/kg showed 71% inhibition of ulcer, which was comparable to that of ranitidine, the anti-ulcer drug used, which had 78% inhibition, while 200 and 400 mg/kg doses showed 48 and 53% inhibition

respectively.

DISCUSSION

The present study revealed some of the pharmacological basis for the ethnomedicinal use of ginger in the treatment of inflammation. The ethanol extract of ginger showed a good anti-inflammatory activity against acute inflammation, suppressing the rat paw oedema both at the early and later phases, though not dose dependently. Oedema results from the action of inflammatory mediators such as histamine, serotonin and bradykinin at the site of a local inflammatory insult (Harriot et al., 2004).

The early phase of oedema, beginning from 1 h after the administration of the irritant, is due to the release of histamine and serotonine, while the later phase, occurring from 3 to 5 h after the administration of the irritant is induced by bradykinin, protease, prostaglandin and lysosome (Wallace, 2002; Harriot et al., 2004). The reduction in oedema evinced by ginger extract in this study suggests that it contains active constituents which block the release of histamine and serotonin from mast cells and inhibit the activity of other inflammatory mediators. This report agree with earlier reports of Suekewa and Yuasa (1986) which showed that (6)-shogaol isolated from ginger extract inhibited experimentally- induced swelling of the hind paw in rats. This, they reported may be due to the ability of (6)-shogaol to inhibit cyclooxygenase enzyme.

Sharma and Srivastava (1994) also reported that ginger inhibited paw oedema in an experimentally induced arthritis in the right knee and paw of rats. Srivastava and Mustafa (1992) reported that 75% of patients suffering from arthritis, osteoarthritis or muscular discomfort experienced relief in pain and swelling to varying degrees after powered ginger treatment for 3 months to 2.5 years. Shen et al. (2005) also reported the anti-inflammatory effect of ginger roots on osteoarthritic cow chondrocytes showing its strong inhibition of COX-2 enzyme, pro-inflammatory cytokines and prostaglandins which are all components of the inflammatory response. Middleton and Kandaswami (1992) and Read (1995) reported that plant flavonoids, apart from their many pharmacological actions, also have potent anti-inflammatory activities. Phytochemical results of this study showed that ginger is abundantly rich in flavonoids. This suggests that the flavonoids in ginger may be one of its main active anti-inflammatory constituents.

From this study, ginger extract had significant (p < 0.05) protective effect against indomethacin - induced gastric ulcer for all the doses. Some drugs such as indomethacin, ibuprofen and aspirin known to have effective anti-inflammatory activity (NSAIDs); inhibiting the various changes leading to inflammation are associated with some side effects such as gastric erosions and abdominal ulcers after prolonged use (Ogbru, 2006). This is believed to be due to the inhibition by these drugs of the cyclooxygenase 1 enzyme which synthesises prostaglandin (PG) needed for haemostasis and the maintenance of the gastric lining of the stomach (Wallace, 2002). The concern over the severe side effects of these anti-inflammatory drugs have led to the search for new anti-inflammatory agents from plants and plant products with low toxicity and minimal side effects.

In this study, the ethanol extract of ginger exhibited anti-ulcerogenic effect against indomethacin induced gastric ulcer, with percent ulcer inhibition comparable with that obtained for ranitidine, an antiacid used to neutralize intraluminal acid, improve gastric microcirculation and reduce the absorption and concomitant adverse drug interactions of many NSAIDs (Derle et al., 2006). Earlier reports by Agrawal et al. (2000) and Mohsen et al. (2006) on the anti-ulcerative activities of ginger suggest that ginger extract possess its anti-ulcerative properties through a mechanism related to acid and pepsin secretory inhibition. Although the exact mechanism of action of the anti-ulcer activities of ginger has not been clearly delineated, the plant contains some active constituents whose ulcer protective properties have been identified (Yamahara et al., 1988). The results of this present study

show that ginger extract possess good potential as an antioedema and antiulcer agent. This suggests that the extract of ginger is both anti-inflammatory and anti-ulcerogenic.

REFERENCES

Afzal M, Al-Hadidi B, Menon M, Pesek J, Dhami MS (2001). Ginger: an ethnomedicinal, Chem. Pharmacol. Rev. Drug Metabol. Drug Interact. 18(3-4): 159-190.

Agrawal AK, Rao CV, Sairam K, Joshi VK, Goel RK (2000). Effect of Piper longum Linn, Zingiber officinale Linn and Ferula species on gastric ulceration and secretion in rats. Indian J. Exp. Biol. 38(10): 994-998.

Akah PA, Njike HA (1990). Some Pharmacological effects of rhizome aqueous extracts of Anchomanes diformis. Fitoterapia 61: 368-370.

Akah PA, Nwambie AL (1994). Evaluation of Nigerian traditional medicines; plants used in rheumatic disorder. J. Ethnopharmacol. 42: 179-182.

Azu NC, Onyeagba RA. Okoro N (2007). Antibacterial activity of Allium cepa and Zingiber officinale (Ginger) on Staphylococcus aureus and Pseudomonas aeruginosa Isolated from High Vaginal Swab. The Internet J. Trop. Med. 3 (2): 1-12.

Backon J (1991). Ginger in preventing nausea and vomiting of pregnancy: a caveat due to its thromboxane synthetase activity and effect on testorone binding. Eur. J. Obstet. Gynaecol. Res. Biol. 43: 163-164.

Dahanuka SA, Kulkarni RA, Rege NN (2002). Pharmacology of medicinal plants and natural products. Indian J. Pharmacol. 32: 508-512.

Derle OV, Guijar KN, Sagar B (2006). Adverse Effects Associated with the Use of Non-Steroidal Anti-inflammatory Drugs: An Overview. J. Pharm. Indian Sci. 68: 409-414.

Ernest E, Pittler MH (2000). Efficacy of ginger for nausea and vomiting: A systematic review of randomised clinical trials. Br. J. Anaesth. 84: 367-371.

Grzanna R, Linmark L, Frondoza CG (2005). Ginger-an herbal medicine product with broad anti-inflammatory actions. J. Med. Food. 8(2): 125-132.

Harborne JB (1984). Phytochemical Methods. A Guide to Modern Technique of Plant Analysis. London: Chapman and Hall

Harriot M, Marion E, Martha A, Wellford S, William A (2004). Inflammation induced by histamine, serotonine, bradykinin and compound 48/480 in the rat. Antagonists and mechanisms of action. J. Pharmacol. Exp. Therapeutics 191: 300- 302

Kim EC, Min JK, Kim TY, Lee SJ, Yang HO, Han S, Kim YM, Kwon YG (2005). [6]- Gingerol, a pungent ingredient of ginger, inhibits angiogenesis in vitro and in vivo. Biochem. Biophys. Res. Commun. 335(2): 300-308.

Lorke D (1983). A new approach to practical acute toxicity testing. Arch. Toxicity. 54: 275 - 287.

Mahady GB, Pendland SL, Yun GS, Lu ZZ, Stoia A (2003). Ginger (Zingiber officinale Roscoe) and the gingerols inhibit the growth of Cag A' strains of Helicobacter pylori. Anticancer Res. 23(5A): 3699-3702.

Main IHM, Whittle BJR (1975). Investigation of vasodilator and antisecretory role of prostaglandins in the rat gastric mucosa by use of non-steroidal anti-inflammatory drugs. Br. J. Pharmacol. 53: 217-224.

Middleton E, Kandaswami C (1992). Effect of flavonoids on immune and inflammatory cell function. Biochem Pharmacol. 43: 1167-1179.

Moshen M, Alireza G, Alireza K (2006). Anti-ulcerogenic effect of ginger (rhizome of Zingiber officinale Roscoe) on cystemine induced duodenal ulcer in rats. DARU. 14: 97-101.

Ogbru O (2006). Nonsteroidal anti-inflammatory drugs (NSAIDS) Jay W. Marks eds. pp 232-233.

Perez GRM (1996). Anti-inflammatory activity of Ambrosia artemisaefolia and Rheo spathacea. Phytomed. 3(2): 163-167.

Raji Y, Udoh US, Oluwadara OO (2002). Anti-inflammatory and Analgesics Properties of the Rhizome Extract of Zingiber officinale. Afr. J.

Biomed. Res. 5: 1-11.

Read MA (1995). Flavonoids: naturally occurring anti-inflammatory agents. Am. J. Pathol. 147: 235-237.

Sharma P, Srivastava K (1994). Suppressive effects of eugenol and ginger oil on arthritic rats. Pharmacol. 49: 314-318.

Shen CL, Hong KJ, Kim SW (2005). Comparative effects of ginger root (*Zingiber officinale*) on the production of inflammatory mediators in normal and osteoarthrotic cow chondrocytes. J. Med. Food 8(2): 149-153.

Srivastava K, Mustafa T (1992). Ginger (*Zinger officinale*) in rheumatism and musculoskeletal disorder. Med. Hypothesis 39: 342-348.

Suekewa M, Yuasa K (1986). Pharmacological studies on ginger IV: effect of (6) - shogoal on the arachidonic acid cascade. Nippon. Ya. Kruigaku. Zasshi. 88: 263-269.

Surn YJ, Park KK, Chun KS, Lee LJ, Lee E, Lee SS (1999). Anti-tumor promoting activities of selected pungent phenolic substances present in ginger. J. Environ. Pathol. Toxicol. Oncol. 18(2): 131-139.

Trease GE, Evans WC (1989). Phenols and Phenolic glycosides. In: Textbook of Pharmacognosy. (12th ed.). Balliese, Tindall and Co Publishers, London pp. 343-383

Urushidani T, Kasuya Y, Okabe S (1979). The mechanism of aggravation of indomethacin –induced ulcers by gastric adrenalectomy in the rat. Jpn. J. Pharmacol. 29: 775-780.

Verma SK, Singh M, Jain P, Bordia A (2004). Protective effect of ginger (*Zingiber officinale* Roscoe) on experimental atherosclerosis in rabbits. Indian J. Exp. Biol. 42: 736-738.

Wallace JM (2002). Nutritional and botanical modulation of the inflammatory cascade: eicosanoids, cyclooxygenase and lipoxygenase- as an adjunct in cancer therapy. Integr. Cancer Ther. 1: 7-37.

Winter EA, Risley EA, Nuss GV (1962). Carrageenan- induced oedema in hind paw of rats as an assay for anti-inflammatory drugs. Proc. Soc. Exp. Biol. Med. 111: 544-547.

Winter EA, Risley EA, Nuss GV (1963). Anti-inflammatory and antipyretic activities of indomethacin. J. Pharm. Exp. Ther. 141: 369-376.

Yamahara J, Mochizuki M, Rong HQ, Matsuda H, Fujimura H (1988). The anti-ulcer effect in rats of ginger constituents. J. Ethnopharmacol. 23(2-3): 299-304.

8

Anti-atherogenic effects of supplementation with vitamin B6 (Pyridoxine) in albino rats

Adekunle Adeniran S. and Adedeji Adebayo L.

Department of Biochemistry, Ladoke Akintola University of Technology, Ogbomoso, Oyo State, Nigeria.

Elevation of serum lipids have been implicated to predispose to cardiovascular disorders which includes hypertension, stroke, atherosclerosis etc. Various studies have reported links between supplementation with vitamin B complex and reduction in oxidative stress and inflammatory reactions, two events associated with cardiovascular disorders. Data on possible direct regulation on lipid profile by vitamin B6 is very scanty. This study is therefore designed to assess role of administration of vitamin B6 in regulation of serum lipids such as total cholesterol, phospholipids, triglycerides, and high density lipoprotein cholesterol (HDL-C). Results showed that serum total cholesterol and triglyceride were significantly reduced ($p \leq 0.05$) in rats placed on vitamin B_6 supplements compared with control group. Serum phospholipids and high density lipoprotein cholesterol were significantly elevated ($p \leq 0.05$) in rats placed on vitamin B_6 supplements when compared with control group. The data showed anti-hyperlipideamic effects of vitamin B6 supplementation in rats.

Key words: Pyridoxine, lipids, cardiovascular disorder, supplement.

INTRODUCTION

Cardiovascular diseases (CVD) are caused by disorder of the heart and blood vessels and include the coronary heart disease, raised blood pressure that is, hypertension etc. Major traditional risk factors of CVD include elevated serum levels of total cholesterol, triglyceride, low density lipoprotein and reduced serum concentration of high density lipoprotein among other things. The disease is the most common cause of sudden death (Thomas et al., 1988) and is also the most common reason for death of men and women over 20 years of age (American Heart Association, 2007). According to present trends in the United States, half of healthy 40-year-old males will develop coronary artery disease (CAD) in the future, and one in three healthy 40-year-old women (Rosamond et al., 2007). Traditionally, these conditions are considered to result from lipid abnormalities, and other risk factors such as hypertension, smoking, hyperhomocysteinemia and diabetes (Niessen et al., 2003).

The conditions have caused lots of losses in both human and material resources. Among recommended

antidote to this include adjustment in lifestyle which involves nutritional modifications, slight physical exercise and in some instances use of drugs (Djousse et al., 2009).

A connection between homocysteine (a sulphur containing amino acid) and cardiovascular disease was proposed when it was observed that people with a rare hereditary condition called homocysteinuria are prone to develop severe cardiovascular disease in their teens and twenties and this was comfirmed by the study of David et al. (2002). In this condition an enzyme deficiency causes homocystiene to accumulate in the blood and to be excreted in the urine. Elevations in plasma homocystiene level promote oxidative damage, inflammation and endothelial dysfunction and are independent risk factor for cardiovascular disease.

Furthermore, epidemiological studies have shown plasma homocysteine levels are inversely related to plasma levels of folate, B12 and B6- the three vitamins involved in the conversion of homocystiene to methionine and cysteine.

This study is designed to assess possible lipid-lowering effect of administration of vitamin B6 and also the protective effect of the administration towards development of cardiovascular disease.

---

*Corresponding author. E-mail: kunleniran@yahoo.com.

Table 1. Effect of vitamin B_6 supplement on total cholesterol, triglyceride, phospholipid and HDL-cholesterol.

Biochemical parameters	Control group	Vitamin B6 group
Total cholesterol	130.96 ± 19.84	109.62 ± 19.64*
Triglyceride	160.32 ± 50.15	104.93 ± 13.04*
Phospholipids	103.33 ± 28.45	137.04 ± 47.12*
HDL-cholesterol	124.03 ± 62.79	150.60 ± 84.05*

Significant at *$p < 0.05$ when compared with control values.

EXPERIMENTAL DESIGN

Experimental animals

Sixteen 14-week old albino rats with an average weight of 136 g were purchased from commercial breeder in Ilorin, Kwara State. They were kept in a well-ventilated cage in the animal house of the Department of Anatomy, Ladoke Akintola University of Technology, Nigeria. The animals have unrestricted access to clean water and were fed commercial normal feed as described by Kong et al. (2009).

They were separated into 2 groups, each group consisting of eight rats. Group one were not given vitamin B supplement (control) while group two were given a therapeutic dose of 0.2 mg/kg body weight of vitamin B6 for 28 days. All animal procedures were in strict accordance with the NIH Guide for the Care and Use of Laboratory Animals.

Sample collection

On the 28th day, the rats were sacrificed and blood samples were obtained through cardiac puncture (Yin et al., 2008). The blood was collected into appropriately labeled sample bottles and centrifuged at 4000 rev/s for 5 min (Kong et al., 2008; Deng et al., 2009). The supernatants were decanted and stored at -2°C for analyses of biochemical parameters (Wu et al., 2010).

Determination of biochemical parameters

The biochemical parameters determined included total cholesterol, triglyceride, high density lipoprotein, and phospholipid.

Determination of total cholesterol

Total cholesterol was determined using enzymatic method described by Allain et al. (1974). Cholesterol esterase hydrolyses cholesterol esters to free cholesterol. The free cholesterol produced is oxidized by cholesterol oxidase to cholesten-4-ene-3-one with simultaneous production of hydrogen peroxide which couples with 4-aminoantipyrine and phenol in the presence of peroxidase to yield chromogen with maximum absorption at wavelength 510 nm, The colour intensity is proportional to the cholesterol concentration.

Determination of triglycerides

Triglyceride was determined using enzymatic method described by Buccolo and David (1973). Triglycerides are hydrolyzed by lipases to yield glycerol and fatty acids. The glycerol produced is oxidized

to dihydroxylacetone phosphate with the production of hydrogen peroxide which couples with 4-aminophenazone and 4-chlorophenol to produce a chromogen referred to as quinoneimine. The reaction is catalyzed by peroxidase. The degree of absorbance of the chromogen is directly proportional to the concentration of triglyceride measured at 505 nm.

Determination of high density lipoprotein

The precipitation method by Assmann et al. (1983) was used to determine HDL-cholesterol. The addition of phosphotungistic acid in the presence of magnesium ions precipitates quantitatively low density lipoprotein, very low density lipoprotein and chylomicron fractions from whole plasma, leaving the HDL fraction in the supernate. The cholesterol in the HDL which remains in the supernatant after centrifugation is estimated using the enzymatic method of Allain et al. (1974).

Statistical analysis

Quantitative data were presented as mean ± SD. Triglyceride, total cholesterol, phospholipids and high density lipoprotein between the two groups were compared using student's 't' test. A value of $p < 0.05$ was considered statistically significant.

RESULT

Table 1 shows the mean plasma concentrations of selected biochemical parameters (total cholesterol, triglyceride, phospholipids, HDL-cholesterol) in different experimental groups that is, control and group given vitamin B6.

The mean concentrations of total cholesterol and triglyceride were significantly decreased in group given vitamin B6 as compared with the values in the control group, while there were increases in the mean concentrations of phospholipids and HDL-cholesterol when compared with the values obtained in the control group.

DISCUSSION

Cholesterol plays a major role in human heart health and high cholesterol is a leading risk factor for the development of human cardiovascular disease. It was observed that there was a significant decrease in the level of cholesterol in animals that were administered with vitamin B6 as compared to control animals. High plasma cholesterol has been linked with hyperlipidemia which is associated with increased risk of cardiovascular disease (Naito, 1984). Studies have proved that low cholesterol is a desirable level in the body for normal and proper function (Zuhani et al., 2010).

Triglyceride is a fat in the blood stream and high levels of triglycerides has been linked to atherosclerosis' (hardening of arteries) and by implication the risk of heart disease and stroke. It was observed that there was a significant decrease in the level of triglycerides in animals that were administered with vitamin B6 as compared with control animals. Studies have shown that low concentration of triglyceride is normal for the body (Zuhani et al., 2010). High triglyceride level does indicate a defect in the system and recent evidence strongly suggests that high serum concentration is significantly associated with cardiovascular disease (Altan et al., 2006).

High density lipoprotein-cholesterol (HDL-C) is referred to as the good cholesterol because of its relevance to the cardiovascular system. HDL-C helps to remove extra cholesterol from the body. Study had shown that when HDL-C is higher, there is lower chance of heart disease and that higher level of HDL-C predicts longevity (Zuliani et al., 2010). It was observed that there was a significant increase in the levels of HDL-C in animals that were placed on vitamin B6 compared to control animals. The observation is consistent with the findings of Balch (2006), who observed significantly elevated serum HDL-cholesterol in vitamin B6 administered rats.

Phospholipids are compound lipids that participate in the lipoprotein complexes which are thought to constitute the matrix of cell walls and membranes, the myelin sheath, and of such structure as mitochondria. It was observed that there was a significant increase in the level of phospholipids in animals that were administered with vitamin B6 compared to control animals. For the future study, the factional amino acids, such as argnine also should be considered to be used by combined with B_6. Recently, leading findings told us that arginine can enhance blood flow, antioxidant activity, protein synthesis, immune cell proliferation, and intestinal development, thereby improve animal health (Tan et al., 2009; Yin and Tan, 2010; Yao et al., 2008, 2011; Geng et al., 2011).

From this study, it was observed that the supplementation with vitamin B6 resulted in an increased serum concentration of HDL-cholesterol and phospholipids and a reduction in the serum level of total cholesterol and triglyceride. High levels of HDL-cholesterol and low levels of total cholesterol and triglyceride are indications of a good cardiovascular health. It may be suggested that administration of vitamin B6 can be encouraged as this may help in reducing the rate of

accumulation of total cholesterol and triglyceride, which is the two major factors of atherogenicity.

REFERENCES

Allain CC, Poon LS, Chan CSG (1974). Enzymatic determination of total serum cholesterol. Clin. Chem., 20: 470-475.

Altan O, İbrahim S, Mehmet Y, Günay C, Gülay H, Günsel ŞA (2006). Plasma triglycerides, an independent predictor of cardiovascular disease in men: A prospective study based on a population with prevalent metabolic syndrome. Int. J. Cardiol., 19(1): 89-95.

American Heart Association (2007). Heart Disease and Stroke Statistics-2007 Update. AHA, Dallas, Texas.

Assmann G, Schriewer H, Schmitz G, Hagele EO (1983). Quantification of HDL-C by precipitation with phosphotungstic acid and $MgCl_2$. Clin. Chem., 29(12): 2026-2030.

Balch PA (2006). Prescription for nutritional healing. 4th ed. New York: Avery, p. 54.

Buccolo G, David H (1973). Quantitative determination of serum triglyceride by the use of enzymes. Clin. Chem., 19: 476-482.

David SW, Malcolm L, Joan KM (2002). Homocysteine and cardiovascular disease: evidence on causality from a meta-analysis. BMJ, 325(7374): 1202.

Djousse L, Driver JA, Gazioano JM (2009). Relation between modifiable lifestyle factors and lifetime risk of heart failure. JAMA, 302: 394-400

Geng MM , Li TJ, Kong XF, Song XY, Chu WY, Huang RL, Yin YL , Wu GY (2011). Reduced expression of intestinal N-acetylglutamate synthase in suckling piglets: a novel molecular mechanism for arginine as a nutritionally essential amino acid for neonates. Amino Acids, 40: 1513-1522.

Kong X.F, Yin YL, He QH, Yin FG, Liu HJ, Li TJ, Huang RL, Geng MM, Ruan Z, Deng ZY, Xie MY. Wu G (2008). Dietary supplementation with Chinese herbal powder enhances ileal digestibilities and serum concentrations of amino acids in young pigs. Amino Acids, 37: 573-582.

Kong XF, Zhang YZ, Yin YL, Wu GY, Zhou HJ, Tan ZL, Yang F, Bo MJ, Huang RL, Li TJ, Geng MM (2009). Chinese Yam polysaccharide enhances growth performance and cellular immune response in weanling rats. J. Sci. Food Agric., 89(12): 2039-2044.

Naito K (1984). Lipids. Clin. Chem., The C.V; 918-919 and 570.

Niessen HW, Krijnen PA, Visser CA, Meijer CJ, Erik HC (2003). Type II secretory phospholipase A2 in cardiovascular disease: a mediator in atherosclerosis and ischemic damage to cardiomyocytes? Cardiovasc. Res., 60(1): 68-77.

Rosamond W, Flegal K, Friday G (2007). "Heart disease and stroke statistics--2007 update: a report from the American Heart Association Statistics Committee and Stroke Statistics Subcommittee". Circulation, 115(5): 169-171.

Tan B, Yin YL, Liu ZQ, Li XG, Xu HJ, Kong XF, Huang RL, Tang WJ, Shinzato I, Smith SB, Wu GY (2009). Dietary L-arginine supplementation increases muscle gain and reduces body fat mass in growing-finishing pigs. Amino Acids, 37: 169-175.

Tan BE, Li XG, Kong XF, Huang RL, Ruan Z, Deng ZY, Xie MY, Shinzato I, Yin YL, Wu G (2009). Dietary L-arginine supplementation enhances the immune status in early-weaned piglets. Amino Acids, 37: 323-331.

Thomas AC, Knapman PA, Krikler DM, Davies MJ (1988). "Community study of the causes of "natural" sudden death. BMJ, 297(6661): 1453-1456.

Wu X, Yin YL, Li TJ, Wang L, Ruan Z, Liu ZQ, Hou YQ (2010). Dietary supplementation with l-arginine or N-carbamylglutamate enhances intestinal growth and heat shock protein-70 expression in weanling pigs fed a corn- and soybean meal-based diet. Amino Acids, 39: 831-839.

Yao K, Guan S, Li TJ, Huang RL, Wu GY, Ruan Z, Yin YL (2011). Dietary L-arginine supplementation enhances intestinal development and expression of vascular endothelial growth factor in weanling piglets. Br. J. Nutr., 105: 703-709.

Yao K, Yin YL, Chu WY, Liu ZQ, Dun D, Li TJ, Huang RL, Zhang JS, Tan B, Wang WC, Wu GY (2008). Dietary Arginine Supplementation

Increases mTOR Signaling Activity in Skeletal Muscle of Neonatal Pigs. J. Nutr., 138: 867-872.

Yin YL, Tan BE (2010). Manipulation of dietary nitrogen, amino acids and phosphorus to reduce environmental impact of swine production and enhance animal health. J. Food Agric. Environ., 8: 447-462.

Yin YL, Tang ZR, Sun ZH, Liu ZQ, Li TJ, Huang RL, Ruan Z, Deng ZY, Gao B, Chen LX, Wu GY, Kim SW (2008). Effect of galacto-mannan-oligosaccharides or chitosan supplementation on cytoimmunity and humoral immunity response in early-weaned piglets. Asian-Aust. J. Anim. Sci., 21:723-731.

Zuhani G, Cavalieri M, Galvani M, Volpato S, Cherubim A, Bandinelli S, Corsi M, Lauretain I, Guranik J, Fellin R, Ferrucci L (2010). Relationship between low levels of high density impoprotein cholesterol and dementis in the elderly. The inchianti study. J. Garentol. Sries A, 65A: 559-564.

9

Antifeedant and antimicrobial activity of *Tylophora indica*

B. Krishna Reddy[1], M. Balaji[2], P. Uma Reddy[1], G. Sailaja[2], K. Vaidyanath[1] and G. Narasimha[3]*

[1]Department of Genetics, Osmania University, Hyderabad, A.P, India.
[2]Department of Biochemistry, Sri Venkateswara University, Tirupati, A.P, 517502, India.
[3]Department of Virology, Sri Venkateswara University, Tirupati, A.P, 517502, India.

Crude and pure extracts of *Tylophora indica* were investigated in view of antifeedant, antibacterial and antifungal properties. Leaf crude extract showed more antifeedant activity than stem and root against *Spodoptera litura*, a polyphagous pest on wide ranging crops. Among the pure compounds isolated, Tylophorine showed the highest antifeedant activity followed by Septicine, O-Methyl Tylophorinidine and simple aliphatic acid. Similarly the crude extracts of leaf has exhibited higher antibacterial activity than root and shoot against *Basillus subtilis*, *Staphylococcus aureus*, *Mycrococcus luteus* and *P. aergenosa*. In contrast, *Escherichia coli* was not inhibited even at higher concentrations of either crude extracts or extracted pure compounds of *T. Indica*. Pure compounds displayed strong antibacterial activity at lower concentrations in all tested bacterial strains except *E. coli*. While all the crude and pure compounds showed antifungal activity against *Aspergillus niger*, *Aspergillus fumigatus* and *Trichoderma viridae*, the pure compounds had strong antifungal activity compared to crude extracts.

Key words: *Tylophora indica*, antifeedant activity, antimicrobial activity.

INTRODUCTION

A considerable concern has been raised to adverse affects of pesticides affecting environment and resistance development. Hence, there is imperative need for development of safe alternative plant protections by botanical insecticides and antifeedants. The use of plants for medicinal and insecticidal purposes dates back to antiquity (Sofowora, 1984; Devanand and Usharani, 2008). Recent studies have focused on natural plant products as alternatives for disease control. Majority of rural dwellers in developing countries still depend on medicinal plants to prevent or eliminate diseases (Parekha and Chanda, 2008). Medicinal plants are cheaper, more accessible in the world. Thus, it is needed to encourage the use of medicinal plants as potential sources of new drugs. There has been an upsurge interest in herbal remedies, many of which with the herbal remedial being incorporated in to orthodox medical practice in several parts of the world (Satyanarayana et al., 1991; Ogbulie et al., 2007). Micro-

organisms and insect pests cause massive damage to the crops, horticultural plants, animals as well as humans. In tropical countries like India the damage potential of microorganisms and insects is immense due to congenial atmospheric factors such as temperature and humidity contributing to the growth of microorganisms and insect pests. Although chemical control measures are highly effective and have been in fact employed with tremendous success, there has been a renewed interest for botanicals possessing antimicrobial antifeedant and antibiotic properties (Makinde et al., 2007; Parekh and Chanda, 2008).

Whilst several natural insecticides were used in agriculture, only recently systematic investigations on antifeedant and other physiological, pharmacological and antibiotic activity of plant based compounds have been initiated. Several botanicals have been tested for their antifeedant activity (Dreyer and Jones, 1981; Devanand and Usharani, 2008). Compounds with antifeedant and medicinal properties have been identified from plants like *Reseda luteola*, *Trifolium incarnatum* (Robinson and Venkatachalam, 1929), *Morus alba* (Montgomery and Arn,

---

*Corresponding author. E-mails: gnsimha123@rediffmail.com.

1974), *Vitex negundo* and *Zingiber officinale* (Sahayaraj, 1998). Most of them displays antifeedant activity ranging strong to moderate, that this case opens a new eco-friendly source of plant based compounds for pest management.

Antimicrobial activities of several plant products have gained importance in recent times. Plant derived second-dary metabolites like alkaloids, terpenoids and flavonoids have shown to interfere with many biological activities. They possess antibacterial, antifungal, cyotoxic or anti-tumour, antifeedant and insecticidal activities (Purohit et al., 1995; Muhammad, 2009). Folklore and Ayurvedic literature assert that some plants possess antiseptic and antimicrobial properties (Chatarjee et al., 1991). Satyanarayana et al. (1991) reported that crude extracts of *Flacourtia ramonthi* inhibited *S. aureus* and *E. coli*. Hiremath et al. (1993) also demonstrated antibacterial and antifungal activity from crude and different solvent extracts of *Acalypha indica*. The evaluation of solvent extracts of *Evolvulous alsinoids* against representative bacteria and fungi in *in vitro* conditions was reported by Purohit et al. (1995). Flavonoids are major groups of normal compounds due to their biological activity (Giesman, 1962). Antibacterial activity of some flavonoids was reported earlier by Sharma (1970). Alkaloids isolated from Rutaceae members such as Furoquinoline alkoloids, skimmianine isolated from *Fagara* species have shown antimicrobial activity (Tan et al., 1991). Although *T. indica* is a versatile medicinal plant, placing in restricted localities in Indian sub continents and parts of Africa, the information on the antifeedant, antimicrobial and antifungal activity of *Tylophora* species is insufficient. Hence the present study was carried out on antifeedant, antibacterial and antifungal activity of *T. indica*.

MATERIALS AND METHODS

Preparation of methanolic extracts

Fresh leaves, stem and roots of *T. indica* were collected from forests of Telangana region, Andhra Pradesh, India and these were shade dried and powdered. Nearly 10 gr of each crude powders were extracted with methanol. The methanolic extract was distilled in a rotation-vapour to obtain a concentrated sample. A yield of 6 - 9% was obtained and this was used as sample for further tests to be carried out.

Purification of secondary metabolites from methanolic extracts

About 2 kg of shade dried and powdered plant material was extracted with 20 L of methanol in a soxhlet-apparatus, filtered and concentrated. The semisolid dark colored methanolic extract was macerated thrice with 2N HCl (100 ml) and allowed to stand for about 15 min. The aqueous HCl layer was collected, filtered and extracted with ethyl acetate in a separating funnel. The aqueous acidic solution was treated with NH_4OH until the solution was alkaline and extracted thrice with ethyl acetate in separating funnel. The upper ethyl acetate fraction was collected, dried over anhy-drous Na_2SO_4 and decanted the ethyl acetate layer into a clean dry china dish, concentrated under reduced pressure. The ethyl acetate

soluble part of the methanolic extract of the leaves of *T. indica* was fractioned by column chromatography on neutral alumina (200 mesh, ACME). A total of 278 fractions were collected by eluting with increasing order of solvents like petroleum ether, (Fraction 1 - 33), petroleum ether and Benzene 1:1 (Fraction 34 - 49), benzene (fraction 50 - 69), Benzene and ethyl acetate 9:1 (fraction 70 - 110), Benzene and ethyl acetate 8:2 (fraction 111 - 141), Benzene and ethyl acetate 7:3 (142 - 202), ethyl acetate (fraction 203 - 252) and ethyl acetate and methanol (fraction 253 - 278). All the fractions with uniform RF values upon TLC were pooled together. The IR, UV, NMR and Mass spectra revealed the presence of simple aliphatic acid in fractions 50 - 69, Septicine in 70 - 110, Tylophorine in 111 - 141, O-Methyl Tylophorinidine in 142 - 202 (Data not shown here).

Culture medium

Nutrient broth /agar medium for bacterial cultures and potato dextrose agar medium for fungal cultures was prepared and sterilized as instructed by the manufacturers (Himedia, India).

Microorganisms

The bacterial and fungal cultures were obtained from IMTECH, Chandigarh, India.

Insect antifeedant activity

The antifeedant activity was evaluated by non-choice test method of Debey et al. (1991) with a modification. The pre-starved larvae for six hours have been employed instead of unstarved larvae used in the leaf disc method. The test insect *Spodoptera litura*, a polyphagous pest on wide ranging crops was maintained in the laboratory conditions, at 27 ± 2°C and 70 ± 5% Relative humidity. The IV instar larvae were fed on their natural food, castor leaves. In non-choice test method, leaf discs of 10 cm diameter were cut from fresh-castor leaves and treated with acetone solution of test compounds at 250, 500, 750 and 1000 ppm. These leaf discs were air dried for 3 to 5 s and placed in separate Petri dishes and one preserved IV instar larvae were released simultaneously into the jars containing test leaf discs maintained independently. The consumption of leaf was evaluated at the end of 24 h. The leaf area consumed by the insect in both control and treated was measured by planimeter. The mean percentage of damage and protection was calculated and expressed as percentage of protection (antifeedant activity) using the formula of Singh and Pant (1980).

Antimicrobial activity

Antimicrobial activity was tested against three gram positive and two gram negative bacterial cultures obtained from IMTECH, Chandigarh, India. They include *B. subtilis, S. aureus, M. luteus, E. coli, P. aerginosa*. Antifungal activity was assayed against *A. niger, A. fumigat* and *T. viridae* (from IMTECH). The standard method of paper disc diffusion on agar plates was employed using a concen-tration range of 50 to 1000 µg /ml of test compound (Mathew, 2006). The presence or absence of growth inhibition zone around each disc was recorded by comparing with the standard antibiotic disc (streptomycin). Formation of a clear zone around the disc indicated the inhibition of microbial growth. The compounds tested were viz., (1) leaf crude extract (2) Stem crude extract (3) Root crude extract (4) Simple aliphatic acid (5) Septicine (6) Tylophorine (7) O-methyl tylophorinidine.

Table 1. Antifeedant activity $^\varphi$ of crude and pure extracts of *T. indica* of different concentrations.

Compound	250 ppm	500 ppm	750 ppm	1000 ppm
Leaf crude extract	45.36 ± 2.45 ***	71.85 ± 1.21 ***	93.34 ± 1.83 **	95.85 ± 0.91 **
Stem crude extract	40.46 ± 2.20 ***	62.90 ± 1.67 ***	90.12 ± 1.32 **	90.82 ± 1.21 **
Root crude extract	38.38±1.14 ***	56.00 ± 2.92 ***	80.64 ±1.31 ***	81.75 ± 1.43 **
Simple aliphatic extract	55.21 ± 1.38 ***	72.68 ± 1.55 ***	92.28 ± 1.25 **	93.34 ±1.28 **
Septicine	70.69 ±2.15 ***	90.35 ± 1.39 **	98.51 ± 1.03	98.88 ± 0.99
Tylophirine	95.63 ±1.09	100 ± 0.59	100 ± 0.04	100 ± 0.12
O- Methyl Tylophorinidine	85.68 ± 1.34 ***	99.43 ± 0.53	100 ± 0.57	100 ± 0.62

*** p < 0.005 Values are significant at 5% level when compared to control value, ** P < 0.001 Values are significant at 1% level when compared to control value, $^\varphi$ Antifeedant activity measured in terms of area of leaf remained unconsumed by insect.

Statistical analysis

The standard deviation and analysis of variance (ANOVA) was calculated where ever necessary from the data obtained in the study.

RESULTS AND DISCUSSION

The antifeedant activity of crude extracts and pure compounds of *T. indica* was tested against *Spodoptera litura* and listed in the Table 1. With ascending concentration of crude or pure compounds, antifeedant activity also increased. Among the crude extracts tested in the present study, leaf showed maximum antifeedant activity by 71.85% followed by stem (62.90%) and root extracts (56.04%) at 500 ppm at 24 h interval. These three crude extracts, however, showed antifeedant activity of 95.85, 90.82 and 81.75 per cents respectively at 1000 ppm. Of the pure compounds used in the study Tylophorine and O-methyl tylophorinidine have shown cent per cent antifeedant activity followed by Septicine (90.35%) and simple aliphatic acid (72. 68%) at 500 ppm at 24 h interval (Table 1). Similar reports on the insect antifeedant activity of Tylophorine was observed by Verma et al. (1986), Thripathi et al. (1990) against *Spilosoma oblique walker*. Arivudainambi and Nachiappan (1993) observed that extracts of *Ipomoea* have shown antifeedant property against the semilooper, *Achaea janata Linn*. The antifeedant properties of indigenous medicinal plants against the larvae of *Heliothis armigera* (Hubner) was reported by Dubey et al. (1991).

The bacterial cultures in Petri plates were incubated along with test compounds, which were checked for growth inhibition zone of organisms after 24 h. The antibacterial activity of crude extracts and pure compounds of *T. indica* was studied and listed in Table 2. Among the pure compounds used in the present study, Tylophorine and O-Methy Tylophorinidine showed higher antibacterial activity (10 - 20 mm diameter) than other compounds. Of the five bacterial cultures used in the study, except *E. coli* all strains resulted in inhibition by *T. indica* (Table 2). Pure compounds exhibited maximum antibacterial activity compared to the crude compounds. Antibacterial activities

tof *D. stemonium* and *T. indica* were evaluated on bacterial strains *S. aureus*, *P. vulgaris*, *P. aergenosa* and *E. coli*. (Uma, 2009). These extracts exhibited significant zone of inhibition and good antimicrobial activity. Similar results were obtained with the crude ethanol extracts of *Euphorbia hirta* showing antibacterial activities against a variety of species (Ogbulie et al., 2007). Garg and Jain (1998) reported that, essential oils extracted from *Curcuma caesia* have showed significant antibacterial activity.

The antifungal activity of *T. indica* was studied against three fungal species, *A. niger*, *A. fumigatus* and *T. viride* and listed in Table 3. Both crude extracts and isolated pure compounds showed antifungal activity. However, except stem crude extract against *A. niger* and root crude extract against *A. fumigatus*, antifungal activity was shown by all the extracts. Compared to crude extracts, isolated pure compounds exhibited maximum antifeedant activity. Of the pure compounds tested in the study, Tylophorine and O-Methy Tylophorinidine showed maximum antifeedant activity (10 - 15 mm diameter of zone of inhibition) against *A. niger* and *T. viride* followed by Septicine and simple aliphatic acid (5 - 10 mm zone of inhibition). *A. fumigatus* was less inhibited even by pure compounds. Similar report of antifungal activity was earlier observed from the crude extracts of *A. indica* (Hiremath et al., 1993). Antibacterial and antifungal activity of the aqueous and methanol extracts of *C. alata* leaves was also evaluated (Makinde et al., 2007). According to studies of Uma Reddy (2009), the crude extract of *T. indica* effetly inhibited the growth of fungal strains *A. niger* and *Fusarium* species.

Conclusion

The present work clearly indicates that crude and pure extracts of *T. indica* showed potent antifeedent and antimicrobial activity. Leaf crude extracts showed antifeedent, antibacterial and antifungal activity at higher concentrations; where as pure compounds are highly effective at lower concentration against tested organisms, except *E. coli* which inhabits human intestine. It suggests that

Table 2. Anti bacterial activity of crude and pure extracts of *T. indica*.

Compound (120 µg/ml)	*B. subtilis*	*S. aureus*	*M. luteus*	*E. coli*	*P. aergenosa*
Leaf crude extract	+	+	+	-	+
Stem crude extract	-	+	-	-	+
Root crude extract	+	+	+	-	-
Simple aliphatic acid	+ +	+ +	+	-	+
Septicine	+ +	+ +	+ +	-	+ +
Tylophorine	+ + +	+ + +	+ +	-	+ + +
O-Methyl Tlophorinidine	+ ++	+ + +	+ +	-	+ +
Streptomycin	+ ++	+ ++	+ +	+	+ ++

- = No inhibition, + = ≤ 5 mm diameter of zone of inhibition, + + = 5 - 10 mm diameter of zone of inhibition, + + + = 10 - 20 mm diameter of zone of inhibition.

Table 3. Anti fungal activity of crude and pure extracts of *T. indica*.

Compound (120 µg/ml)	*A. niger*	*A. fumigatus*	*T. viridi*
Leaf crude extract	+	+	+
Stem crude extract	-	+	+
Root crude extract	+	-	+
Simple aliphatic acid	+ +	+	+ +
Septicine	+ +	+	+ +
Tylophorine	+ + +	+	+ + +
O-Methyl Tlophorinidine Streptomycine (Control)	+ ++	+	+ + +

- = No inhibition, + = ≤ 5 mm diameter of zone of inhibition, + + = 5-10 mm diameter of zone of inhibition, + + + = 10-15 mm diameter of zone of inhibition.

these extracts can be employed for therapeutic purposes as oral medicine without having any adverse affects on normal bacterial strains present in human gut. Hence the extracts of *T. indica* would also serve as novel antibacterial in addition to anti fungal and antifeedant agent.

REFERENCES

Arivudainambi S, Nachiappan RM (1993). Evaluation of antifeedant property of extracts of *Ipomea carnea Jacquin* against the semilooper, *Achaea janta* L. J. Ent. Res. 17(3): 225-226.

Chaterjee S, Vijaykumar EKS, Franco CMM, Borde UP, Blumach J, Ganguli BN, Fehlhaber HW, Kogler H (1991). Butalactin: A new Butanolide antibiotic from *Streptomyces corchosii*. Tetrahedron Lett. 32(1): 44.

Devanand P, Usharani P (2008). Biological potential of certain plant extracts in management of lepidopteran pests of *Ricinus communi L*. J. Biopest. 1(2): 170-176

Dreyer DL, Jones KC (1981). Feeding deterrency of flavonoids and related phenolics towards *schizaphis graminum* and *myzus persicae*: Aphid feeding deterrents in wheat. Phytochem. 20: 2489-2493.

Dubey OP, Odak SC, Gargava VP (1991). Evalualtion of antifeedant properties of indigenous medicinal plants against the larvae of *Heliothis armiger* (Hubner). J. Entomol.Res. 15 (3): 208-211.

Garg SC, Jain RK (1998). Antimicrobial efficacy of essential oil from *Curcuma caesia*. Ind. J. Microbial. 38: 169-170.

Giesman TA (1962). The chemistry of flavonoid compounds Pergamon press, London.

Hiremath SP, Shrishilappa B, Swamy HKS, Biradar, JS (1993). Antimicrobial activity of various extracts of *Acalypha indica* (Euphorbiaceae). Ind. J. Microbial. 33 (1): 75-77.

Makinde AA, Igoli JO, TAAma L, Shaibu SJ, Garba A (2007). Antimicrobial activity of *Cassia alata*. Afr.J.Biotechnology. 6(13): 1509-1510.

Mathew AW, Donald EL, Franklin RC, Daniel JS, William AC, Fred CT, Michael ND, John DT, George ME, Melvin PW, David WH, Barbara LZ, Janet FH, Mary JF, Jana MS (2006). Performance standards for antimicrobial disc susceptibility tests; Approved standard.9th edition, 26(1): 9-11.

Montgomery ME, Arn H (1974). Feeding response of Aphis pomi, Myzus persicae and Amphorophora agathonica to phlorizin. J. Insect Physiol. 20: 414-421.

Muhammad Abubakar EM (2009). Efficacy of crude extracts of garlic (*Allium sativum L.*) against nasocomial *Escheria coli*, *Staphylococcus aureus*, *Streptococcus pneumoniea* and *Pseudomonas aeruginosa*. J.Med.Plants. 3(4): 179-185.

Ogbulie JN, Ogueke CC, Okoli IC, Anyanwu BN (2007). Antibacterial activities and toxicological potentials of crude ethanolic extracts of *Euphorbia hirta*. Afr. J. Biotechnol. 6(13): 1544-1548.

Parekha J, Chanda SV (2008). Antibacterial activity of aqueous and alcoholic extracts of 34 Indian medicinal plants against some *Staphylococcus* species. Turk. J. Biol. 32: 63-71.

Purohit MG, Santhaveerappa BK, Shrisailappa B, Swamy HKS (1995). Anti microbial activity of various extracts of *Evolvulus alsinoids* (Ind. J. Microbiol. 35 (1): 77-78.

Robinson R, Venkataraman K (1929).Annual reports on progress of chemistry p .152.

Sahayaraj K (1998). Antifeedant effect of some plant extracts on the Asian army worm, *Spodoptera litura* (Fabricius). Curr. Sci. 74(6): 523-525.

Satyanarayana V, Gopal reddy S, David Krupadanam GL, Srimannarayana G (1991). Anti microbial activity of some natural and synthetic organo heterocyclic compounds. Ind. J. Microbiol. 31 (1): 57-60.

Sharma PN, Srimannarayana G, Subbarao NV (1970). The medicinal plant industry p. 205.

Singh RP, Pant NC (1980). Hymenocallis littoralis salisb as antifeedant to desert locust, Schistocera gregaria forsk. Ind. J. Ent. 42 (3): 460-464.

Sofowora A (1984). Medicinal plant and traditional medicine in Africa. Johnwiley, New York pp. 256-257.

Tan GT, John PM, Kinghorn AD (1991). Medical botany, plants affecting human health p 126.

Thripathi AK, Singh D, Jain DC (1990). Persistency of Tylophorine as an insect antifeedant against Spilosoma oblique walker. Phytotherapy Res. 4(4): 144-147

Uma Reddy P (2009). Antimicrobial activity of Datura stramonium (L) and Tylophora indica (Buru L). New Pharmacology online 1: 1293-1300.

Verma GS, Ramakrishnan V, Mulchandani NB, Chadha M.S (1986). Insect feeding deterrants from the medicinal plant Tylophora asthmatica. Entomol. Exp. Appl. 40: 99-105.

10

In vitro and in vivo evaluation of free radical scavenging potential of ethanolic extract of Podophyllum hexandrum

Showkat Ahmad Ganie[1], Mohmmad Afzal Zargar[1], Akbar Masood[1] and Ehtishamul Haq[2]*

[1]Department of Biochemistry University of Kashmir, Srinagar, 190006, India.
[2]Department of Biotechnology, University of Kashmir, Srinagar, 190006, India.

The study was aimed at evaluating the antioxidant activity of ethanolic extract of rhizome of *Podophyllum hexandrum* under *in vitro* and *in vivo* situations. The extract was found to contain a large amount of polyphenols and also exhibit an immense reducing ability. At a concentration of 250 µg/ml, 48% of H_2O_2 radicals could be scavenged by the extract. The extract also inhibited hydroxyl radical ($^\bullet$OH) induced oxidation of protein (BSA). The ethanolic rhizome extract of *P. hexandrum* also exhibited a significant antioxidant activity in acute oxidative tissue injury animal model constituted by CCl_4 induced hepatotoxicity. Oral administration of the extract at a dose of 20 and 50 mg/kg bw significantly protected from CCl_4 induced elevation in aspartate aminotransferase (AST), alanine aminotransferase (ALT) and lactate dehydrogenase (LDH) in the serum, depletion of hepatic protein and GSH content, decrease in the activities of hepatic antioxidant enzymes: glutathione peroxidase (GPx), glutathione reductase and glutathione-S-transferase.

Key words: *Podophyllum hexandrum*, CCl_4, antioxidant activity, free radical scavenging.

INTRODUCTION

In biological systems the generation of free radicals is a normal phenomenon. Sometimes these free radicals are generated to such an extent that the body's defense mechanism is not able to remove them and as a result stress develops in the body. This process is called oxidetive stress and it is defined as a shift in the prooxidant-antioxidant balance towards a prooxidant environment. The free radicals are the chemical species which have unpaired electrons and are thus very unstable and reactive. In order to attain stability they react with their neighboring atoms to gain the electrons and as a result new free radicals are generated, which in turn attack the other nearby molecules causing a cascade of reactions (Okezie, 1996).

Aerobic organisms use oxygen to oxidize food and obtain the energy, a phenomenon essential for their sustenance. But during this oxidation process the oxygen molecule themselves get reduced and form intermediates called reactive oxygen species (ROS). The intermediates that are formed during the oxidizing process are hydrogen peroxide radicals ($H_2O_2^\bullet$) and hydroxyl radicals ($OH^\bullet$) and superoxide radicals (O_2^{-}) (McCord et al., 1971). Free radicals are also formed exogenously due to interplay of factors external to the body. Certain pesticides, drugs, hepatotoxins, sunlight, ionizing radiations and pollutants including cigarette smoke are some of the known exogenous factors. The free radicals generated in the body cause several types of damages including peroxidation of unsaturated fatty acids in membranes.

Mitochondria and microsomal membranes contain relatively large amounts of polyunsaturated fatty acids and

*Corresponding author. E-mail: haq@kashmiruniversity.net.

hence are susceptible to the damage (Fleischer et al., 1965). It is already known that the membrane lipids being rich in unsaturated fatty acids undergo peroxidation both in vitro and in vivo (Witting, 1965). Free radicals are also responsible for causing the denaturation of proteins, carbohydrates and nucleic acids and are intermediates in the induction of cardiovascular diseases, inflammatory conditions, autoimmune disorders and cancer pathology (Hogg, 1998; Pong, 2003). Free radicals are continuously formed in the body but the aerobic organisms employ a battery of defense mechanisms such as antioxidant enzymes glutathione reductase (GR), glutathione peroxidase (GPx), glutathione–S-transferase (GST), superoxide dismutase (SOD) and catalase (CAT) to prevent or mitigate oxidative tissue damage (Halliwell et al., 1989). When the liver cell plasma membrane is damaged, many of the enzymes normally located in the liver cell cytosol are released into the blood stream. Their estimation in the blood is a useful quantitative marker of the extent and type of hepatocellular damage (Mitra et al., 1998). In addition, perturbation of the GSH status of a biological system has been reported to increase the lipid peroxidation (Uday et al., 1999). Thiobarbituric acid reactive substances, TBARS, are produced as by-products of lipid peroxidation that occurs in the hydrophobic core of biomembranes (Fraga et al., 1987). At other sites, intake of compounds that induce antioxidant enzyme activity or scavenging of free radicals prevents oxidative damage (Hochstein et al., 1988). Antioxidants are the substances that when present at a low concentration compared with those of the oxidizable substances considerably delay or inhibit the oxidation of the substrate. Antioxidants act as a major defense against radical mediated toxicity by protecting the damage caused by free radicals (Nayan and Janardhanan, 2000). Further-more medicinal plants are used as 'antioxidants' in traditional medicine, their claimed therapeutic properties could be, in part, due to the presence of organic compounds being able to scavenge oxygen free radicals.

P. hexandrum belongs to the Berberidaceae family, it is locally known as Banwangon in the Kashmiri region of J and K, North India. It is a fibrous, juicy herb, 35 - 60 cm high with perennial rhizome (tubers) bearing numerous roots. P. hexandrum grows in the inner range of Himalayas from Kashmir to Sikkim (India) at an altitude of 3000 – 4200 m over sea level. The dried rhizomes and roots of this plant are traditionally used for medical purposes. Podophyllin a resin (derived from P. hexandrum) has cholagogue, purgative and emetic pro-perties. The rhizome powder is locally used as a laxative, to treat intestinal parasites (worms), warts and tumorous growths on the skin." Application of podophyllum resin 25% solution is efficacious in producing significant short-term

resolution of HIV related oral hairy leukoplakia (Cobb, 1990; Gowdey et al., 1995). Podo-phyllatoxin isolated from P. hexandrum is a natural lignin that is currently being used as a precursor to semi-synthetic anti-cancer drugs like etoposide, teniposide and etopophos. These compounds have been used for the treatment of lung and testicular cancers as well as certain leukemias (Stahelin and Wartburg, 1991; Imbert, 1998). Carbon tetrachloride (CCl_4) has been widely used in animal models to induce acute liver injury (Mizuoka et al., 1999; Rao et al., 1997; Czaja et al., 1995). It is generally believed that the toxicity of CCl_4 results from its reductive dehalogenation by the cytochrome P_{450} enzyme system into the highly reactive free radical trichloromethyl radical (Recknagel et al., 1989). The present study was carried out to examine free radical scavenging properties of an ethanolic rhizome extract of P. hexandrum and its protective effect in an animal model of hepatotoxicity induced by carbon tetrachloride.

MATERIAL AND METHODS

Plant materials and preparation of plant extract

The rhizome of P. hexandrum were collected from the higher reaches of Aharbal (J and K, North India) during the months of May - June of 2006 and authenticated by Dr. Irshad Nawchoo, Associate Professor of the Department of Botany, University of Kashmir Srinagar, India. A voucher specimen with herbarium number (KASH- bot/Ku/PH- 702- SAG) has been retained for future reference at the Taxonomy Centre of the University of Kashmir. The rhizome material was shade dried at 30 ± 2°C. The dried material was grinded to powder using mortar and pestle and sieved with a sieve of 0.3 mm aperture size. The powder obtained was successively extracted in hexane, ethyl acetate, absolute ethanol, 70% ethanol by using soxhlet extractor (Borosil New Delhi India) (60 - 80°C). The 70% ethanolic extract was then concentrated with the help of rotary evaporator under reduced pressure and the dried extract was stored at 4°C until further use.

Animals

Wistar male albino rats, weighing 200 – 250 g, were purchased from the Indian Institute of Integrative Medicine (IIIM), Jammu J and K India. The animals were fed on a pellet diet (Hindustan Lever, Ltd., Mumbai, India) and water ad libitum. The animals were maintained in a controlled environment under standard conditions of temperature and humidity with an alternating 12 h light and dark cycle, in accordance with the guidelines prescribed by the National Institute of Nutrition, Indian Council of Medical Research. The use of animals for the current study was duly approved by the Animal Ethic Committee of the University of Kashmir.

Determination of phenolic content

The total phenolics in 70% ethanolic extracts of P. hexandrum rhizome were determined by using Folin- Ciocalteau reagent according to the protocol of (Chandler et al., 1993). Quantitation was based on the standard curve of gallic acid (10 mg%), which was dissolved in methanol/water (60:40, v/v, 0.3% HCl). The concentration of polyphenols was expressed in terms of mg/100 ml of sample.

Reducing power

The reducing power of *P. hexandrum* rhizome extract was evaluated according to Oyaizu (1986). Different concentrations of the plant extracts were mixed with 2.5 ml of 0.2 M phosphate buffer (pH 6.6), and 2.5 ml of 1% potassium hexacyanoferrate (11). The mixture was incubated at 50°C for 20 minutes, 2.5 ml of 10% TCA was added to the mixture and centrifuged at 3000rpm for 10 minutes. The upper layer of the solution (2.5ml) was mixed with distilled water (2.5ml) and $FeCl_3$ (0.5 ml, 0.1%), and the absorbance was measured at 700nm by using spectrophotometer. Butylated hydroxyltolune (BHT; Sigma Aldrich) was used as standard.

Protein oxidation

Bovine serum albumin (BSA) was oxidized by a Fenton- type reaction. BSA (1 mg/ml) was incubated at 25°C in solution with 2.5 mM H_2O_2, 1.0 mM ascorbic acid and 3.0 mM EDTA in the presence or absence of 70% ethanolic rhizome extract of *P. hexandrum*. After incubation for 45 min, protein was precipitated with 10% TCA, centrifuged at 5000 rpm (Remi C-24 India), at 4°C for 10 min and the supernatant was decanted, protein pellets were dissolved in minimum amount of 50 mM potassium phosphate buffer, pH 7.5. Total sulphydryl (-SH) group determinations were performed according to the method of Moren et al. (1979) using Ellman's reagent (DTNB). The absorbance was measured at 412 nm spectrophotometrically (Elico India), and total sulphydryl groups were expressed as nmoles per mg protein using 5, 5- Dithiobis (2-nitrobenzoic acid) (DTNB) molar extinction coefficient of 13,100.

Assessment of hydrogen peroxide scavenging activity

The ability of *P. hexandrum* extracts to scavenge hydrogen peroxide was evaluated according to the method of Ruch et al. (1989). A solution of H_2O_2 (2 mmole) was prepared in phosphate buffer (pH = 7.5). Plant extract (50 – 250 µg/ml) were added to the hydrogen peroxide solution (0.6 ml). Absorbance of hydrogen peroxide at 230 nm was determined after 15 min against a blank solution containing only phosphate buffer without hydrogen peroxide. BHT was used as standard.

Biochemical analysis

Rats were divided into six groups containing seven animals each. The plant extract was employed at oral doses of 20 and 50 mg/kg body wt./day. The extract was suspended in normal saline such that the final volume of extract at each dose was 1 ml and was given to rats through gavage.

Treatment groups

Group I- Received olive oil only (vehicle) 5.0 ml/kg and served as normal control. Group II- Received only CCl_4 1.0 ml/Kg body weight (suspended in olive oil). Group III- Animals were administrated with Vitamin E (α-tocopherol; Sigma Aldrich) 50 mg/Kg body weight.

Group IV- Received 20 mg/Kg body weight of *Podophyllum* extract orally for all fifteen days. Group V- Received 50 mg/kg body weight plant extract orally for all fifteen days. On the thirteenth day, animals in the groups II - V were treated with CCl_4 at the dose of (1 ml/Kg body weight) by means of an intraperitoneal injection. After 24 h of CCl_4 administration (that is, 15th day), the rats were sacrificed and liver tissue was isolated and post mitochondrial supernatant (PMS) were prepared. The blood was collected from retro-orbital plexus without the use of anticoagulant. The blood was allowed to stand for 10 min at room temperature before being centrifuged at 2,000 rpm for 10 min to obtain serum for analysis of alanine aminotransferase (ALT), aspartate aminotransferase (AST) and serum lactate dehydrogenase (LDH).

Enzyme activity estimation

The estimation of enzymes activities were performed as indicated in the respective references: ALT and AST activity were carried out by the method of (Reitman and Frankel, 1975), LDH by (King, 1965), Glutathione peroxidase (Lawrence et al., 1976), Glutathione reductase (Mannervik et al., 1985), Glutathione-S-transferase (Habig et al., 1974), GSH (Hissin et al., 1976). Protein estimation was done by the method of (Lowry et al., 1951).

Statistical analysis

The values are expressed as mean ± S.D. The results were analyzed statistically by using Graphpad Prism 5 software using one-way ANOVA followed by Bonferroni t-test.

RESULTS

The yield of extract obtained from *P. hexandrum* rhizome using 70% ethanol as solvent was found to be 30% (w/w). The extract was found to contain 153 ± 12 mg/g, total phenolics expressed as gallic acid equivalent (mg/g of gallic acid). Since polyphenols are responsible for the antioxidant activity, the obtained amount of total polyphenols in the extract indicates the extract to possess a high antioxidant activity.

Reducing power is a measure of reductive ability of antioxidants and is evaluated by the transformation of Fe^{3+} to Fe^{2+} in the presence of sample extract. The reducing capacity of a compound may serve as a significant indicator of its potential antioxidant activity. The reducing power of 70% ethanolic extract of *P. hexandrum* is shown in Figure 1. The data shows that the reducing power of extract increased in a dose dependent manner. The ability of reducing power of 70% ethanolic extract was almost comparable with the synthetic antioxidant, butylated hydroxyl toluene (BHT). At a high concentration of 500 µg/ml, the reducing power of 70% ethanolic extract was found to be 77% as compared to 98% inhibition seen

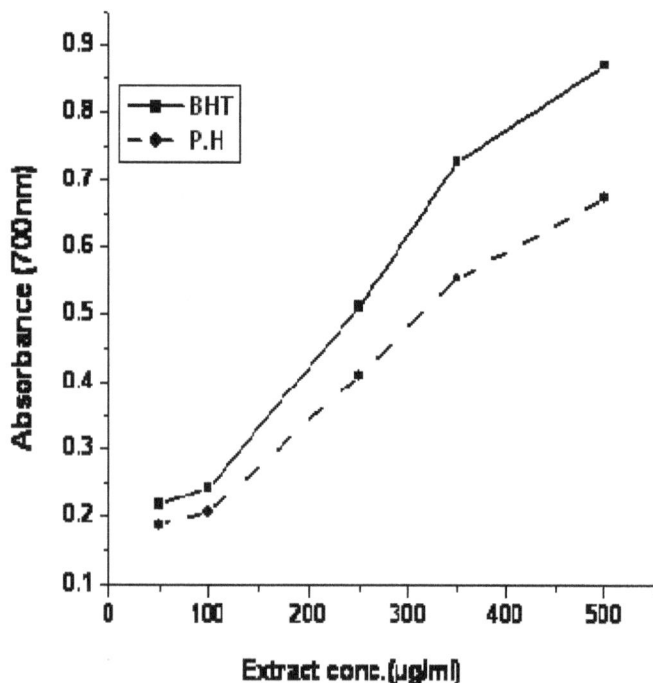

Figure 1. Reducing power (Fe^{3+} to Fe^{2+} conversion) shown by ethanolic extract of *P. hexandrum* and known antioxidant BHT; Butylated hydroxyltolune. IC_{50} values BHT=187, E.E = 266. The data are presented as means ± S.D of three independent experiments. E.E; ethanolic extract of *P. hexandrum*.

with BHT. The 50% inhibition of plant extract was found at a concentration of 266 µg/ml as compared to that of BHT that was 187 µg/ml (Figure 1).

Ethanolic extract of *P. hexandrum* effectively inhibited BSA oxidation induced by Fe- ascorbate- H_2O_2 system that generates $OH^\bullet$ radicals. BSA oxidation was determined in terms of – SH group loss by Ellman reagent (5, 5- dithiobis- (2–nitrobenzoic acid). The incubation of BSA with Fe- ascorbate- H_2O_2 complex caused the oxidation of 62% of the –SH groups, in the absence of any extract. The ethanolic extract of *P. hexandrum* rhizome dose dependently reversed this –SH oxidation (Figure 2). As can be seen in Figure 2, the 500 µg/ml extract was able to revert this oxidation to 36%, which was a significant change as compared to Fe-ascorbate- H_2O_2 complex.

The ability of *P. hexandrum* extracts to scavenge hydrogen peroxide is represented in Figure 3. This was assessed by taking hydrogen peroxide, under *in vitro* conditions and then adding increasing concentrations of *P. hexandrum* extract. The absorbance was taken at 230 nm, this is where H_2O_2 absorbs maximally and it was seen that the plant extract was effective in scavenging H_2O_2 in a concentration dependent manner as was

evident by the decrease in absorbance. BHT which was used as a positive control also scavenged H_2O_2 in concentration dependent manner (Figure 3).

Studies using an animal model of hepatotoxicity

Effect on liver marker enzymes

The effect of *P. hexandrum* on serum marker enzymes is presented in Table 1. The levels of serum AST, ALT and LDH after 24 h of CCl_4 administration were markedly elevated in CCl_4 treated animals, indicating liver damage. Adminstration of *P. hexandrum* extract protected the livers from CCl_4 damage. The effect by 50 mg/Kg bw of the extract was similar to that provided in the presence of vitamin E, as no significant difference existed between these two groups, in the activities of ALT, AST and LDH (Table 1).

Enzymes involved in maintaining redox

The effect of *P. hexandrum* treatment on maintaining the machinery involved in maintaining redox is shown in Table 2. The damage to liver was also supported by decreased protein concentration in CCl_4 treated animals, again the level was restored by *P. hexandrum* treatment. Reduced glutathione content in liver homogenate was significantly ($P < 0.001$) decreased in CCl_4 treated animals in comparison to control group. The *P. hexandrum* treatment appreciably restored the GSH levels. Glutathione reductase (GR) and Glutathione peroxidase (GP_X) activity were significantly decreased ($P < 0.001$) in Group II CCl_4 treated rats in comparison to control. A dose dependent restoration of both GR and GPx activities was observed with increasing concentration of plant extract (Table 2). Similar trend was observed with Glutathione-S-transferase (GST). Treatment with vitamin E, a known antioxidant also significantly increased the above mentioned activities.

DISCUSSION

Free radicals formed in the body react with variety of biomolecules creating an undesirable situation known as oxidative stress, resulting ultimately in disturbances of prooxidant/antioxidant equilibrium status. The equilibrium could be restored back by supplementing with exogenous antioxidant and or activating endogenous antioxidant system. It has long been recognized that naturally occurring substances in plants have antioxidant activities.

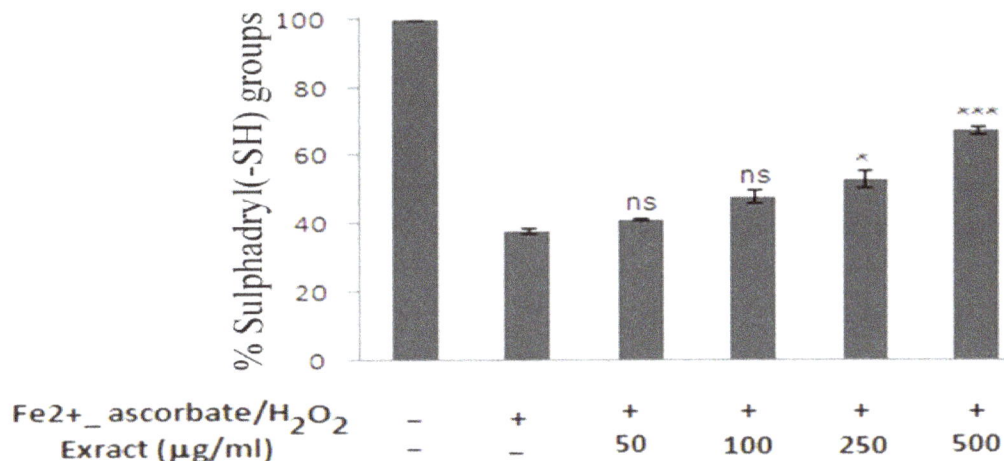

Figure 2. Inhibitory effect of ethanolic extract of *P. hexandrum*x on BSA oxidation induced by Fe^{2+}-ascorbate/ H_2O_2 system. Each value is the mean of three determinations. ***$P < 0.001$, *$P < 0.05$, ns-non significant as compared to without extract but with Fe2+ - ascorbate/H_2O_2.

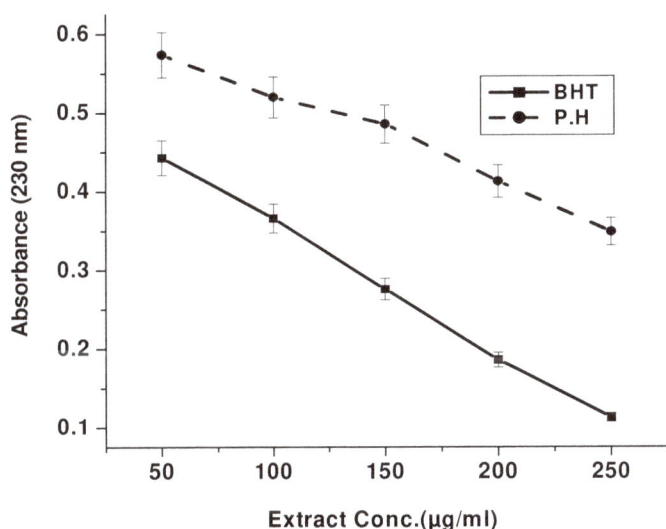

Figure 3. Hydrogen peroxide radical scavenging activity of ethanolic extract of Podophyllum hexandrum and known antioxidant BHT, Butylated hydroxyltolune. Absorbance of control = 0.671 ± 0.017, IC_{50} values BHT=109, E.E = 323.The data are presented as mean ± S.D of three independent experiments. E.E; ethanolic extract of *P. hexandrum*.

In the present study, we investigated the antioxidant potential of 70% ethanolic extract of *P. hexandrum*. Antioxidant activity of the plant extracts is often ascribed to the phenolic compounds present in them. Phytochemicals, especially plant phenolics constitute a major group of compounds that act as primary antioxidants (Hatano et al., 1989). The phenolic content of 70% ethanolic *P. hexandrum* rhizome extract was 153 ± 12 mg/g gallic acid. In various studies that evaluated the antioxidant activity of medicinal plants and fruits, a linear relationship between the total phenolic content and the antioxidant activity has been found indicating that the phenolic compounds might be the major contributors to the antioxidant activities of these extracts (Banerjee et al., 2005).

Glutathione is one of the most abundant tripeptide, non-enzymatic biological antioxidant present in liver. It removes free radicals species such as H_2O_2, $^\bullet O_2$ and maintains protein thiols. Is is a substrate for GPx also. Hydrogen peroxide can attack many cellular energy producing system e.g. glycolytic enzymes. It has been reported that removal of hydrogen peroxide as well superoxide anion is very important for protection of pharmaceutical and food systems (Gulcin et al., 2004). The extract used during this study, also scavenged H_2O_2, and also restored the levels of antioxidant enzymes viz., GPx, GR and the level of GSH (reduced), which had otherwise been significantly decreased in Group II CCl4 treated rats (Table 2). Similar findings were reported by Palanivel et al. (2008) for *Pisonia aculeate L.* against CCl4 induced hepatic damage in rats. The sulphydryl (SH) groups of proteins are crucial for several important functions. They maintain the functional conformation of proteins and also participate in catalytic activity of several enzymes. –SH groups, due to their ability to be reversibly oxidized, are recognized as key components involved in the mainte-nance of redox balance. 70% ethanolic extract of *P. hexandrum* showed appreciable protection against protein oxidation. Only few of plant extracts are reported to have this property (Martinez et al., 2001), pointing to the fact that the extract used during this study may have future beneficial applications in food and pharmaceutical

Table 1. Effect of ethanolic extract of *Podophyllum hexandrum* on serum hepatic markers in CCl4 induced hepatotoxicity in albino rats.

Treatment	Dosage	ALT (U/L)	AST (U/L)	LDH (U/L)
I. Control group (Olive oil only)	5 ml/Kg bw	20 ± 4	32 ± 12	46 ± 8
II. CCl4 treated group	1 ml/Kg bw	137 ± 2***	115 ± 8***	253 ± 13***
III. CCl4 treated + vitamin E	50 mg/Kg bw	76 ± 5***$$$	67 ± 7***$$$	181 ± 5***$$$
IV. CCl4 treated + *P. H* extract	20 mg/Kg bw	104 ± 1***	105 ± 7***	224 ± 4***
V. CCl4 treated + *P. H* extract	50 mg/Kg bw	87 ± 3 NS	75 ± 4 NS	193 ± 6 NS

$$$; $p < 0.001$ compared to CCl4,; ***$p < .001$ compared to control group, NS-non significant when compared to CCl4 + vitamin E. The data were presented as means ± S.D of six parallel measures and evaluated by the Bonferroni t – test. bw: body weight; ALT :alanine aminotransferase; AST: aspartate aminotransferase; LDH: lactate dehydrogenase; P.H: *Podophyllum hexandrum*.

Table 2. Effect of 70% ethanolic extract of *P. hexandrum* on antioxidant enzymes and protein levels of liver tissue in CCl4 treated rats.

Parameters	Group I (Olive oil only)	Group II CCl4 treated	Group III CCl4 + V.E	Group IV 20 mg/kg *P. hexandrum* extract	Group V 50 mg/kg *P. hexandrum* extract
Protein Content (mg/100 mg tissue)	51.2 ± 0.2	12 ± 0.8	34.1 ± 0.4	$13 \pm 1.$	$27 \pm 1.$
Glutathione Reduced (nm/g protein)	128 ± 21	34 ± 0.7***	$93 \pm 8$$$$	60 ± 3***	70 ± 2#
Glutathione reductase (µg GSSG utilized/minute/mg protein)	51 ± 20	2.6 ± 0.7***	$42 \pm 10$$$$ns	8 ± 0.8***	16 ± 1###
Glutathione peroxidase (µg GSH utilized/minute/mg protein)	50 ± 9	5.9 ± 0.7***	42 ± 6 $$$ns	7.4 ± 0.6***	19 ± 0##
Glutathione- S- transferase (nmoles of CDNB conjugated/min/mg protein)	44 ± 1	11.4 ± 0.5***	$39 \pm 1$$$$*	18 ± 2***	34 ± 2#

* $p < 0.05$, ** $p < 0.001$, ns-nonsignificant as compared to normal group, #p,0.05, ## $p < 0-01$, ###$p < 0.001$as compared with CCl4 +V.E, $$$ $p < 0.001$ to CCl4 induced group. The data represent the means ± SD for 7 animals in each group and evaluated by one-way ANOVA following Bonferroni t-test. Differences were considered to be statistically significant if $p < 0.05$. V.E: Vitamin E. P.H, *P. hexandrum*.

industry.

The reductive capacity of the extract was further studied using the Fe^{3+} to Fe^{2+} reduction assay. In this method, polyphenols reduce ferrocyanide ions i.e. $[Fe (CN)_6]^{3-}$ to ferric ferrocyanide Fe_4 [Fe

$(CN)_6]_3$ which in turn give rise to Prussian blue coloured complex. It is a known fact that phenolic acids and phenols having more number of reactive OH groups attached to ring act as more powerful reducing agents. This ultimately results

in the neutralization of free radical chain reactions. Thus the most powerful reducing agents are in general the most efficient radical scavengers (Andersen et al., 2003). Our results suggest that polyphenolic components within the 70% ethanolic extract of *P. hexandrum* may play a critical role in radical scavenging properties under *in vitro* and *in vivo* situations. Similar results were reported by Wang et al., (2009) for marine red alga, *Rhodomel confervoides* with high relationship between phenolic compounds and reducing power of the extract.

CCl_4 administration to rats causes changes in the serum levels of marker enzymes for liver damage and hepatic antioxidant enzymes, which is due to the CCl_4 damage to the liver parenchymal cells (Singh, 1980).When there is hepatopathy, these enzymes leak into the blood stream in conformity with the extent of liver damage (Nkosi et al., 2005). Accordingly the assessment of the level of AST, ALT and LDH provides a good and simple tool to measure the protective activity of the target drug against the hepatic damage (Hewawasan et al., 2004). The elevated level of these marker enzymes observed in the group II CCl4 treated rats in this present study corresponded to the extensive liver damage induced by CCl_4. The reduced concentrations of ALT, AST and LDH as a result of plant extract administration observed during this study (Table 1), indicated hepato-protection. Similar results were reported by different authors, when they used different plant extracts to study CCl_4 induced hepatic damage (Samudram P et al., 2008; Palanivel et al., 2008; Lima et al., 2010). Our results demonstrate that P. *hexandrum* ethanolic extract treatment prevents CCl_4 induced hepatotoxicity in rats by strengthening the antioxidant defense system and by scavenging free radicals. Detailed studies are warranted to look for the active ingredient in the extract that could be of possible therapeutic use.

REFRENCES

Andersen ML, Lauridsen RK, Skibsted LH (2003). Optimizing the use of phenolic compounds in foods. In: Johson I, Williamson G, eds. phytochemical functional foods. Cambridge: Woodhead Publishing Ltd. 315-346.

Banerjee A, Dasgupta N, De B (2005). *In vitro* study of antioxidant activity of *Syzygium cumini* fruit. Food Chem. 90: 727-733.

Chandler SF, Dodds JH (1993). The effect of phosphate, nitrogen and sucrose on the production of phenolics and solasidine in callus cultures of *Solanum laciniatum*. Plant Cell Rep. 2: 1005-110.

Cobb MW (1990). Human Papilloma virus infection. J. Am. Acad. Dermatol., 22: 547.

Czaja MJ, Xu J, Alt E (1995). Prevention of carbon tetrachloride induced rat liver injury by soluble tumor necrosis factor receptor. Gastroenterol. 108: 849-54.

Fleicher S, Rouser G (1965). Lipid of subcellular particles. J. Am. oil chemists Soc. 42: 588.

Fraga C, Leibovitz B, Tappel A (1987). Halogenated compounds as inducers of lipid peroxidation in tissue slices. Free Rad. Biol. Med. 3: 119-123.

Gowdey G, Lee RK, Carpenter WM (1995). Treatment of HIV- related hairy leukoplakia with Podophyllum resin 25% solution. Oral Surg. Oral Med. Oral Pathol. Oral Radiol. Endocrinol., 79: 64.

Gulcin IG, Sat S, Beydemir SM, Elmasta, Kufrevioglu OI (2004). Food Chem. 87:393.

Habig VH, Pabst MJ, Jakoby WB (1974). Glutathione-S-transferase. The first enzymatic step in mercapturic acid formation. J. Biol. Chem. 249: 7130-7139.

Halliwell B, Gutteridge JMC (1989). Free Radicals in Biology and Medicine, 2nd ed. Oxford University Press. Oxford. pp. 78-93.

Hatano T, Edamatsu R, Mori A, Fujita Y, Yasuhara E (1989). Effects of tannins and related polyphenols on superoxide anion radical and on 1, 1-diphenyl-2-picrylhydrazyl. Chem. Pharm. Bull. 37: 2016-23.

Hewawasan RP, Jayatilaka KAPW, Pathirana C, Mudduwa LKW (2004). Hepatoproctective effect of *Epaltes divaricata* extract on carbon tetra chloride induced hepatotoxicity in mice. Ind. J. Med. Res. 120: 30-34.

Hissin PJ, Hilf R (1976). A fluorometric method for determination of oxidized and reduced glutathione in tissues. Anal. Biochem. 74: 214-226.

Hochstein P, Atallah AS (1988). The nature of oxidants and antioxidant systems in the inhibition of mutation and cancer. Mutation Res. 202: 363-37.

Hogg N (1998). Free radicals in disease. Seminars in reproductive endocrinology. 16: 241-288.

Imbert F (1998). Discovery of Podophyllatoxin. Bio.Chimie. 80: 207. *In vivo*. J. Am. Oil Chem. Soc. 42(11): 908.

King J (1965). The dehydrogenase of oxidoreductase- Lactate dehydrogenase. *In Practical Clinical Enzymology* (King JC and Van D, Eds.) Nostrand Co. Lundon. 83-93.

Lawrence RA, Burk RF (1976). Glutathione peroxidase activity in rat liver. Biochem. Biophys. Res. Commun. 71: 952-8.

Lima TB, Suja A, Jisa OS, Sathyanarayanan S, Remya KS (2010). Hepatoprotective activity of LIV-first against carbon tetra chloride-induced hepatotoxicity in albino rats. Int. J Green Pharm. 4(2): 71-74.

Lowry OH, Rosenbrough NJ, Farr AI, Randall RJ (1951). Protein estimation with the Folin-Phenol reagent. J. Biol. Chem. 193: 265-275.

Mannervik B, Carlberg I (1985). Glutathione Reductase. Methods in Enzymol. 113: 484-490.

Martinez G, Giuliani A, Leon OS, Perez G, Nunez, Selles AJ (2001). Effects of *Magnifera indica* L. extract (QF808) on protein and hepatic microsome peroxidation. Phytother. Res. 15: 581-585.

McCord JM, Keele BB, Fridovich I (1971). An enzyme base theory of obliate anaerobiosis: the physiological function of superoxide dismutase. PNAS. 68: 1024-1027.

Mitra SK, Venkataranganna MV, Sudaram R, Gopumadhavan S (1998). Protective effect of HD -03, a herbal formulation, against various hepatotoxic agents in rats. J. Ethnopharmacol. 63: 181-186.

Mizuoka H, Shikata N, Yang J, Takasu M, Inoue K, Tsubura, A (1999). Biphasic effect of colchicine on acute liver injury induced by carbon tetrachloride or by dimethylnitrosamine in mice. J. Hepatol. 1: 825-33.

Moren MA, Depierre JW, Mannervick B (1979). Levels of glutathione, glutathione reductase and glutathione S- transferase activities in rat lung and liver. Biochem. Biophys. Acta. 582: 67-78.

Nayan J, Janardhanan KK (2000). Antioxidant and antitumor activity of Pleurotus florida. Current Science. 79: 941-943.

Nkosi CZ, Opoku AR, Terblanche SE (2005). Effect of pumpkin seed (*Cucurbita pepo*) protein isolate on the activity levels of certain plasma enzymes in CCl4-induced liver injury in low-protein fed rats. Phy. Res. 19: 341-345.

Okezie IA (1996). Characterization of drugs as antioxidant prophylactic. Free radical Biology and Medicine. 20(5): 675-705.

Oyaizu M (1986). Studies on products of browning reaction prepared from glucosamine. Jap. J. Nutr. 44: 307-315.

Palanivel MG, Rajkapoor B, Kumar RS, Einstein JW, Kumar EP, Kumar MR, Kavitha K, Kumar MP, Jayakar B (2008). Hepatoprotective and Antioxidant Effect of *Pisonia aculeata* L. against CCl4- Induced Hepatic Damage in Rats Sci. Pharm., 76: 203-215.

Pong K (2003). Oxidative stress in neurodegenerative diseases: therapeutic implications for superoxide dismutase mimetics. Exp. Opin. Boil. Ther., 3: 127-139.

Rao PS, Mangipudy RS, Mehendale HM (1997). Tissue injury and repair as parallel and opposing responses to CCl4 hepatotoxicity: a novel dose-response. Toxicology., 118: 181-93.

Recknagel RO, Glende EA, Dolak JA, Waller RL (1989). Mechanisms of carbon tetrachloride toxicity. Pharmacol Ther. 43:139-54.

Reitman S, Frankel AS (1975). A Colorimetric method for the determination of serum glutamic oxaloacetic and glutamic pyruvic transaminases. Am. J. Clin. Pathol., 28: 56-63.

Ruch RJ, Cheng SJ, Klaunig JE (1989). Carcinogenesis. 10: 1003-1008.

Samudram P, Rajeshwari H, Vasuki R, Geetha A, Sathiya-moorthi P (2008). Hepatoprotective activity of Bi - herbal ethanolic extract on CCl$_4$ induced hepatic damage in rats. Afr. J. Biochem. Res. 2(2): 61-65.

Singh ID (1980). In: Text book of Biochemistry and Human biology (Talwar, G.P., ed), Prentice Hall of India. New Delhi

Stahelin HF, Wartburg AV (1991). The chemical and biological route form Podophyllatoxin glucoside to etoposide. Cancer Res. 51: 5.

Uday B, Das D, Banerjee KR (1999). Reactive oxygen species. Oxidative damage and pathogenesis, Curr. Sci. 77: 658-666.

Wang BW, Zhang Z, Duan, Li X (2009). In vitro antioxidative activities of extract and semi-purified fractions of the marine red alga, *Rhodomela confervoides* (Rhodomelaceae). Food Chem. 113: 1101-1105.

Witting LA (1965). Lipid peroxidation in vivo. J. Am. Oil Chem. Soc. 42 (11): 908.

11

Enhancing antioxidant availability in grains of wheat plants grown under seawater-stress in response to microalgae extracts treatments

Hanaa H. Abd El-Baky

Plant Biochemistry Department, National Research Centre, Dokki, Cairo, Egypt. E-mail: Abdelbaky@hotmail.com.

This study investigated the antioxidant capacity and the levels of enhanced total carotenoids (TCAR), tocopherols (TOC) and phenolic (TPC) and protein (PC) contents in whole grains of wheat plants irrigated 10 and 20% (v/v) seawater (SW) in response to water extracts of microalgae *Spirulina maxima* (SME) and *Chlorella ellipsoida* (CEE) and exogenous plant growth enhancers of ascorbic acid (Vit. C) and benzyladinin (BA) treatments. Significant differences ($P < 0.05$) in amounts of TCAR (ranged 80 to 140 µg/g), TOC (ranged 50.4 to 115 µg/g), TPC (ranged 0.80 to 2.96 mg/g) and PC (ranged 9.34 to 13.79 %) in wheat grains among all treated plants were observed. The levels of their compounds increase related to irrigation-SW combined with algal treatments. The ethanolic extracts of grains of SW-stress plants treated with algal extracts exhibited high antioxidant capacity based on scavenging of DPPH and ABTS radicals than other samples. This activity remarked correlation with levels of antioxidant compounds present in these extracts. The electrophoretic profiles (SDS-PAGE fingerprint) of grains protein of treated samples exhibited similar pattern that in controls samples. It is concluded that the application of algal extracts to wheat plants irrigated SW lead to increase antioxidative components and protein content; hence consumption of these whole grains may render beneficial health effects.

Key words: Microalgae, antioxidant activity, phenolics, proteins, seawater.

INTRODUCTION

Wheat is a major agriculture commodity and dietary component across the world. It is one the most important cereals in view of nutrition values. It serves as rich sources of fiber, vitamins, carbohydrate, proteins and mineral (Fardet et al., 2008). Furthermore, wheat grains contain unique phytochemicals that complement those in fruits and vegetables when consumed together. In general, wheat grains have been known to contain high amounts of various classes of phenolics compound includes phenolic acids, anthocyanidins, quinones, flavonoids and amino phenolic compounds that render potential health benefits (Maillard and Berset, 1995; Shahidi and Naczk, 1995; Lloyd et al., 2000). However, some of these phytochemicals such as ferulic acid and diferulates are generally predominantly found in wheat varieties (about 50 - 67%, of total phenolic acids), but are not present in significant quantities in some fruits and vegetables (Bunzel et al., 2001; Zhou et al., 2004).

Epidemiological studies have shown that regular consumption of whole grains and whole grain products is positively associated with reduced risk of various type of chronic diseases such as cardiovascular disease (Liu, 2007; Anderson et al., 2000), type 2 diabetes (Meyer et al., 2000; Venn and Mann, 2004) some cancers (Kasum et al., 2002) and stroke (Keli et al., 1996). However, wheat grain possesses significant antioxidant activity, which implies the potential for utilizing and promoting the health benefits of wheat (Iqbal and Ashraf, 2006; Fardet et al., 2008). Phenolic compounds found in wheat grains (e.g., phenolic acid, flavoionds and tocopherols) are the main antioxidant compounds that is believed to be responsible for the antioxidant properties (Zhou et al., 2004; Liu 2007 and Fardet et al., 2008). Furthermore, many of these compounds show diverse of bioactivities, such as antimitotic, antiviral, antiallergic, antimutagenicity and antiageing effects (Stavric, 1994; CooK and Samman, 1996; Abd El Baky et al., 2008; Liyana-Pathirana and Shahidi, 2007).

In Egypt, human overpopulation becomes a serious constraint for crop production such as maize, rice and wheat. Thus, improving overall growth and performance of agriculture crops is an important goal to improve productivity. This is driven by the need to provide food for steadily growing population. Egypt also is present in semiarid region; seawater therefore, has been a resent effort, the possibility of obtaining reasonable yield and quality to products from whole grains (Abd El-Baky et al., 2008). In a previous study involving wheat plants, the cultivated plants were irrigated seawater (10 and 20% levels) and treated with algal extracts enrich in antioxidant compounds such as Vitamin C, carotenoids, tocopheroles and phenolic acids (Abd El-Baky et al., 2008). Due to their inherent antioxidant potential, the wheat plants appear to be enhancing in growth as reflected in both biochemical and agronomic response. Therefore, the present study was carried out, based on hypothesized that the treated of wheat plants with algae extracts may results in an increase of photochemical compounds in grains that possess high antioxidant properties. Thus, the antioxidant contents and antioxidant capacity of different wheat grains was determined. In addition, the protein content and protein profile was investigated in order to determine the bread-making quality of their wheat grains.

MATERIALS AND METHODS

Samples

The different samples were obtained from harvest wheat crops after cultivation under different treatments. Controls samples of the wheat grains (*Triticum aestivum* L., cv. Giza 94) were obtained from plants irrigated either 10 and 20% seawater (SW-stress, v/v) or natural water (NW non-stress) though with different growth stages (GS). Treated samples were obtained from wheat plants irrigated 10 and 20% seawater and treated intervals at 40 and 70 d of GS, with either microalgae water extracts of *Chlorella ellipsoida* and *Spirulina maxima* (at concentration of 5g /L in 0.1% tween 20) or standard plant growth enhancers (ascorbic acid and benzyladinine, at concentration of 200 mg/L). The data of biochemical parameters of treated samples were compared with those data of either 10 or 20% SW-stress and NW non-stress plants.

Extraction of crude phenolics of wheat

The crude phenolic compounds of whole grains of different samples were extracted with 80% aqueous ethanol (1:10, w/v) at 4°C for 16 h. The resulting slurries were centrifuged at 6000 xg for 5 min and the supernatants were saved. The residues were re-extracted (1:5 w/v; 80% ethanol) under the same conditions. The supernatant of both extractions were combined and was concentrated under vacuum at 40°C to give a semisolid. Yields of the crude phenolic extracts were reported as percentage of defatted materials (Liyana-Pathirana and Shahidi, 2007). All samples were protected permanently from light.

Determination of total phenolics content (TPC)

Total phenolic contents of crude ethanolic extracts were determined following the method by Singleton et al. (1999). A 100 µl aliquot of sample (2 mg of extract/ 1 ml of ethanol) was added to 1 mL of 10%

Folin–Ciocalteu phenol reagent. After 4 min incubation at room temperature, 2 mL of 5% sodium carbonate solution was added. The reaction mixture was incubated for 45 min in a dark-cupboard, the absorbance at 725 nm was then determined. Ferulic acid (10 - 100 µg/mL of 95% ethanol) was used as phenolic standard for preparation of calibration curve. Phenolic contents are expressed as micrograms of ferulic acid equivalents (FAE) per gram.

Determination of tocopherols by HPLC

Tocopherols were analyzed by HPLC method. HPLC system equipped with Spectra system UV2000 detector at 290 nm and separated on Vydac analytical column (25 cm X 4.6 mm i.d., 5 µm particle sizes). Tocopherols were eluted with acetonitrile: methanol (9:1 v/v) at a flow rate of 1 mL min^{-1}. Standard of α-tocopherol was run under the same conditions (Abd El-Baky et al., 2003).

Determination of total carotenoids

The total carotenoids in wheat grains samples were spectophotometrically determined at 450 nm according to AOAC standard methods (1995). A standard curve was established using β-carotene in hexane.

Antioxidant assays

DPPH (2,2-diphenyl-1-picrylhydrazyl) radical scavenging assay

The method described by Tagashira and Ohtake (1998) was used in order to assess the DPPH radical scavenging of ethanolic wheat extracts. A 0.1 mM (final concentration) DPPH in ethanol solution was mixed with wheat extracts and vortexed thoroughly. The absorbance of the mixture at ambient temperature was measured at 519 nm, for 60 min at 10 min intervals. The scavenging of DPPH was calculated according to the following equation: scavenging percentage (%) = [(A_{517} control - A_{517} sample) / A_{517} control] X 100; where: A control = absorbance of DPPH radical + methanol; A sample = absorbance of DPPH radical + wheat extract/ standard. The scavenging capacity was expressed as I mol DPPH radical scavenged/g of defatted material.

Measurement of total antioxidant activity

Total antioxidant activity was determined according to the Trolox (6-hydroxy-2, 5, 7, 8-tetramethylchroman-2-carboxylic acid) equivalent antioxidant capacity (TEAC) assay described by Re et al. (1999). The extracts and reagents were prepared in a 0.1 M phosphate buffer saline (PBS, pH 7.4). A ABTS^{+} solution (2,2'-azinobis-(3-ethylbenzthiazoline-6-sulfonate) was prepared by mixing 2.5 mM potassium persulfate with 7.0 mM ABTS^{+} in a 1:1 (v/v) ratio, and leaving the mixture for 8 h. The absorbance of the radical solution at 743 nm was 0.7 ± 0.03. The solution was stored at room temperature and protected from light. Trolox standard curve (ranged 0.5 - 20 µg/mL) was prepared. The reduction in the absorbance of the ABTS^{-2} solution (1.9 mL) at different concentrations of Trolox (2 - 30 µg/mL) over a period of 6 min was measured and plotted. The TEAC values of wheat extracts (5 mg/mL) were determined in the same way and expressed as µM Trolox equivalents.

Determination of total protein content

A known weight of fine powdered seeds (Ca, 0.2 g) was digested using a micro Kjeldahl apparatus. The total protein content was calculated by multiplying the total nitrogen by 5.75 (AOAC, 1995).

Table 1. Changes in antioxidant compounds and total protein contents of wheat grains   irrigated seawater in response to algal extracts and plant growth enhancer's treatments.

Treatments	µg /g D.W	Ratio[a]	µg/ g D.W	Ratio[a]	mg /g D.W	Ratio[a]	% D.W
Irrigation natural water (NW) only	80.39		50.21		0.80		11.25
NW+S. maxima	125.37	1.56	98.12	1.95	1.43	1.80	13.79
NW +C. ellipsoida	110.35	1.37	91.25	1.82	1.33	1.70	13.23
NW +vit C	90.11	1.12	72.11	1.44	0.82	1.03	11.45
NW +BA	85.17	1.06	65.14	1.30	0.95	1.20	11.93
Irrigation 10% sea water (SW) only	84.78	1.05	55.14	1.1	1.02	1.30	9.95
SW+S. maxima	134.10	1.67	110.25	202	2.31	2.90	13.21
SW +C. ellipsoida	117.38	1.4	98.14	1.95	1.72	2.15	13.12
SW +vit C	95.17	1.18	79.35	1.58	1.21	1.52	11.96
SW +BA	89.15	1.11	68.27	1.35	1.43	1.80	10.29
20% sea water only	90.84	1.13	58.36	1.16	1.53	1.92	9.34
SW+S. maxima	140.98	1.75	115.14	2.30	2.96	3.71	13.23
SW +C.ellipsoida	124.32	1.55	105.24	2.10	2.14	2.70	13.21
SW +vit C	98.35	1.22	82.21	1.60	1.45	1.81	11.11
SW +BA	92.36	1.15	73.25	1.45	1.92	2.40	10.53
LSD at level (P < 0.01)	2.50		1.64		0.12		0.95

Ratio[a]: Treatment / Negative control (irrigated only by natural water)
All values are significant at (P ≤ 0.05), ± S.D
Data present the mean of three experiments with replicated measurements.

Separation of grains protein by SDS-PAGE

Protein extracted by grinding 0.5 g of wheat grains mortar in liquid nitrogen and 5 ml buffer solution (containing 250 mM sucrose and 25 mM Tris, pH 7.2). SDS-PAGE was performed based on the method described previously by Laemmli (1970).

Statistical analysis

All analyses were performed in triplicate and data reported as mean ± standard deviation, unless otherwise stated. Analysis of variance was done using the COSTAT computer package (Cohort Software, CA, USA). The mean values were compared with LSD test.

RESULTS AND DISCUSSION

The amounts of total carotenoids (TCAR), tocopherols (TOC) and phenolic content (TPC) of whole-wheat grains of plants irrigated either 10 and 20% seawater (SW-stress plants) or irrigated natural water (NW non-stressed) in response to algal water extracts, Vitamin C and BA treatments, are shows in Table 1. The concentration of these components in whole-wheat grains showed a significant difference (P < 0.05) among all treatments. Irrigation of wheat plants with 10 and 20% SW caused significant increase in accumulation of TCAR, TOC and TPC

in yielded grains. The levels of those compounds being about 1.05, 1.1 and 1.3 and 1.13, 1.16 and 1.92 times as high as that in grains of plants irrigated NW, respectively. Thus, irrigation with SW increased concentration low molecular mass antioxidant compounds in yield wheat crops. Application of extracts of blue green algae, *S. maxima* and green algae, *C. ellipsoida* on wheat plants irrigated SW led to accumulation of high amounts of antioxidant compounds in yielded grains as compared to that in plants irrigated 10 and 20% SW. The highest levels of TCAR, TOC and TPC in wheat grains were found in plants irrigated 20% SW and treated with extracts of *S. maxima* (124.32, 105.24 and 2.1 mg/g of defatted wheat grains (DWG), respectively), followed by *C. ellipsoida* (124.32, 105.24 and 2.1 mg/g DWG). Similar trained was observed in grains of plants irrigated 10% SW and treated with *S. maxima* (134.1, 110.25 and 2.3 mg/g, respectively) and *C. ellipsoida* (117.38, 98.14 and 1.72 mg/g, respectively). On the other hand, the concentration of TCAR, TOC and TPC in yielded grains of wheat plants irrigated either 10 or 20% SW were affected by treated with Vitamin C and BA when compared to plants irrigated NW values, and there was no effect as compared to those values found in plants irrigated SW only. Thus, the concentration of antioxidant compounds was significantly

Table 2. DPPH Scavenging Capacity % of wheat grains extracts of plants irrigated sea water combined with algal extract treatments.

Treatments	$IC_{50}{}^b$ ($\mu g\ mL^{-1}$)	DPPH Scavenging Capacity %
BHA	13.8	92.00
BHT	15.6	94.00
α-Tocopherol	19.0	82.00
Irrigation natural water (NW) only	105.5	13.25
NW +S. maxima	30.8	55.21
NW +C.ellipsoida	35.2	42.31
NW + vit. C	40.9	29.32
NW +BA	50.8	23.52
Irrigation 10% sea water (SW) only	90.5	16.24
SW +S. maxima	25.4	59.21
SW +C.ellipsoida	32.4	46.21
SW +vit. C	38.6	35.27
SW +BA	42.1	28.31
20% sea water (SW) only	85.9	19.21
SW + S. maxima	24.2	62.12
SW +C. ellipsoida	33.5	48.21
SW + vit. C	37.3	37.85
SW +BA	39.6	31.24
LSD at level (P< 0.01)	1.45	

$IC_{50}{}^b$: Concentration ($\mu g/ml$) for a 50% inhibition was calculated from the plot of inhibition (%) against wheat grains extracts concentration
Tests were carried out in triplicate

increased in yielded grains of wheat plants irrigated SW in response to application of algal extracts, when compared with all controls plants include: plants irrigated only NW and either 10 and 20% SW. Furthermore, application of algal extracts had a significant greater effect than standard growth enhancers (SGE, with Vitamin C or BA) in increasing antioxidant contents. However, the order of antioxidant compounds content in yielded grains of wheat plants irrigated SW in response to application with algae extracts and SGE was S. maxima > C. ellipoida > Vitamin C > BA. This finding clearly suggests that antioxidant compounds in grain of plants irrigated SW were significantly influenced in response to S. maxima and C. ellipsoida algae extract treatments. In previous studies with wheat, an increase in concentration of low molecular mass antioxidant compounds includes GSH, carotenoids, tecopherols and phenols compounds in wheat leaves of plants irrigated seawater up to 20% correlated with treated with microalgale extracts enrich in antioxidant constituents (Abd El-Baky et al., 2008). Generally, this study showed that the levels of phenolic, carotenoids and tocopherols content in Giza-94 wheat grains were comparable to previous findings in several varieties of wheat located in Asia and North America (Iqbal and Ashraf, 2006). However, it is know that grain types, varieties, agronomic, the part of the grain sampled and environmental factors had significant affect on the concentrations of antioxidant compounds in whole grains (Adom et al., 2005).

Radical scavenging capacity

Free radical scavenging ability of various wheat grains ethanolic extracts of SW-stressed plants in response of treatments was measured with the change of absorbance caused by the reduction of DPPH radical, and results of percentage scavenging activity (% SC) and the values of IC_{50} are shown in Table 2. High %SC was an indication of high degree of scavenging DPPH radical and high antioxidant activity. It was clear that the grains ethanolic extracts showed significant scavenging activities with various degrees (IC_{50} values ranged from 24.2 to 105.5 $\mu g/mL$). The highest scavenging activity (P < 0.5%) was found for grains extracts of plants irrigated 10 and 20% SW combined with treated by extracts of S. maxima (% SC, 59.21 and 62.12%), followed by C. ellipsoida (% SC, 46.21 and 48.21%) and then that treated with Vitamin C (% SC, 35.27 and 37.85%) and BA (% SC, 28.31 and 31.24%). Thus, scavenging activities of extracts of SW-stressed plants treated with algal extracts were apparently higher than those treated with BA and Vitamin C. However, scavenging activity from wheat grains of stressed plants treated by algal extracts (% SC, 46.21 – 62.12%) was lower compared with that of commercial antioxidant BHT (94%) and BHA (92%).

ABTS$^+$ scavenging activity: As shows in Table 3, the ethanolic extracts of wheat grains of plants irrigated SW

Table 3. ABTS[.+] Scavenging capacity % of wheat grains extracts of plants irrigated sea water combined with algal extract treatments.

Treatments	ABTS$^+$ scavenging activity
	µmol trolox /g grain
Irrigation natural water (NW) only	8.74
NW+ *S. maxima*	17.36
NW + *C. ellipsoida*	15.66
NW +vit. C	12.35
NW +BA	10.36
Irrigation 10% sea water (SW) only	10.25
SW+ *S. maxima*	18.24
SW + *C. ellipsoida*	16.94
SW +vit. C	13.65
SW +BA	11.57
Irrigation 20% sea water (SW) only	12.54
SW+ *S. maxima*	20.14
SW + *C. ellipsoida*	18.35
SW +vit. C	15.14
SW +BA	13.57
LSD at level (P< 0.01)	1.21

combined with treated by algal extracts and PGEs exhibited appreciable ABTS[.+] scavenging activity. These activities were varied significantly from one anther. The ABTS[.+] scavenging activity was in the range of 20.14 and 8.74 µM of trolox / g grains. The highest ABTS[.+] scavenging activity were observed for extracts of wheat grains of SW-stressed plants treated with *S. maxima* (ranged 17.36 to 20.14 µmol of trolox/ g grains), followed by *C. ellipsoida* (ranged 15.66 to 18.35 µmol of trolox/ g grains) and then Vitamin C (ranged 12.35 to 15.14 µmol of trolox/ g grains) and BA (ranged 10.36 to 13.57 µmol of trolox/ g grains). In general, the ability to scavenge both DPPH and ABTS radicals by ethanolic extracts of grains of SW-stressed wheat plants in response to algae extracts and reference PGEs treatments was in the order of *S. maxima* > *C. ellipsoida* > Vitamin C > BA.

This finding was in accordance with that study on alcoholic extracts of a wheat variety grown in different location (Canadian and Pakistanis), which showed good antioxidant activity with various degrees (Iqbal and Ashraf, 2006). Moreover, in a series of *in vitro* antioxidant assays, the alcoholic extracts of some wheat varieties (whole-grain) and their constituent fractions (such as wheat germ, bran and flour) exhibited significant antioxidant properties against many free radicals scavenging models (Zhou et al., 2005; Fardet et al., 2008). Iqbal and Ashraf (2006) and Liyana-Pathirana and Shahidi (2007) reported that the wheat ethanolic extracts contains large amounts of phenolic compounds possessed high antioxidant activity due to their hydrogen-donating ability. Therefore, it could be possess hydroxyl radical scavenging properties in both non-enzymatic lipid peroxidation and

deoxyribose assays. Again, the present results suggested that alcoholic extracts of wheat grains contains high amounts of antioxidative components included TCAR, TOC and TPC (Table 2). Their compounds having a potent antioxidant activity (Adom, et al., 2003; Zhou et al., 2005; Abd El Baky et al., 2007). Recently, positive correlation between free radical scavenging activity of wheat grains and their fraction and phenolic contents was reported (Zhou et al., 2005; Choi, et al., 2007; Liu, 2007). However, in this study, ethanolic extracts of wheat grains of SW-stressed plant treated with growth enhancer (Vitamin C and BA) possess a week antioxidant activity than that treated with algal extracts. Although, their extracts contains a significant amounts of phenolic compounds compared to those of the others extracts. It is though that other components in wheat ethanolic extracts, such as carotenoids and tocopherols, may be affected in the antioxidant activity.

Consequently, antioxidant activity may vary depending on the actual composition of these extracts. Finally, these findings suggest that wheat grains of SW-stressed wheat plants exhibited a marked antioxidant potential and consequently, can be uses as a rich sources of antioxidant compounds, which play a significant role in protective our bodies against oxidative radicals, which cause various types of chronic diseases.

Protein contents and protein profile

As show in Table 1, the amount of total proteins content (TPs) varied significantly among whole wheat grains of non-stressed and SW-stressed plants treated with either

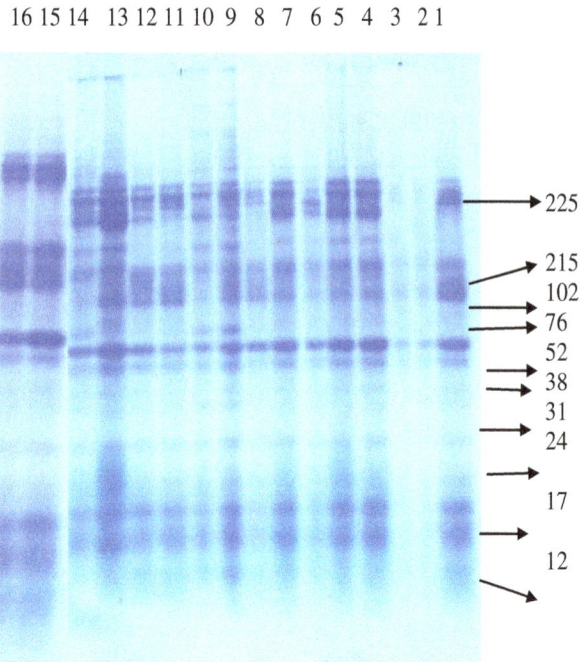

Figure 1. SDS-PAGE pattern of wheat grains as affected by algal antioxidant spraying and irrigated with sea water.

1. Protein marker; 2. Natural water only; 3. Sp. antioxidant; 4. Chl. antioxidant; 5. Vit. C. 6. BA; 7. 10% sea water only; 8. Sp. antioxidant; 9. Chl. antioxidant; 10. Vit. C; 11. BA. 12. 20% sea water only; 13. Sp. Antioxidant; 14. Chl. antioxidant; 15. Vit. C; 16. BA

algae extracts or PGEs. The differences were also significantly (p < 0.5) between algal extracts and PGE treatments. However, the grains of plants irrigated 10 and 20% SW combined with application by algal extracts of *S. maxima* (13.21 and 13.23%) and *C. ellipsoida* (13.12 and 11.21%) had higher TPs contents compared with both that in plants irrigated 10 and 20% SW only (9.95 and 9.34%), and that in SW-stressed plant treated by PGEs (either with Vitamin C: 11.96 and 11.11% or BA, 10.29 and 9.53%). Thus, the ability to increase protein content in wheat grains of SW-stressed plants was in the order of *S. maxima* > *C. ellipsoida* > Vitamin C > BA. Furthermore, the grains of non-stressed plant treated with algal extracts or PGE had higher levels of protein content than that in grains of Sw-stress plants in response to the same treatments, but was not significantly (Table 1). Therefore, these results suggest that the treatment of wheat plants with algal extracts and PGE have significant effect on stimulation of protein synthesis. This finding is compatible with that found by Abd El Baky et al. (2008), which is the application of algal extracts on SW-stressed plants during the growth stages leading to increased of endogenous protein synthesis.

SDS-Polyacrylamide gel electrophoresis

The electrophoretic profiles (SDS-PAGE fingerprint) of

grains protein of SW-stress wheat plants treated either with algal extracts or PGE compared to those of the (controls) non-stressed, 10 and 20% SW- stressed plants are shown in Figure 1. As expected the treated of SW-stress plants had an approximate similar protein profile [among all protein groups, high (> 80 kDa, HMW), medium (<80 - >40 kDa, MMW) and low molecular weight (<40 kDa, LMW)] that was found in all controls plants (Figure 1, lanes 2 - 16), This finding indicated that no recognizable losses of bands in protein grains of stressed plants due to application of algal extracts through growth stages. However, there were some new protein bands (Figure 1, lanes 12 - 14) corresponding to molecular of approximate weights from 225 to 215 kDa (lanes 13 and 14). In addition, the strong relative intensity of some bands in LMW proteins was present in the wheat grains of 20% SW-stressed plants treated with algal extracts. This phenomena indicating that the new HMW proteins were induced in grains of stressed plants in response to algal application. According to Huang and Khan (1997) HMW glutenin subunits are the most important components in determining wheat grains quality. That HMW and LMW proteins may be randomly linked leading to increase strength of the gluten polymer network. Therefore, the wheat grains contain high amounts of HMW glutenin had good bread-making quality (Payne et al., 1979). Finally, it could be concluded that the application of algal extracts to wheat plants irrigated SW showed a positive effects on antioxidative components and protein contents; hence consumption of these whole grains may render beneficial health effects.

REFERENCES

Abd El-Baky, H. Hanaa, El Baz FK, El-Baroty GS (2003). *Spirulina* Species as a Source of Carotenoids and α-Tocopherol and its antiTCARinoma factors. Biotechol. 2(3): 222-240.

Abd El-Baky H H, El Baz FK, El-Baroty G S (2007). Production of carotenoids from marine microalgae and its evaluation as safe food colorant and lowering cholesterol agents. Am. Eurasian. J. Agric. Environ. Sci., 2 (6): 792-800.

Abd El-Baky H H, Hussein M M, El-Baroty G S (2008). Algal extracts improve antioxidant defense abilities and salt tolerance of wheat plant irrigated with sea water. Afr. J. Biochem. Res. 2 (7), pp. 151 –164

Adom K K, Sorrells M, Liu R H, (2005). Phytochemicals and antioxidant activity of milled fractions of different wheat varieties. J. Agric. Food Chem. 53: 2297–2306.

Anderson JW, Hanna TJ, Peng X. Kryscio RJ (2000). Whole grain foods and heart disease risk. J. Amer. Coll .Nutrition 19: 291S–299S.

A.O.A.C (1995). Official Methods of Analysis. Association of Official Analytical Chemists, 16 th ed., K Hlrich. Arlington, Virginia.

Bunzel M, Ralph J, Martia JM, Hateld RD, Steinhart H (2001). Diferulates as structural components in soluble and insoluble cereal dietary fiber. J. Sci. Food. Agric. 81, 653–660.

Choi Y, Jeong HS, Lee J (2007). Antioxidant activity of methanolic extracts from some grains consumed in Korea. Food Chemistry, 103: 130-138.

Cook NC, Samman S (1996). Flavonoids-chemistry, metabolism, cardioprotective effects and dietary sources, Nutrition and Biochemistry, 7:66-76.

Fardet A, Rock E. Christian R (2008). Is the in vitro antioxidant potential of whole-grain cereals and cereal products well reflected in vivo. J. Cereal Sci., 48: 258-276.

Huang Y D, Khan K (1997). Quantitative determination of high molecular weight glutenin subunits of hard red spring wheat by SDS-PAGE. II. Quantitive effects of individual subunits on bread-making quality characteristics Cereal chem.., 74 (6): 786-790.

Iqbal M M, Ashraf (2006). Wheat seed priming in relation to salt tolerance, growth, yield and level of free salicylic acid and polyamines. Ann. Bot. Fennici., 43(4): 250-259.

Kasum CM, Jacobs DRJ, Nicodemus K, Folsom AR (2002). Dietary risk factors for upper aerodigestive tract cancers. Inter. J. Cancer 99: 267–272.

Keli S O, Hertog M G, Feskens E J, Kromhout D (1996). Dietary flavonoids, antioxidant vitamins, and incidence of stroke: the Zutphen study. Arch. Int. Med., 156: 637–642.

Laemmli U K (1970). Cleavage of structural proteins during the assembly of the head bacteriophage T4. Nature, 227:680-685.

Liyana-Pathirana MC, Shahidi F (2007). Antioxidant and free radical scavenging activities of whole wheat and milling fractions. Food Chem. 101: 1151–1157

Liu RH (2007). Whole grain phytochemicals and health. J. Cereal Sci., 46: 207-219.

Lloyd BJ, Siebenmorgen TJ, Beers KW (2000). Effect of commercial processing on antioxidants in rice bran. Cereal Chemistry 77: 551–555.

Maillard MN, Berset C (1995). Evolution of antioxidant activity during kilning: role of insoluble bound phenolic acids of barley and malt. J. Agric. Food. Chem. 43: 1789–1793.

Meyer K A, Kushi L H, Jacob D R, Jr Slavin J, Sellers T A, Folsom A R (2000). Carbohydrates, dietary fiber, incident type 2 diabetes mellitus in older women. Am. J. Clin. Nutr. 71: 921-930.

Payane PI, Corfield KG, Blackman JA (1979). Identification of a high molecular weight subunit of glutenin whose presence correlates with breadmaking quality in wheats of related pedigree. Theor. Appl. Genet. 55: 153-159.

Shahidi F, Naczk M (1995). Food Phenolics: sources, Chemistry, Effects, Applications. Technomic Publishing Company Inc., USA.

Re R, Pellegrini N, Proteggente A, Pannala A, Yang M, Rice-Evans C (1999). Antioxidant activity applying an improved ABTS radical cation decolorization assay. Free Radic. Biol. Med. 26: 1231–1237.

Singleton VL, Orthofer R, Lamuela-Raventos R M (1999). Analysis of total phenols and other oxidation substrates and antioxidant by means of Folin-Ciocalteu reagent. Methods Enzymol. 299: 152- 178.

Stavric B (1994). Role of chemopreventers in human diet clinical. Biochem. 27: 5: 319 – 332.

Tagashira M, Ohtake Y (1998). A new antioxidative 1,3- benzodioxole from *Melissa officinalis*. Planta Med., 64: 555-558.

Venn BJ, Mann JI (2004). Cereal grains, legumes and diabetes. European .J. Clinical. Nutr. 58: 1443-1461.

Zhou K, Laux J J, Yu L (2004). Comparison of Swiss red wheat grain and fractions for their antioxidant properties. J. Agric. Food. Chem. 52: 1118–1123.

Zhou K, Yin J J, Yu L (2005). Phenolic acid, tocopherol and carotenoid compositions, and antioxidant functions of hard red winter wheat bran. J. Agric. Food. Chem.. 53: 3916–3922.

12

Assessment of the potency of some selected anti-malaria drugs on the supplements of vitamin B2 and orange fruit juice (combination therapy)

Adumanya O. C.[1], Uwakwe A. A.[2], Odeghe O. B.[2*], Essien E. B.[2] and Okere T. O.[1]

[1]Department of Nutrition and Dietetics, Imo State Polytechnic, Umuagwo, Imo State, Nigeria.
[2]Department of Biochemistry, University of Port Harcourt, Rivers State, Nigeria.

Current practice in treating cases of malaria is based around the concept of combination therapy, since this offers several advantages - reduced risk of treatment failure, reduced risk of developing resistance, enhanced convenience and reduced side-effects. The effect of the supplements vitamin B2 (Riboflavin) and orange fruit juice on the potency and efficacy of some selected anti-malaria drugs (Armact, Coartem, Waipa and Fansider) as a combination therapy were investigated. 80 patients (adults) infected with malaria parasites were used. The study showed that the simultaneous administration of the drugs with vitamin B2 did not alter the potency of the drugs, while orange fruit juice altered the efficacy of the drugs. Therefore, the concomitant administration of these anti-malaria drugs (combination therapies) with orange fruit juice should be avoided during the period of malaria treatment for the effectiveness of such drugs. The result of this study also showed that concomitant administration of Riboflavin with antimalarial drugs may possess potent antimalarial effects and may therefore offer a potential drug lead for development of a safe, effective and affordable antimalarial.

Key words: Combination therapy, orange fruit juice, riboflavin, antimalarial.

INTRODUCTION

Malaria is a mosquito-borne infectious disease of humans and other animals caused by *Plasmodia*. The disease results from the multiplication of Plasmodium parasites within red blood cells, causing symptoms that typically include fever and headache, in severe cases progressing to coma or death. Five species of *Plasmodium* can infect and be transmitted by humans. Severe disease is largely caused by *Plasmodium falciparum* while the disease caused by *Plasmodium vivax*, *Plasmodium ovale* (Sutherland et al., 2010) and *Plasmodium malariae* is generally a milder disease that is rarely fatal. *Plasmodium knowlesi* is a zoonosis that causes malaria in macaques but can also infect humans (Fong et al., 1971; Singh, et al., 2004).

Malaria transmission can be reduced by preventing mosquito bites by distribution of mosquito nets and insect repellents, or by mosquito-control measures such as spraying insecticides and draining standing water (where mosquitoes breed). Despite a clear need, no vaccine offering a high level of protection currently exists. Efforts to develop one are ongoing (Kilama and Ntoumi, 2009). A number of medications (anti-malaria drugs) are also available to prevent malaria in travelers to malaria-endemic countries (prophylaxis).

A variety of anti-malaria medications are available. Severe malaria is treated with intravenous or intramuscular quinine or, since the mid-2000s, the artemisinin derivative artesunate (Dondorp and Day, 2007), which is superior to quinine in both children and adults (Dondorp et al., 2010). Resistance has developed to several anti-malaria drugs, most notably chloroquine (Kirby, 1989). There were an estimated 225 million cases of malaria worldwide in 2009 (WHO, 2011). An estimated 655,000 people died from malaria in 2010 (WHO, 2011),

---

*Corresponding author. E-mail: bensandym@yahoo.com.

Table 1. Effects of Armact only on patients infected with malaria parasite.

Patients	Weight(kg) before treatment	Malaria parasite before treatment	Drug/supplements	Malaria parasite/after treatment	Weight(kg) after treatment	Remark
Female	60	++	Armact only	−	58	Cleared
Female	65	+++	Armact only	−	64	Cleared
Male	70	++	Armact only	−	65	Cleared
Male	70	++	Armact only	−	67	Cleared

+ = Positive (Malaria parasite present), ++ = Moderately severe parasite present, +++ = Severe malaria parasite, - = Negative (malaria parasite absent).

a decrease from the 781,000 who died in 2009 according to the World Health Organization's 2011 World Malaria Report, accounting for 2.23% of deaths worldwide. However, a 2012 meta-study from the University of Washington and University of Queensland estimates that malaria deaths are significantly higher. Published in *The Lancet*, the study estimates that 1,238,000 people died from malaria in 2010 (Christopher et al., 2012). Ninety percent of malaria-related deaths occur in sub-Saharan Africa, with ~60% of deaths being young children under the age of five (Christopher et al., 2012). *P. falciparum*, the most severe form of specie, is responsible for the vast majority of deaths associated with the disease (Snow, 2005). This work looked at the effects of some supplements (grape fruit juice, orange fruit juice, multivitamin and vitamin C) on the efficacy and potency of some selected anti-malaria drugs-combination therapy (Armact, Coartem, Waipa and Fansider).

MATERIALS AND METHODS

Experimental animals

A total of 80 persons (40 males and 40 females) infected with malaria parasite residing in Umuguma in Owerri west local government area of Imo state, Nigeria were used during the experiment after a general malarial test on all the individuals and their body weights were taking before and after drug administration (treatment).

Collection of blood sample

The methanol was used as a disinfectant to swab the big thumb and a lancet used to puncture it for blood collection. Two drops of blood was placed on free grease slide, a thick film was made and allowed to air-dry. The dried thick blood film slide was laid on a staining rack, and Giemsa stained and allowed for 30-40 min, washed off with clean water, drained and allowed to dry at room temperature. Then viewed under the microscope using 10x objectives for focusing and 40x objective for identifying the plasmodium involved. Blood samples of subjects were all confirmed to be malaria parasite infected via malaria parasite test as described by Sibley (2001). The research had the approval of the concerned institutional medicinal ethics boards.

Drugs and supplements administered

The drugs used were Armact (Artesunate and Amodiquine), Coartem (Artemether and Lumefantrine), both purchased from Novartis pharmaceutica, Waipa (Dihydroartemisinin and Piperaquine) and Fansider (Sulfadoxin and Pyrimethamine) both purchased from Swiss Pharma Nigeria limited. The supplements used were vitamin B2 and orange fruit juice.

RESULTS

The results of the test on the blood samples before and after administration of the anti-malaria drugs to the patients are shown in Tables 1 to 12.

DISCUSSION

From the assessment of the potency of some selected anti-malaria drugs on the supplements of orange fruit juice and vitamin B2 (combination therapy), the result of the effects of the administration of antimalarial drugs such as Armact only, Coartem only, Waipa only and Fansider on patients infected with malaria parasite showed that the malaria parasite in all the groups were absent. The absence of malarial symptoms or death in the oral administration of those antimalarial drugs observed in the patients suggests that the drug is practically non-toxic acutely (Salawu et al., 2009; Russell, 2008). This could also explain the safe use of the drugs by the local people, for the treatment of malaria, in the eastern part of Nigeria. This also suggests the findings of Ajaiyeoba et al. (2006) that the use of these drugs for the treatment of malaria was due to the presence of alkaloids. Also, this is similar to the effect of the extract reported by previous studies on Alstonia boonei (Iyiola et al., 2011). From Tables 1, 5, 8 and 11, it showed that the concomitant administration of the antimalarial drugs (Armact, Coartem, Waipa and Fansider) and orange fruit juice indicated the presence of the Plasmodium in all the treated groups. This could be as a result of the anti-oxidant properties present in the fruit which may increase plasma concentrations of the drug and delays reaching

Table 2. Effects of Armact and orange juice (OJ) on patients infected with malaria parasite.

Patients	Weight (kg) before treatment	Malaria parasite before treatment	Drug/Supplements	Malaria parasite/after treatment	Weight (kg) after treatment	Remark
Female	85	++	Armact /OJ	+	85	Cleared
Female	80	++	Armact /OJ	+	80	Cleared
Male	55	+	Armact /OJ	+	55	Cleared
Male	65	+++	Armact /OJ	+	65	Cleared

Table 3. Effects of Armact and vitamin B2 on patients infected with malaria parasite.

Patients	Weight(kg) before treatment	Malaria parasite before treatment	Drug/Supplements	Malaria parasite/after treatment	Weight(kg) after treatment	Remark
Female	60	++	Armact/Vit B2	−	60	Not cleared
Female	60	++	Armact / Vit B2	−	60	Not cleared
Male	85	++	Armact / Vit B2	−	85	Not cleared
Male	85	++	Armact / Vit B2	−	85	Not cleared

Table 4. Effects of Coartem (Coart) only on patients infected with malaria parasite.

Patients	Weight (kg) before treatment	Malaria parasite before treatment	Drug/supplements	Malaria parasite/after treatment	Weight (kg) after treatment	Remark
Female	65	++	Coart only	−	60	Cleared
Female	65	+	Coart only	−	65	Cleared
Male	60	+	Coart only	−	60	Cleared
Male	60	+	Coart only	−	60	Cleared

Table 5. Effects of Coartem and orange juice (OJ) on patients infected with malaria parasite.

Patients	Weight (kg) before treatment	Malaria parasite before treatment	Drug/supplements	Malaria parasite/after treatment	Weight (kg) after treatment	Remark
Female	60	++	Coart /OJ	+	60	Cleared
Female	65	+	Coart /OJ	+	65	Cleared
Male	70	++	Coart /OJ	+	70	Cleared
Male	70	+++	Coart /OJ	+	70	Cleared

Table 6. Effects of Coartem and vitamin B2 on patients infected with malaria parasite.

Patients	Weight (kg) before treatment	Malaria parasite before treatment	Drug/supplements	Malaria parasite/after treatment	Weight(kg) after treatment	Remark
Female	70	+++	Coart /Vit B2	−	70	Not cleared
Female	55	+	Coart / Vit B2	−	55	Not cleared
Male	75	++	Coart / Vit B2	−	75	Not cleared
Male	75	+	Coart / Vit B2	−	75	Cleared

Table 7. Effects of WAIPA (Wp) only on patient infected with malaria parasite.

Patients	Weight (kg) before treatment	Malaria parasite before treatment	Drug/supplements	Malaria parasite/after treatment	Weigh t(kg) after treatment	Remark
Female	60	+	Wp only	−	60	Cleared
Female	60	++	Wp only	−	58	Cleared
Male	70	++	Wp only	−	68	Cleared
Male	75	+	Wp only	−	72	Cleared

Table 8. Effects of WAIPA (Wp) and orange juice (OJ) on patients infected with malaria parasite.

Patients	Weight (kg) before treatment	Malaria parasite before treatment	Drug/supplements	Malaria parasite/after treatment	Weight (kg) after treatment	Remark
Female	75	+	Wp /OJ	+	75	Cleared
Female	65	++	Wp /OJ	+	65	Cleared
Male	70	+	Wp /OJ	+	70	Cleared
Male	75	++	Wp /OJ	+	73	Cleared

Table 9. Effects of WAIPA (Wp) and vitamin B2 on patient with malaria parasite.

Patients	Weight (kg) before treatment	Malaria parasite before treatment	Drug/supplements	Malaria parasite/after treatment	Weight (kg) after treatment	Remark
Female	60	+	Wp /Vit B2	−	60	Not cleared
Female	68	+	Wp / Vit B2	−	68	Not cleared
Male	75	+	Wp / Vit B2	−	75	Not cleared
Male	70	++	Wp / Vit B2	−	70	Cleared

Table 10. Effects of Fansider (Fans) only on patients infected with malaria parasite.

Patients	Weight (kg) before treatment	Malaria parasite before treatment	Drug/supplements	Malaria parasite/after treatment	Weight (kg) after treatment	Remark
Female	75	+	Fans only	−	70	Cleared
Female	70	+	Fans only	−	68	Cleared
Male	65	+	Fans only	−	62	Cleared
Male	60	+	Fans only	−	58	Cleared

Table 11. Effects of Fansider and orange fruit Juice (G.J) on patients infected with malaria parasite.

Patients	Weight (kg) before treatment	Malaria parasite before treatment	Drug/supplements	Malaria parasite/after treatment	Weight (kg) after treatment	Remark
Female	70	+	Fans /GJ	+	68	Cleared
Female	70	+	Fans /GJ	+	67	Cleared
Male	60	+++	Fans /GJ	+	58	Cleared
Male	55	+	Fans /GJ	+	53	Cleared

Table 12. Effects of Fansider and vitamin B2 on patients with malaria parasite.

Patients	Weight (kg) before treatment	Malaria parasite before treatment	Drug/supplements	Malaria parasite/after treatment	Weight (kg) after treatment	Remark
Female	78	+++	Fans /Vit. B2	−	78	Not cleared
Female	65	+	Fans /Vit. B2	+	65	Not cleared
Male	60	++	Fans /Vit. B2	−	60	Not cleared
Male	65	+	Fans /Vit. B2	−	65	Cleared

peak drug concentration (Owira and Ojewole, 2010). Also it may be due to the presence of orange fruit enzyme that break down medications in the digestive system and cause more of the medications to stay in the body which may increase the risk of serious malarial problems (Stump, 2006).

The concomitant administration of the antimalarial drugs (Armact, Coartem, Waipa and Fansider) and vitamin B2 (Riboflavine) from Tables 2, 6, 9 and 12 showed no malaria parasite presence in all the patients in the various treated groups. This infers that vitamin B2 may play a significant role in antimalarial activity which is similar to the report of Adesokan and Akanji (2010). This could be as a result of its ability to promote appetite, quick recovery and do not hinder the activity of the antimalarial drug (Makarchikov, 2003). This report supports the finding of Basu et al. (2007) that this vitamin may possess health promoting effects, at least under some circumstances.

Conclusion

Successful malaria control depends greatly on treatment with efficacious anti-malarial drugs. The ability of the four drugs (Armact, Coartem, Waipa and Fansider) to reduce the presence of malaria parasite may be due to presence of phytochemically-active components in the drugs which might be responsible for their therapeutic activity as antimalarial drugs. Also, the use of vitamin B2 (Riboflavin) with antimalarial drugs (combination therapy) has potential health promoting effects. Multiple-drug therapies that include a nonantimalarial drug like vitamin E and orange fruit juice to enhance the antimalarial effect of a blood schizontocidal drug are not considered combination therapy.

This finding supports the use of vitamin B2 and antimalarial drugs as a combination therapy which is safe and possess potent antimalarial activity as found in its ability to suppress Plasmodium infection in patients.

ACKNOWLEDGEMENT

The authors acknowledged the assistance from the World Bank and the Federal Republic of Nigeria with the World Bank Step B projects.

REFERENCES

Adesokan AA, Akanji MA (2010). Antimalarial Bioactivity of *Enantia chlorantha* stem bark. Medical Plants: Phytochem. Pharmacol. Ther. 4(1):441-447.

Ajaiyeoba E, Falade M, Ogbole O, Okpako L, Akinboye D (2006). *In vivo* antimalarial and cytotoxic properties of *Annona senegalensis* extract. Afr. J. Trad. Complementary altern. Med. 3(1):137-141.

Basu SK, Thomas JE, Acharya SN (2007). Prospects for Growth in Global Nutraceutical and Functional Food Markets: A Canadian Perspective. Aust. J. Basic Appl. Sci. 1(4):637-649.

Christopher JL, Murray LC, Rosenfeld S, Kathryn GA, Kyle J, Diana H, Nancy F, Mohsen N, Rafael L, Alan DL (2012). "Global malaria mortality between 1980 and 2010: a systematic analysis". Lancet 379(9814):413-431.

Dondorp AM, Day NP (2007). "The treatment of severe malaria". Trans. R. Soc. Trop. Med. Hyg. 101(7):633-634. doi:10.1016/j.trstmh.2007.03.011.

Dondorp AM, Fanello CI, Hendriksen IC (2010). Artesunate versus quinine in the treatment of severe falciparum malaria in African children (AQUAMAT): an open-label, randomised trial. Lancet 376(9753):1647-1657.

Fong YL, Cadigan FC, Coatney GR (1971). A presumptive case of naturally occurring *Plasmodium knowlesi* malaria in man in Malaysia. Trans. R. Soc. Trop. Med. Hyg., 65(6):839-840. doi:10.1016/0035-9203(71)90103-90109. PMID 5003320.

Iyiola OA, Tijani AY, Lateef KM (2011). Antimalarial Activity of Ethanolic Stem Bark Extract of *Alstonia boonei* in Mice. Asian J. Biol. Sci. 4:235-243.

Kilama W, Ntoumi F (2009). Malaria: a research agenda for the eradication era. Lancet 374(9700):1480-1482. doi:10.1016/S0140-6736(09)61884-5.

Makarchikov AF, Lakaye B, Gulyai E, Czerniecki J, Coumans B, Wins P, Grisar T, Bettendorff L (2003). Thiamine triphosphate and thiamine triphosphatase activities: from bacteria to mammals. Cell. Mol. Life Sci. 60(7):1477-1488.

Owira PM, Ojewole JA (2010). The Grapefruit: An Old Wine in a New Glass? Metabolic and Cardiovascular Perspectives. Cardiovasc. J. Afr. 23:2-7.

Russell B (2008). Determinants of *in vitro* drug susceptibility testing of *Plasmodium vivax*. Antimicrob. Agents Chemother. 52:1040-1045.

Salawu OA, Chindo BA, Tijani AY, Obidike IC, Akingbasote JA (2009). Acute and sub-acute toxicological evaluations of the methanolic stem bark extract of *Crossopteryx febrifuga* in rats. Afr. J. Pharm. Pharmacol. 3:621-626.

Sibley CH (2001). Pyrimethamine-sulfadoxine resistance in *Plasmodium falciparum*: what next? Trends Parasitol. 17:582-588.

Singh B, Kim Sung L, Matusop A (2004). A large focus of naturally acquired *Plasmodium knowlesi* infections in human beings. Lancet 363(9414):1017–1024. doi:10.1016/S0140 6736(04)15836-4.

Snow RW, Guerra CA, Noor AM, Myint HY, Hay SI (2005). The global distribution of clinical episodes of *Plasmodium falciparum* malaria.

Nature 434(7030):214-217.

Stump AL (2006). Management of Grapefruit-Drug Interactions. Am. Family Phys. J. 12:45-52

Sutherland C, Tanomsing N, Nolder D, Oguike M, Jennison C, Pukrittayakamee S, Dolecek C, Hien TT, do Rosário VE, Arez AP, Pinto J, Michon P, Escalante A, Nosten F, Burke M, Lee R Blaze M, Otto T.D, Barnwell J, Pain A, Williams J, White NJ, Day NPJ, Snounou G, Lockhart PJ, Chiodini PL, Imwong M, Polley SD (2010). Two nonrecombining sympatric forms of the human malaria parasite *Plasmodium ovale* occur globally. J. Infect. Dis. 201(10):1544-1550.

World Health Organisation (2011). World malaria report summary. Geneva.

13

Effects of vitamin E and folic acid on some antioxidant enzymes activities of female Wistar rats administered combined oral contraceptives

Akinsanya, Mushafau A.[1], Adeniyi, Taiwo T.[2*], Ajayi, Gabriel O[1] and Oyedele, Musbau A.[2]

[1]Department of Medical Biochemistry, Faculty of Basic Medical Sciences, Lagos State University College of Medicine (LASUCOM), PMB 21266, Ikeja, Lagos, Nigeria.
[2]Department of Biochemistry, College of Natural Sciences, University of Agriculture, PMB 2240, Abeokuta, Ogun State, Nigeria.

In this study, the effects of vitamin E and folic acid on the superoxide dismutase (SOD), catalase (CAT), malondialdehyde (MDA) production and glutathione-S-transferase (GST) activities in female Wistar rats treated with combined oral contraceptives (COC) containing ethinyl estradiol in combination with levonorgestrel were determined. Twenty female rats were divided into four groups: Group A (control) received distilled water; Group B received combined oral contraceptives (COC) for 15 days with a dosage of 0.667 mg/kg body weight/day; Group C received combined oral contraceptive and vitamin E (0.667 mg/kg body weight COC + 15 mg/kg body weight of vitamin E/day) for 15 days and Group D received combined oral contraceptives and folic acid (0.667 mg/kg body weight of COC + 1 mg/kg body weight/day) for 15 days. Administration of vitamin E and folic acid caused significant decrease ($P < 0.05$) in superoxide dismutase levels by 90 and 69% respectively. In catalase, administration of vitamin E significantly decrease ($p < 0.05$) catalase level by 47% while administration of folic acid has no significant difference ($p > 0.05$) in catalase level. In addition, administration of vitamin E and folic acid caused significant decrease ($P < 0.05$) in malondialdehyde (MDA) concentration by 21 and 11% respectively. Administration of vitamin E and folic acid caused significant decrease ($P < 0.05$) in glutathione-S-transferase by 39 and 23%, respectively.

Key words: Combined oral contraceptives, vitamin E, folic acid, antioxidant enzymes.

INTRODUCTION

Oral contraceptive, or birth control pills, is primarily used to prevent pregnancy and to treat menstrual irregularities and endometriosis (Gaspard et al., 2004). When taken as directed, they prevent ovulation. The female hormones estrogen and progestin are the agents in oral contraceptives that prevent ovulation. The use of oral contraceptive agents has been reported to be associated with a number of metabolic changes. Biochemical changes suggestive of altered nutritional status with regard to several vitamins such as folic acid (Prasad et

al., 1975), vitamin E (Aftergood et al., 1974), ascorbic acid (Princemail et al., 2007) and vitamin A (Gaafar et al., 1973) have been reported among women who use contraceptive agents. Vitamin E (α-tocopherol) is traditionally recognised as the most biological antioxidant in human (vitamin E Fact Sheet). Moreover, hormonal contraceptives are medicines which contain artificially made hormones which regulate women's menstrual cycles (Ross-Flanigan, 1999). Female hormones, such as estradiol have been reported to have strong inhibitory effects on lipid peroxidation and in vivo and in vitro antioxidant effects (Subbiah et al., 1993). In living system and aerobic organism, a complex antioxidant mechanism have been evolved to protect against uncontrolled free radical damage (Murray, 2002). However, there are

---

*Corresponding author. E-mail: ttadeniyi@yahoo.com.

evidences from studies in rats that the administration of contraceptive steroids significantly lowers plasma tocopherol levels and increases dietary requirements for vitamin E (Aftergood et al., 1974). In several cases, women taking oral contraceptive equally developed folic acid deficiency (Hathcock, 1997). The aim of this study was to assess the effects of vitamin E and folic acid supplementations on female Wistar rats administered combined oral contraceptive and to evaluate antioxidant enzymes such as lipid peroxidation, superoxide dismutase, catalase and glutathione-S-transferase.

MATERIALS AND METHODS

Drugs

The contraceptives drugs used were purchased from a family planning clinic in Abeokuta. Combined oral contraceptive pills (COC) DUOFEM® tablets, which contained ethinyl estradiol and levonorgestrel were manufactured by Pfizer, Belgium. Vitamin E was manufactured by Korea United Pharmaceutical Inc. 40410, South Korea and folic acid was manufactured by Emzor Pharmaceutical Industries Ltd. Lagos, Nigeria.

Clinical recommended daily allowance (RDA) dosage of each drug was prepared as concentration adjusted to mg/kg body weight of animals in the groups. Other reagents were of analytical grade and of the purest quality available.

Animals

Inbred of 5 – 6 week old female Wistar albino rats that weighed between 200 g and 240 g were purchased from the Animal House of College of Veterinary Medicine (COLVET), University of Agriculture, Abeokuta, Ogun State, Nigeria. The animals were kept in well-ventilated cages at room temperature (28 – 30 °C) and under controlled light cycles (12 h light: dark) with humidity (54 - 57%). They were maintained on normal laboratory chow (Ola Feed Mills, Asero, Abeokuta, Nigeria) and water was by ad libitum. All experiments were conducted without anaesthesia and the protocol conformed to the guidelines of the National Institutes of Health (NIH publication no. 85 – 23, 1985) for laboratory animal care and use.

Experimental design and administration of drugs

20 female albino rats (Wistar strain) were randomly distributed into four groups of five animals each and were allowed free access to feed and water for a period of 2 weeks for acclimatization before the commencement of the experiment. The first group served as the control and received only distilled water. The second group received combined oral contraceptive (COC) only. The third group received combined oral contraceptive with vitamin E and the fourth group was administered combined oral contraceptive with folic acids. The contraceptive was administered orally for 15 consecutive days. The drug dosages for the rats were 0.667 mg/kg body weight for combined oral contraceptive, 15 mg/kg body weight for vitamin E and 1 mg/kg body weight for folic acid.

Sample collection

Preparation of serum

Rats were sacrificed 24 h after the last dose of drugs and an overnight fast. Blood was collected from the inferior *vena cava* of the heart of the animals into plain centrifuge tubes and was allowed to stand for 1 h. Serum was prepared by centrifugation at 3000 ×g for 15 min in a centrifuge. The clear supernatant was used for the estimation of serum enzymes. All procedures were carried out at temperatures 0 – 4 °C.

Assay methods

Superoxide dismutase, catalase and glutathione S-transferase determination

Superoxide dismutase (SOD) activity was measured by the nitroblue tetrazolium reduction method of McCord and Fridovich (1969). Glutathione S-transferase (GST) activity was determined by the method of Habig et al. (1974); the method is based on the rate of conjugate formation between glutathione (GSH) and 1-chloro-2, 4-dinitrobenzene. Catalase (CAT) activity was assayed by measuring the rate of decomposition of hydrogen peroxide at 240 nm as described by Aebi (1974).

Lipid peroxidation determination

The extent of lipid peroxidation (LPO) was estimated by the method of Buege and Aust (1978). The method involved the reaction between malondialdehyde (MDA), product of LPO and thiobarbituric acid to form a pink precipitate, which was read at 535 nm spectrophotometrically.

0.4 ml of reaction mixture already quenched with 0.5 ml of 30% TCA was added to 1.6 ml of Tri-KCl. Addition of TBA and incubation for 45 min at 80 °C produced pink coloured reaction mixtures which were centrifuged at 14000 g for 15 min. The absorbance of the clear pink supernatant was then read at 535 nm.

Statistical analysis

All values were expressed as the mean ± S.D of five animals per group. Data were analysed using one-way ANOVA test followed by the *post-hoc* Duncan's multiple range test for analysis of biochemical data using SPSS version 10.0 (SPSS Inc., Chicago, IL, USA). Values were considered statistically significant at $P < 0.05$.

RESULTS

Effect of combined oral contraceptives, vitamin E and folic acid supplements on lipid peroxidation in female Wistar rats

The effect of vitamin E and folic acid on lipid peroxidation in combined oral contraceptive treated female rats was assessed. The combined oral contraceptives dose (0.667 mg/kg body weight) produced no significant difference ($p > 0.05$) in MDA level compared to the control while vitamin E (15 mg/kg body weight) produced significant reduction ($p < 0.05$) of MDA level by 21% compared to group B (combined oral contraceptive dose only). The folic acid (1 mg/kg body weight) equally produced significant reduction ($p < 0.05$) of MDA level by 11% compared to group B (combined oral contraceptive dose only) as shown in Figure 1.

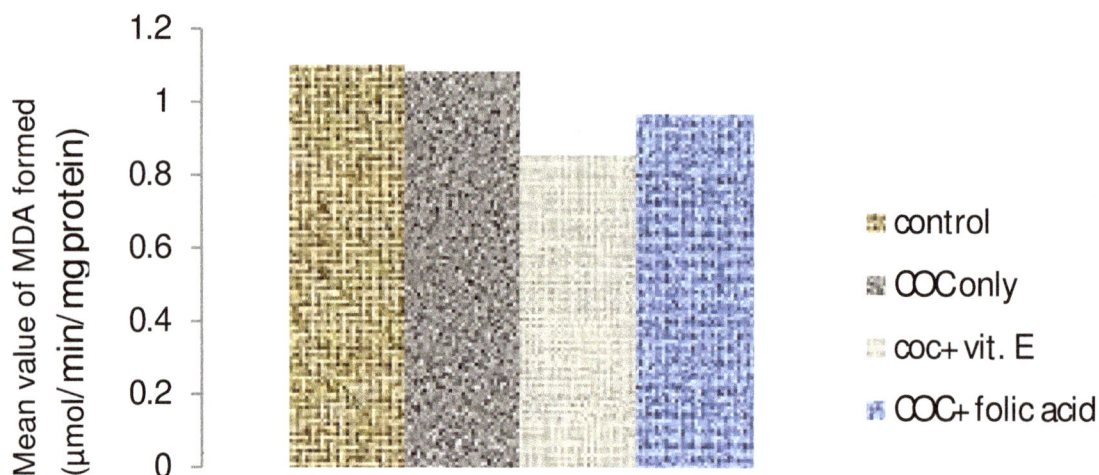

Figure 1. Effect of combined oral contraceptives, vitamin E and folic acid supplements on lipid peroxidation in female Wistar rats.

Effect of combined oral contraceptives, vitamin E and folic acid supplements on superoxide dismutase, glutathione-S-trasferase and catalase enzymes activities in female Wistar rats

The effect of vitamin E and folic acid supplements on superoxide dismutase (SOD), glutathione-S-transferase (GST) and catalase activities in combined oral contraceptives treated female rats were assessed. The combined oral contraceptive dose (0.667 mg/kg body weight) produced significant elevation ($p < 0.05$) of SOD, GST and catalase activities by 87, 25 and 41% respectively compared to the control while vitamin E and folic acid produced significant reduction ($p < 0.05$) in superoxide dismutase (SOD) by 90 and 69% respectively when compared to group B (combined oral contraceptive dose only). Administration of vitamin E and folic acid, significantly decrease ($p < 0.05$) glutathione-S-transferase levels by 39 and 23% respectively when compared to group B. However, administration of vitamin E and folic acid, significantly decrease ($p < 0.05$) catalase level by 47% but there was no significant decrease ($p > 0.05$) in catalase level by folic acid administration when compared to group B as shown in Figures 2, 3 and 4.

DISCUSSION

In this study, one major observation is that combined oral contraceptive pills (COC) containing ethinyl estradiol and levonorgestrel had significant effect ($p < 0.05$) on all the antioxidant markers but in exception to lipid peroxidation and this is in agreement with the observation of Subbiah et al. (1993) and Kose et al. (1993). They both observed that estradiol have strong inhibitory effects on lipid peroxidation. However, the effects of vitamin E and folic acid supplementation on the antioxidant markers after the

treatment of the female rats with combined oral contraceptive are remarkable. Based on the MDA assay, vitamin E and folic acid reduced the effects of the COC significantly ($p < 0.05$) and this is in accordance to the findings that vitamin E is a powerful antioxidant (Obikoya, 2008).

Glutathione-S-transferase (GST) is a family of multifunctional isozymes found in all eukaryotes, catalysing both glutathione dependent conjugation and reduction reactions (Rujurkar et al., 2003; Adaramoye et al., 2008). It can also act as an antioxidant enzyme (Adaramoye et al., 2006). In this study, GST activity was elevated in rats treated with combined oral contraceptives; this also suggested that COC may have elevated oxidative stress in the female rats. Consequently, the administration of vitamin E and folic acid significantly altered ($p < 0.05$) the effect of the COC which equally collaborated with the antioxidant ability of vitamin E.

In the superoxide dismutase (SOD) and catalase results, an equal trend was observed suggesting the corrective ability of vitamin E and folic acid on oxidative stress that may arise following administration of combined oral contraceptives.

Conclusion

The findings suggested that vitamin E and folic acid reduced significantly the effect of the combined oral contraceptives on female treated rats which is in agreement with evidence from previous studies in rats that the administration of contraceptive steroids significantly lowers plasma tocopherol levels and increases dietary requirements for vitamin E. Therefore, it will be suggested that women on combined oral contraceptives should be on vitamin E and folic acid

Table 1. Effect of combined oral contraceptives, vitamin E and folic acid on lipid peroxidation, superoxide dismutase (SOD), catalase and glutathione-S- transferase (GST) activities.

Groups of rats fed with combined oral contraceptive (COC)	Concentration of MDA x10² (μmol/min/mg protein)	Superoxide dismutase activity x10² (U/mg protein)	Catalase activity x10² (μmol/min/mg protein)	Glutathione S -transferase activity x10² (μmol/min/mg protein)
A (Control)	1.105±0.27	0.372±0.06	0.375±0.14	0.884±0.19
B (Combined oral contraceptive)only	1.084±0.13*	2.896±1.41*	0.635±0.06*	1.183±0.81*
C (COC + Vitamin E)	0.854±0.07*	0.289±0.07*	0.335±0.02*	0.715±0.49*
D (COC+ Folic acid)	0.967±0.22	0.897±0.10*	0.594±0.07	0.910±1.07*

COC, Combined oral contraceptive; MDA, malondialdehyde. Values are means ± S.D of five animals per group. *Significantly different from control (P < 0.05).

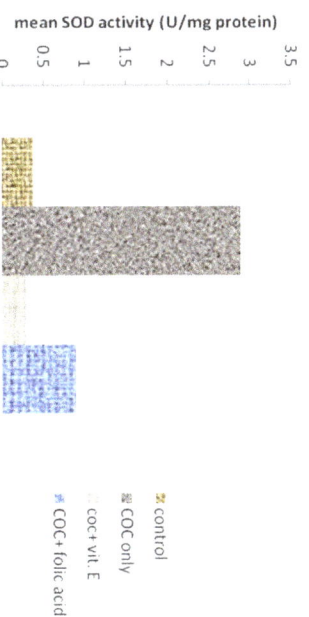

Figure 2. Effect of combined oral contraceptives, vitamin E and folic acid supplements on superoxide dismutase enzyme in female Wistar rats.

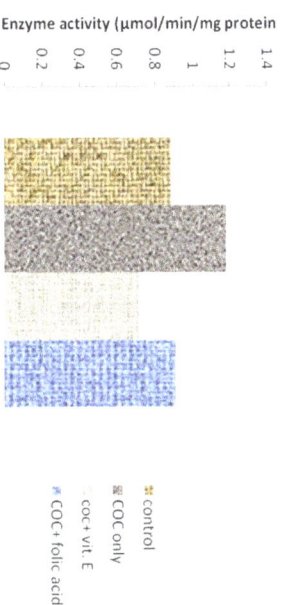

Figure 3. Effect of combined oral contraceptives, vitamin E and folic acid supplements on catalase activity in female Wistar rats.

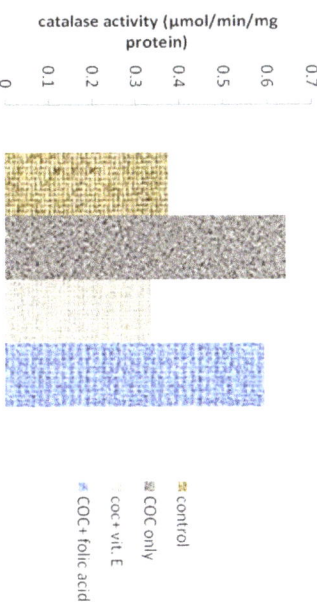

Figure 4. Effect of combined oral contraceptives, vitamin E and folic acid supplements on glutathione-S-transferase activity in female Wistar rats.

supplementation to reduce any oxidative stress that may arise from its use. Further researches on lipids profile components and enzymes activities in human subjects are in progress.

REFERENCES

Adaramoye OA, Adeyemi EO (2006). Hepatoprotection of D galactosamine-induced toxicity in mice by purified fractions from Garcinia kola seeds. Basic Clin. Pharmacol. Toxicol., 98: 135-41.

Adaramoye OA, Osaimeje DO, Akinsanya MA, Nneji CM, Fafunso MA, Ademowo OG (2008). Changes in Antioxidants Status and Biochemical Indices after Acute Administration of Artemether, Artemether-Lumefantrine and Halofantrine in Rats. Basic Clin. Pharmacol. Toxicol., 102: 412-418.

Aebi H (1974). Catalase estimation. In: Bergmeyer HV (Ed.). Methods of Enzymatic Analysis. Verlag Chemic, New York, 673-84.

Aftergood L, Alfin-Slater RB (1974), Oral contraceptive-α-tocopherol interrelationships.Lipids 9: 91.

Buege JA, Aust SD (1978). Microsomal lipid peroxidation. Methods Enzymol, 30: 302-10.

Gaafar A, Toppozada HK, Hozayen A, Abdel-Malek AT, Moghazy M, Youssef M (1973). Study of folate status in long-term Egyptian users of oral contraceptive pills. Contraception, 8: 43.

Gaspard U, Endrikat J, Desager JP, Buicu C, Gerlinger C, Heithecker R (2004). Contraception, 69: 271-279.

Habig WH, Pabst MJ, Jakoby WB (1974). Glutathione-S-transferases. The first enzymatic step in mercapturic acid formation. J. Biol. Chem., 249: 7130-9.

Hathcock JN (1997). Vitamins and minerals: Efficacy and safety. Am. J. Clin. Nutr., 66(2): 427-437.

McCord JM, Fridovich I (1969). Superoxide dismutase, an enzymatic function for erythrocuperin. J. Biol. Chem., 244: 6049-55.

Murray RK (2002). Metabolism of xenobiotic and red white blood cells. In Harpers Biochemistry, 25th ed., Murray RK, Granner DK, Mayes PA, Rodwell VW editors. McGraw-Hill, Appleton and Lange. pp. 763-786.

Obikoya G (2008). Vitamin E: A Powerful Antioxidant. http://www.vitamins-nutrition.org/vitamins/vitamin-e-antioxidant.html accessed on 18/02/2010.

Pincemail J, Vanbelle S, Gaspard U, Collette G, Haleng J, Cheramy-Bien JP, Charlier C, Chapelle JP, Giet D, Albert A, Limet R, Defraigne JO (2007). Effect of different contraceptive methods on the oxidative stress status in women aged 40–48 years from the ELAN study in the province of Lie'ge, Belgium. Hum. Reprod., pp. 1-9.

Prasad AS, Lei KY, Donald O, Kamran SM, Joanne CS (1975). Effect of oral contraceptive agents on nutrients: II. Vitamins, Am. J. Clin. Nutr., 28: 385-391.

Rajurkar RB, Khan ZH, Gujar GT (2003). Studies on levels of

Glutathione-S-Transferase, its Isolation and Purification from *Helicoverpa armingera* Curr. Sci., 85: 1355-60.

Ross-Flanigan N (1999). Oral contraceptives . Gale encyclopaedia of medicine, Gale group. Http//www.findarticles.com. Accessed 18/02/2010.

Subbiah MTR, Kessel B, Agarwal M, Rajan B, Abplanalp W, Rymaszewski Z (1993). Antioxidant potential of specific estrogens on lipid peroxidation. J. Clin. Endocrinol. Metab., 77: 1095-1097.

14

A study on prostate specific antigen (PSA) with the ratio of free to total PSA

Chavan Atish[1], Suman Diggi Prasad[1], Rawal Mukesh[1], Kandasamy Surendran[2], Sivapatham Sundaresan[3*] and Thangarajan Thangapannerselvem[4]

[1]Department of Biotechnology, School of Bioengineering, SRM University, Kattankulathur, Tamil Nadu, India- 603203, India.
[2]Central Laboratory, Department of Biochemistry, SRM Medical College Hospital and Research Centre, SRM University, Kattankulathur, Tamil Nadu, India- 603203, India.
[3]Department of Medical Research, SRM Medical College Hospital and Research Centre, SRM University, Kattankulathur, Tamil Nadu, India- 603203, India.
[4]Department of Biochemistry, SRM Medical College Hospital and Research Centre, SRM University, Kattankulathur, Tamil Nadu, India- 603203, India.

Prostate specific antigen (PSA) is a glycoprotein produced as a marker by prostate gland for prostate cancer, benign prostate hyperplasia and prostatitis. Study objective is to evaluate f/t PSA ratio to distinguish the Benign Prostate Hyperplasia (BPH) and prostate cancer patients in and around SRM University. To define the age specific reference ranges of PSA in control and test group at Chennai, India. Healthy men aged 40 - 75 years in and around SRM Medical College and Research Centre, Chennai, India were selected and grouped as control. Blood samples were collected from patients who attended Cancer Hospital, Adiyar underwent rectal examination revealed prostate enlargement. Results of our study showed that they were diagnosed as BPH and as Cancer, using PSA determination. The free to total PSA ratio were decreased significantly in cancer patients than BPH. PSA was increased linearly with age and observations were associated with the claims of National Academy of Clinical Biochemistry guideline reported that the clinical decisions limits should be decreased for younger patients (age below 50) and should be increased for older patients (age above 50). PSA should be used more appropriately to distinguish (BPH) and prostate cancer and to detect cancer prostate at an early stage. The age specific reference ranges and different forms of PSA have the potential to make serum PSA, a more discriminating tumor marker for detecting cancer prostate significantly in men.

Key words: Prostate specific antigen, free PSA prostate cancer, benign prostate hyperplasia, free to total PSA ratio, complex PSA, percentage of free PSA.

INTRODUCTION

Prostate cancer (CaP) is the common malignancy in men globally and ranked second after lung and bronchus cancer with respect to death (Angelis et al., 2007; Katz and Katz, 2008). Serum prostate specific antigen (PSA) has been widely regarded as the most clinically useful marker for the detection of CaP and BPH (Wu, 1994; Brawley et al., 2009). Tumor markers, measurable either in serum or from tissue specimens are generally useful in the detection, screening, staging, prognosis and monitoring therapy (Loeb and Catalona, 2008). PSA was first described in 1971 and purified in 1979 in seminal plasma and the prostate. PSA is a single chain glycoprotein with 240 amino acids having a molecular weight of approximately 34 KDa (Noldus et al., 1997; Singh, 2009). PSA is synthesized by the epithelial cells of prostatic acini and ducts and is secreted as a normal constituent of seminal fluid.

Free to total ratio of PSA (f/t PSA) has been studied to distinguish BPH and CaP and found more specific and sensitive in detection (Woodrum et al., 1998). Measure-

*Corresponding author. E-mail: sundarsivapatham@rediffmail.com.

Table 1. Shows the distribution levels of free PSA, total PSA, free to total PSA ratio, complex PSA and % free PSA in control and test group.

Groups	Free PSA (ng/ml)	Total PSA (ng/ml)	Free to total PSA ratio	Complex PSA	Percent free PSA
Control	0.22 ± 0.06	0.67 ± 0.08	0.33 ± 0.08	0.44 ± 0.07	33.85 ± 8.85
Test	1.09 ± 0.69*[a]	4.62 ± 2.85*[a]	0.24 ± 0.07*	3.52 ± 2.31*[b]	24.72 ± 7.59*[b]

* indicate values are statistically significant if the p value ≤ 0.05 (t' test). [a] indicates value are statistically correlated at p value of 0.01 level (Spearmen analysis). [b] indicates value are negatively related between complex PSA and mean percent free SPA was 18% in prostate cancer and 29% in BPH.

ment of PSA provides essential information about the efficacy of surgery or radiation therapy helps establish the possibility of residual disease local or distant and provides a useful adjunct in the evaluation of therapeutic response (Monda et al., 1994). The detection of prostate cancer using a blood test has by many standards changed the face of the disease (Leman and Getzenberg, 2009). Virtually all guidelines regarding screening view PSA and DRE as dichotomous test results, namely, either positive or negative. As such, a man with a PSA level of 4.1 ng/ml is recommended to undergo a biopsy whereas another man with a PSA level of 3.9 ng/ml is considered normal. Similarly, a man with a nodule detected on DRE is recommended to undergo a biopsy regardless of whether his PSA is 0.2 ng/ml or 9.8 ng/ml (Brawley et al., 2009).

The worrisome conclusion of observations from a study is that screening with PSA using a single upper limit of normal of 4.0 ng/ml may carry a risk of detecting many cancers too late to enable radiation or surgery to cure the disease.

In order to evaluate the effect of total and free form of PSA, free to total PSA ratio on age and to distinguish BPH and CaP, the study was chosen among SRM Hospital, Kattankulathur and Cancer Institute, Adiyar.

MATERIALS AND METHODS

Sample collection

Healthy men aged 40 - 60 years from the area in and around SRM Medical College Hospital and Research Centre, SRM University, Kattankulathur were selected and grouped as control at 2009. Test group of untreated patients who attended SRM Hospital and Cancer Institute, Adiyar, Chennai were enrolled for the study. Individuals who had no history of previous or concomitant malignancies and no acute illness within the last three months were clinically identified. Serum samples were collected prospectively from untreated patients who attended SRM Hospital and Research Centre, Kattankulathur and Cancer Institute, Adiyar, Chennai. The control group includes the men with ages between 40 to 70 years. Blood samples were allowed to clot for one hour at room temperature, were centrifuged at 2000 rpm for 10 min. The study was approved by inter departmental ethical committee and carried out in accordance with procedure, including informed consent of all participants. Blood sampling was performed before the other diagnostic procedures like imaging technique. Serum samples were stored at -20°C.

Biochemical analysis

Free and total PSA were analyzed with Diagnostic Biochem Canada (DBC) kits. Complexed PSA (cPSA) and percent PSA were estimated from free and total PSA values of control and test groups. The samples were analyzed for free PSA and total PSA by using the ANTHOS ELISA reader and washer made in Austria.

Statistical analysis

Data were expressed as mean ± SD and values are statistically significant if the p value at 0.05 level. Data's were analyzed using the statistical software SPSS 16.0 for student's t- test and correlation was calculated by Spearmen one tailed test and the values are significant if the p value is at 0.01 level.

RESULTS AND DISCUSSION

Table 1 describes the distribution of total PSA, free PSA and free to total ratio of PSA among the control group and test group. The highest total PSA was 10.0 ng/ml and lowest was 1.2 ng/ml in test group. The total and free PSA mean was increased in test group when compared to control group significantly at P value 0.05 level. The highest free PSA mean was 2.48 ng/ml and lowest mean was 0.2 ng/ml in test group. Free to total PSA ratio was decreased in test group when compared to control group significantly at P value 0.05 level. The lowest f/t ratio was 0.11 and highest was 0.33. Total and free PSA were correlated significantly at 0.01 level.

Table 1 also signifies the levels of complexed PSA (cPSA) and percent free PSA in control and test group. The highest value of cPSA was 8.06 and the lowest was 1.03. The levels of cPSA were significantly elevated in test group then control. Percentage of free PSA was found to be decreased among cancer patients than BPH. The mean value of percentage free PSA of cancer patients was 18% and the mean value of percentage of free PSA of BPH was 29%. cPSA was negatively related to percentage of free PSA.

Figures 1 and 2 show the distribution of total PSA, free PSA in test group against age respectively. Serum PSA levels gradually increase with age in men over 40 years old (Chen et al., 1996). The reference range of PSA with age has been proposed with the expectation that their implementation increase cancer detection rates in younger men. PSA plays a cardinal role in all aspects of

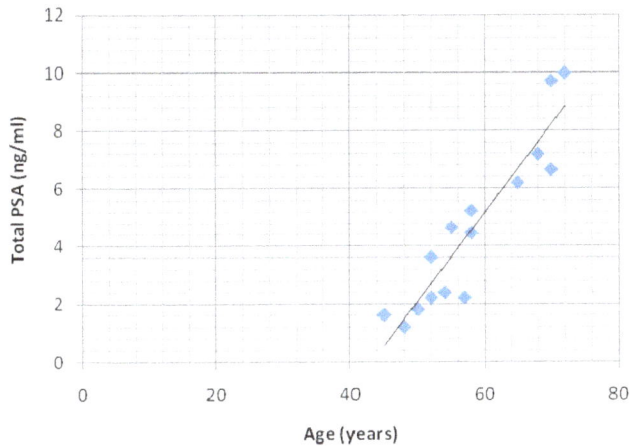

Figure 1. Graph showing age specific total PSA (ng/ml) among test group.

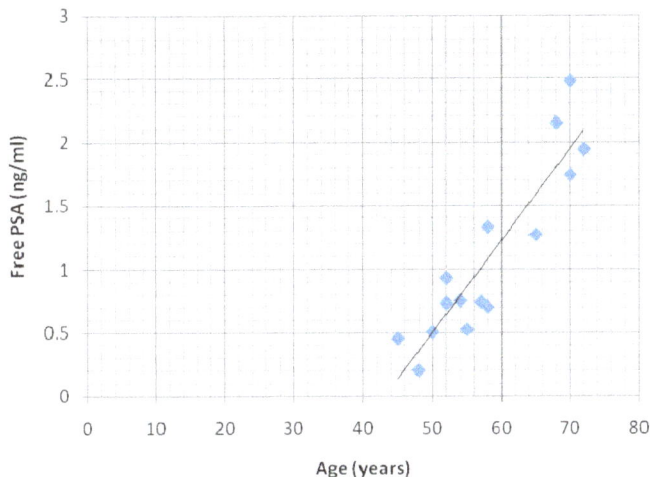

Figure 2. Graph showing age specific free PSA (ng/ml) among test group.

management of prostate cancer (Daniëlle et al., 2008). The recommended follow up testing of high risk individuals initially screened at 40 years of age depends on PSA result. Those with PSA levels < 1 ng/ml would resume testing at 5 years interval and those with levels > 1 but < 2.5 ng/ml would be tested annually, while those with levels ≥ 2.5 ng/ml would be evaluated further and considered for biopsy (Catalona et al., 1995).

When f/t PSA was analyzed among the patients with CaP it showed significantly low f/t PSA levels than those without CaP (Yamamoto and Maruyama, 2008). The use of high cutoff points of f/t PSA resulted in high sensitivity. When the cutoff point of f/tPSA was set at < 15%, sensitivity were 82.0%, while this value increased to 96.0%, at the cutoff point < 20%, indicating that f/t PSA would be useful to improve sensitivity and be able to predict the outcome of prostate cancer (Frempong et al.,

2008; Vutuc et al., 2009).

As data mounted that percent free PSA offered improved specificity over the use of total PSA alone in the range of 4 - 10 ng/ml, it also become evident that percent free PSA might provide improved sensitivity at total PSA values less than 4.0 ng/ml (Yoshimo et al., 2008). Catalona et al. (1998) studied a population of men with PSA values restricted to 2.6 - 4.0 ng/ml are benign prostates on examination.

Percent free PSA predicted cancer in men and that over 80% of the cancers so detected were organ confined (Leman and Getzenberg, 2009). Vashi et al. (1997) examined the use of percent free PSA to trigger biopsy in the range of 3 - 4 ng/ml total PSA. A free PSA cut point of 19% allowed detection of 90% of the cancers in these men and resulted in a 73% biopsy rate and 44% cancer detection rate.

A direct relationship has been demonstrated between preoperative serum PSA and tumor volume as determined from radical prostectomy specimens (Kabalin et al., 1995). As a general rule, as prostate cancer progresses it produces more PSA. Our results confirmed the findings that the f/t PSA ratio is statistically different between control and patients. Gann (1997) have suggested men with PSA between 2 and 3 ng/ml have 5.5 fold higher risks for prostate cancer. National Academy of Clinical Biochemistry recommends validating the medical decision limit for each free and total PSA (Lilja et al., 2004; Vickers and Lilja, 2009). Using more intensive screening in younger men with lower PSA levels will result in the detection of predominantly low–grade, potentially inconsequential cancers. Conversely, using higher levels of PSA to prompt a biopsy in older men will result in significantly higher rates of aggressive cancer going undetected. The risks of using PSA age–related cutoff values for PSA instead of incorporating all risk variables is that younger men are increasingly likely to be diagnosed with inconsequential tumors, whereas older men may ultimately be found to have aggressive, potentially lethal cancers that are diagnosed too late to allow curative treatments to be given (Brawley et al., 2009).

Efforts made to detect cancer in patients with intermediate or low PSA are justified because 40% of confined CaP is expected to occur in patients with PSA from 4 to 10 ng/ml, we conclude that the free to total PSA ratio may be helpful for differential diagnosis of BPH and CaP. Long term multicancer trials to determine the impact of prostate cancer screening on survival are needed to establish the incidence and mortality owing to prostate cancer (Luderer et al., 1995).

REFERENCES

Angelis GD, Rittenhouse HG, Mikolajczyk SD, Shamel LB, Semjonow A (2007). Twenty years of PSA: From prostate Antigen to Tumor Marker, Rev. Urol. 9(3): 113-123.

Brawley OW, Ankerst DP, Thompson IM (2009). Screening for Prostate Cancer. CA Cancer J. Clin., 59(4):264-273. Epub 2009 Jun 29.

Catalona WJ, Partin AW, Slawin KM (1998). Use of the percentage of free prostate-specific antigen to enhance differentiation of prostate cancer from benign prostatic disease: a prospective multicenter Clin. Trial JAMA. 279: 1542-1547.

Catalona WJ, Smith DS, Wolfert R, Wang T, Rittenhouse H (1995).Evaluation of percentage of free serum prostate-specific antigen to improve specificity of prostate cancer screening. JAMA. 274(15): 1214-1220.

Chen YT, Luderer AA, Thiel RP, Carlson G, Cony CL, Soriano TE (1996). Using proportions of free to total prostate-specific antigen, age, and total prostate-specific antigen to predict the probability of prostate cancer. Urology, 47: 518-524.

Daniëlle BP, Andrea L, Monique G, Erik R (2008). Why determine only the total prostate-specific antigen, if the free-to-total ratio contains the information? Ann. Clin. Biochem., 45: 270-274.

Frempong MT, Aboah K (2008). Correlation of serum free/total prostate specific antigen ratio with histological features for differential diagnosis of prostate cancer. J. Med. Sci., 8: 540-546.

Gann PH (1998). Interpreting recent trends in prostate cancer incidence and mortality. Epidemiol., 8: 117-120

Kabalin JN, McNeal JE, Johnstone IM, Stamey TA (1995). Serum prostate specific antigen and the biologic progression of prostate cancer. Urology, 46: 65-70.

Katz A, Katz A (2008). The top 13: what family physicians should know about prostate cancer. Can. Fam. Phys. Rev. 54(2): 198-203.

Leman ES, Getzenberg RH (2009). Biomarkers for prostate cancer. J. Cell. Biochem., Jun 8..

Lilja H, Semjonow A, Sibley P, Babaian R, Dowell B, Rittenhouse H, Sokoll L (2004). NACB: Practice guidelines and recommendations for use of tumor markers in the clinic prostate cancer (Section 3B).

Loeb S, Catalona WJ (2008). What to do with an abnormal PSA Test. Oncologist, 13: 299–305.

Luderer AA, Chen YT, Soriano TF, Kramp WI, Cuny C, Sharp I, Smith W, Petteway J, Brawer MK (1995). Measurement of the proportion of free to total prostate-specific antigen improves diagnostic performance of prostate-specific antigen in the diagnostic gray zone of total prostate-specific antigen. Urology, 46: 187-194.

Monda JM, Barry MJ, Oesterling JE (1994). Prostate specific antigen cannot distinguish stage 1a (A1) prostate cancer from benign prostatic hyperplasia. J. Urol., 151: 1291-1295.

Noldus J, Chen Z, Stamey T (1997). Isolation and characterization of free form prostate specific antigen (f-PSA) in sera of men with prostate cancer. J. Urol., 158: 1606–1609.

Singh JC (2009). Cut-off value for PSA: do we need a change?. J. Postgrad. Med., 55(2): 150-151.

Vashi AR, Wojno KJ, Henricks W, England BA, Vessella RL, Lange PH, Wright GL, Schellhammer PF, Weigand RA, Olson RM, Dowell BL, Borden KK, Oesterling E (1997). Determination of the "reflex range" and appropriate cut points for percent free-PSA in 413 men referred for prostatic evaluation using the AxSYM system. Urology, 49(1): 19-27.

Vickers AJ, Lilja H (2009). Prostate cancer: Estimating the benefits of PSA screening. Nat. Rev. Urol., 6(6): 301-303.

Vutuc C, Waldhoer T, Lunglmayr G, Hoeltl W, Haidinger G (2009). PSA testing in Austria: induced morbidity and saved mortality. Eur. J. Cancer Prev., 18(5): 377-380.

Woodrum DL, Brawer MK, Partin AW, Catalona WW, Southwick PC (1998). Interpretation of free prostate specific antigen clinical research studies for the detection of prostate cancer. J. Urol. (Suppl), 159: 5-12.

Wu JT (1994). Assay for prostate specific antigen (PSA). Problems and possible solutions. J. Clin. Lab. Anal. 8: 51-62.

Yamamoto S, Maruyama T (2008). Diagnostic efficacy of free to total ratio of prostate-specific antigen and prostate-specific antigen velocity, singly and in combination, in detecting prostate cancer in patients with total serum prostate-specific antigen between 4 and 10 ng/ml. Int. Urol. Nephrol., 40: 85–89

Yoshimo K, Yasuhide K (2008). Free-to-total prostate-specific antigen (PSA) ratio contributes to an increased rate of prostate cancer detection in a Japanese population screened using a PSA level of 2.1 -10.0ng/ml as a criterion. Int. J. Clin. Oncol., 13: 229-232.

15

The significance of artemisinin in roll back malaria partnership programmes and cancer therapy

Obimba, Kelechukwu Clarence

Department of Biochemistry, College of Natural and Applied Sciences, Michael Okpara University of Agriculture Umudike. Abia State, Nigeria. E-mail: kccob@yahoo.com.

The role of the natural product, artemisinin, is discussed, with a view to elucidating its importance as an antimalarial, essential to sustainable global development, especially in the health and welfare industry. An estimated 243 million cases of malaria led to an estimated 863,000 deaths in 2008. The Roll Back Malaria (RBM) Partnership is a global network for co-ordinated action against malaria, launched in 1998 by the World Health Organization (WHO), United Nations International Children Emergency Fund (UNICEF), United Nations Development Programme (UNDP), and World Bank. It promotes consensus among key actors in malaria control, harmonizes action, and mobilizes resources to fight malaria in endemic countries. Large scale use of antimalarial monotherapies such as quinoline compounds (for example, chloroquine) and antifolate drugs (for example, sulfonamides), have culminated in cross-resistance, especially of *Plasmodium falciparum,* to these conventional antimalarial drugs. Artemisinin, (a sesquiterpene lactone), isolated from the plant *Artemisia annua*, is a drug used to treat multi-drug resistant strains of falciparum malaria. *Saccharomyces cerevisiae* microbes can produce the precursor artemisinic acid, by a technique of synthetic biology. The total synthesis of artemisinin can also be performed using the organic reagents, isopulegol. The iron-porphyrin complex-moiety, produced during plasmodium infection of the red blood cells, reacts with artemisinin, a potent inhibitor of hemozoin formation, to produce reactive oxygen radicals which damage the parasite leading to its death. Artemisinin acts on the electron transport chain, by causing the depolarization of the parasite's mitochondrial membrane, and kills the asexual forms of plasmodium at the erythrocytic stage. Artemisinin selectively inhibits the production of estrogen receptor-alpha gene and thus, arrests the growth of estrogen responsive breast cancer cells. Artemesinin is not used for malaria prophylaxis because of it's extremely short activity. Artemisinin is fast-acting and poorly bioavailable. The use of semi-synthetic derivatives and analogues of artemisinin, such as artesunate, and artemether, in the production of Artemisinin-based combination therapies (ACTs), for example, lumefantrine-artesunate, increase the therapeutic efficiency of artemisinin to more than 90%, and prevents recrudescence.

Key words: Artemisinin, monotherapies, plasmodium, artemisinin-based combination therapies.

INTRODUCTION

Recent estimates of the global malaria burden have shown increasing levels of malaria morbidity and mortality, reflecting the deterioration of the malaria situation in Africa during the 1990s. Half of the world's population is at risk of malaria. An estimated 243 million cases led to an estimated 863,000 deaths in 2008. Administration of fake malarial drugs has been implicated as a major causative factor of proliferation of drug-resistant malarial parasites leading to large scale deaths, due to malarial infections (Basco, 2004). About 90% of malaria deaths occur in Africa south of the Sahara, and the great majority of them, are children under five (Acton and Roth, 1992). The RBM partnership is a global network for co-ordinated action against malaria, launched in 1998 by WHO, UNICEF, UNDP, and World Bank. It promotes consensus among key actors in malaria

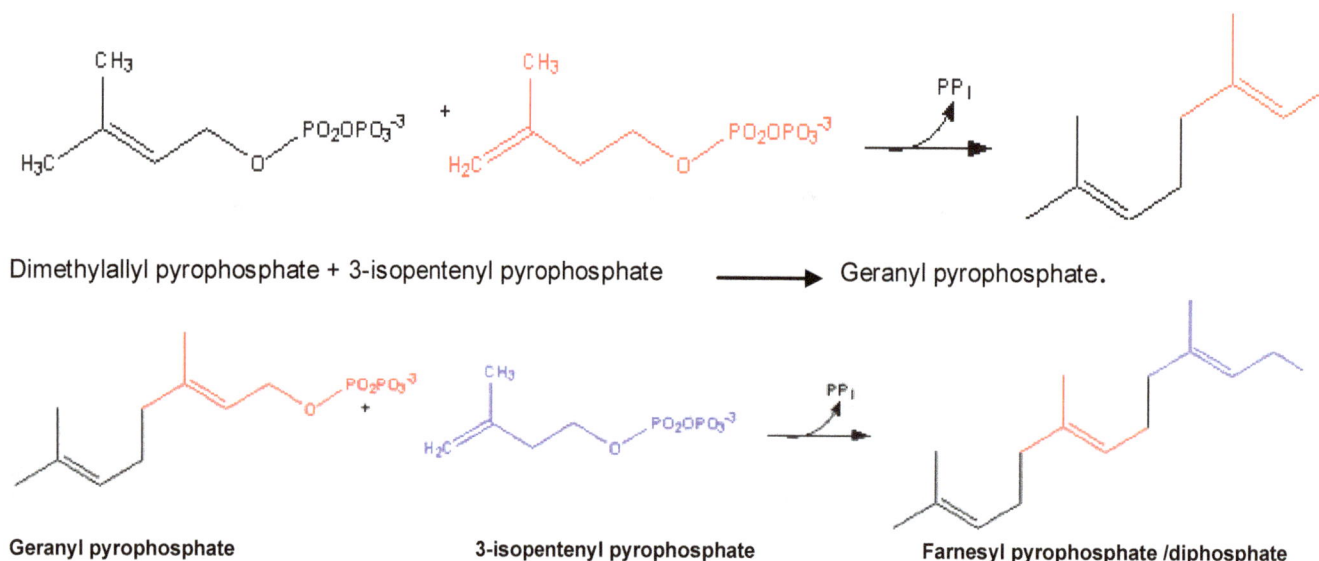

Figure 1. Biosynthesis of farnesyl pyrophosphate (Wikipedia, 2011).

control, harmonizes action, and mobilizes resources to fight malaria in endemic countries. The use of long-lasting insecticidal nets; enlightenment, encouraging indoor spraying of insecticides coupled with artemisinin-based combination therapies has engendered large-scale global malaria control. Antimalarial drugs were deployed on a large scale, always as monotherapies, introduced in sequence, and were generally poorly managed, in that, their use was continued despite unacceptably high levels of resistance.

In addition, there has been over-reliance on both quinoline compounds (that is, quinine, chloroquine, amodiaquine, mefloquine and primaquine) and antifolate drugs (that is, sulfonamides, pyrimethamine, proguanil and chlorproguanil), with consequent encouragement of cross-resistance among these compounds (Mutabingwa et al., 2005). This abuse of antimalarial drugs during the past century, resulting in the widespread resistance of *Plasmodium falciparum* to conventional antimalarial drugs, such as chloroquine, sulfadoxine–pyrimethamine (SP) and amodiaquine, has contributed to the increasing malaria mortality and morbidity (Rowen, 2009). Artemisinin, (a sesquiterpene lactone), is derived from a herb, *Artemisia annua*, and is used as a drug to treat multi-drug resistant strains of falciparum malaria (Parker et al., 1999). Artemisinin is used in Chinese traditional medicine, though it is usually chemically modified and combined with other medications (Acton and Roth, 1992). Physical and chemical data on artemisinin include: Systematic (IUPAC) name: (3R,5aS,6R,8aS,9R,12S,12aR)-octahydro-3,6,9-trimethyl-3,12-epoxy-12H-pyrano[4,3-j]-1,2-benzodioxepin-10(3H)-one; Formula: $C_{15}H_{22}O_5$; Mol.

mass: 282.332 g/mol.; Density: 1.24 ± 0.1 g/cm³; Melt. Point: 152 to 157°C (306 to 315°F); Routes of administration: Oral, rectal, intramuscular, or intravenous uses (Acton and Roth, 1992).

BIOSYNTHESIS OF ARTEMISININ

Saccharomyces cerevisiae microbes can produce the precursor artemisinic acid, by a technique of synthetic biology, via the mevalonate pathway, a pathway for the production of terpenes and terpene products such as cholesterol and plant sterols. The metabolism of the microbe is engineered to produce artemisinic acid, a precursor to artemisinin. Starting from acetyl-CoA (an abundant product of the central metabolism of many microbes), the microbes produce, in turn, mevalonate, farnesyl pyrophosphate (FPP) as shown in Figure 1. Amorphadiene, produced by the enzymatic catalysis of amorphadiene synthase on farnesyl pyrophosphate. A novel cytochrome P450 monooxygenase (hydroxylase) oxidizes artemisinic alcohol to artemisinic acid (Sarpong and Keasling, 2006). The artemisinic acid is released from the microbes, purified from the culture media, and chemically converted to artemisinin. Dihydroartemisinic acid, the final precursor to artemisinin, undergoes photoxidation to produce dihydroartemisinic acid hydroperoxide. Ring expansion by the cleavage of hydroperoxide and a second oxygen-mediated hydroperoxidation furnish the biosynthesis of artemisinin. A three-step oxidation of amorpha-4, 11-diene gives the resulting artemisinic acid (Martin et al., 2001). Once the artemisinin is produced, it must be further chemically

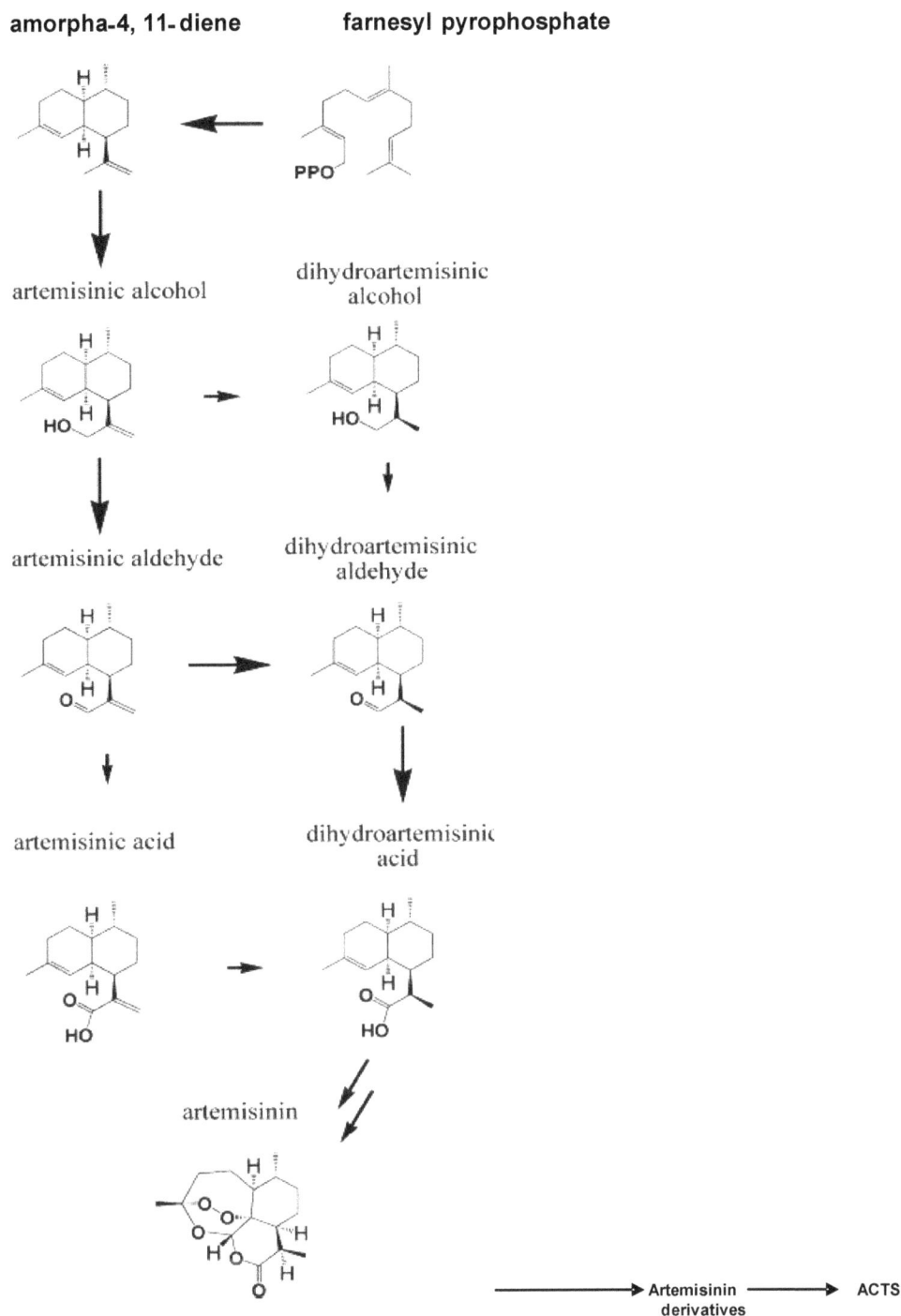

Figure 2. Technique of synthetic biology employed in the microbial synthesis of Artemisinin (Covello et al., 2007).

converted into a derivative such as artesunate or artemether, which are integrated into Artemisinin-based Combination Therapies (ACTs) for the treatment of malaria.

The scheme for the microbial synthesis of artemisinin is shown in Figure 2. Farnesyl pyrophosphate synthase (aprenyl transferase) catalyzes sequential condensation reactions of dimethylallyl pyrophosphate with 2 units of 3-

isopentenyl pyrophosphate to form farnesyl pyrophosphate. The total chemical synthesis of Artemisinin can also be performed using basic organic reagents. The starting material (Isopulegol) is converted to methoxymethyl ether. The ether is hydroborated and oxidized to yield a hydroxylated compound. The primary hydroxyl group is benzylated and the methoxymethyl ether is cleaved, protonated and treated with (E)-(3-iodo-1-methyl-1-propenyl)-trimethylsilane to yield a ketone compound. The resulting ketone is reacted with lithium methoxy(trimethylsily)methylide to obtain two diastereomeric alcohols, one (the l-stereoisomer) which is debenzylated using (Li, NH_3) to yield a lactone. The vinylsilane is oxidized to a ketone which is reacted with fluoride ion that causes it to undergo desilylation, enol ether formation, and carboxylic acid formation. A hydroperoxide function is introduced at C(3) of the resulting compound, photooxygenated and then treated with acid to produce artemisinin (Schmid and Hofheinz, 1983).

PHARMACOKINETICS AND PHARMACODYNAMICS OF ARTEMISININ

Artemisinin and artemisinin derivatives function to destroy plasmodium parasites by alkylation of host heme by carbon-centered free radicals, interference with proteins such as the sarcoplasmic/endoplasmic calcium ATPase (SERCA), as well as damaging of normal mitochondrial functions (Li and Zhou, 2010). The plasmodium parasite consumes hemoglobin and liberates free heme, an iron-porphyrin complex- moiety, during plasmodium infection of the red blood cells. The complex, produced, reacts with artemisinin to produce reactive oxygen radicals which damage the parasite leading to its death. Artemisinin is a potent inhibitor of hemozoin formation activity of malaria parasite. Artemisinin acts on the electron transport chain, generates local reactive oxygen species, and causes the depolarization of the parasite's mitochondrial membrane. Artemisinin kills the asexual forms of plasmodium at the erythrocytic stage (Miller et al., 2002). Artemisinins have also been shown to inhibit PfATP6, a SERCA-type enzyme (calcium transporter) (Jambou et al., 2005), and thus affects adversely, the calcium metabolism of malarial parasites.

USE OF ARTEMISININ IN CANCER THERAPY

The antimalarial artesunate exerts profound cytotoxicity toward tumor cells. The cytostatic and apoptotic effects of artesunate are not diminished by concomitant immunosuppression (Ramacher et al., 2009). Treatment of human breast cancer cells with artemisinin, disrupts estrogen responsiveness and stops cell growth. Artemisinin acts in breast cancer cells by inhibiting the production of the estrogen receptor-alpha (ERα) gene without altering the level of the related estrogen receptor-beta gene (ERβ). Artemisinin-regulated cellular pathways selectively inhibits the production of ERα and arrests the growth of estrogen responsive breast cancer cells by altering the function of nuclear cellular proteins (transcription factors) that are used by breast cancer cells to enhance the synthesis of the ERα gene (Firestone, 2006). Artemisinin selectively kills cancer cells which have more intracellular free iron than do normal cells. Combined HBO_2 and artemisinin exposure may be an effective anticancer chemotherapeutic strategy (Ohgami et al., 2010).

The pleiotropic response elicited in cancer cells by artemisinin and artemisinin derivatives include growth inhibition by cell cycle arrest, apoptosis, inhibition of angiogenesis, disruption of cell migration, and modulation of nuclear receptor responsiveness (Firestone and Sundar, 2009). The anti-cancer potential of artemisinin and artemisinin derivatives has been demonstrated in various cancer cells including those of leukemia and other cancer cells of breast, ovary, liver, lung, pancreas and colon (Lu et al., 2008). The anti-cancer mechanism of artemisinin and artemisinin derivatives is likely to be related to the cleavage of the iron- or heme-mediated peroxide bridge, followed by the generation of reactive oxygen species (ROS) (Efferth et al., 2003). Gao et al. (2011) showed that dihydroartemisinin (DHA)-induced apoptosis in human leukemia cells in vitro and exhibited an anti-leukemic activity in vivo through a process that involves of mitogen-activated protein kinase (MEK)/ extracellular signal-regulated protein kdve4ycinase (ERK) inactivation, Induced myeloid leukemia cell differentiation protein (Mcl-1) down-regulation, culminating in cytochrome c release and caspase activation.

Dosing and contra-indications

The WHO approved adult dose of co-artemether (artemether-lumefantrine) for malaria is 4 tablets at 0, 8, 24, 36, 48 and 60 h (six doses). This has been proven to be superior to regimens based on amodiaquine Vugt et al. (1999); Lefevre et al. (2001), Sutherland et al. (2005) and Jansen (2006). Artemesinin are not used for malaria prophylaxis (prevention) because of the extremely short activity of the drug. The adverse side effects from Artemsinin are similar to the symptoms of malaria: nausea, vomiting, anorexia, and dizziness. The combination drugs may have additional side effects. The drug should not be prescribed for pregnant women less than 3 months, except in the event of cerebral or pernicious malaria. Use of artemisinin by itself as a monotherapy is explicitly discouraged by the WHO as there have been signs that malarial parasites are developing resistance to the drug (WHO, 2001a, b, 2008) (Table 1).

Table 1. Adoption of artemisinin combination therapies (ACTs) by countries of the world (Bosman and Mendis, 2007).

Parameter	Number of countries	
	Africa	Rest of the world
Changed treatment policy to ACT[a]	14[b]	14[c]
Changed treatment policy to CT	3	1
In process of treatment policy review	11	5
Studying efficacy of ACT options	4	1

[a]Adoption does not immediately translate into implementation: In Africa only 5 out of the 14, and outside Africa 10 out of 14 countries which have adopted ACTs are deploying these drugs in the public sector. [b]Burundi, Cameroon, Comoros, Cote d'Ivoire, Eq. Guinea, Gabon, Ghana, Kenya, Mozambique, Sao Tome and Principe, Senegal, South Africa, Zambia, Zanzibar; [c]Bhutan, Bolivia, Cambodia, Ecuador, Guyana, Indonesia, Lao PDR, Myanmar, Papua New Guinea, Peru, Philippines, Surinam, Thailand, Vietnam (WHO, 2008).

Table 2. How access to ACTs is being ensured.

Purpose	Effort
Quality assurance, prequalification and sourcing project	Establishment by WHO in collaboration with other United Nations agencies, of an international mechanism to pre-qualify manufacturers of artemisinin compounds and ACTs [for example, the Global Fund to Fight AIDS, Tuberculosis and Malaria (GFATM)], on the basis of compliance with internationally recommended standards of manufacturing and quality
WHO-UNICEF call for tenders of ACTS	WHO and UNICEF have called for tenders of co-blistered combinations of the following products for which there are not yet pre-qualified manufacturers: (i) artesunate plus amodiaquine; (ii) artesunate plus sulfadoxine/pyrimethamine; iii) artesunate plus mefloquine; and iv) amodiaquine plus sulfadoxine/pyrimethamine
Negotiated prices and centralized procurement artemether/lumefantrine (Coartem®)	WHO and Novartis, the manufacturer of artemether–lumefantrine (Coartem®), have entered into a special pricing agreement: Novartis provides the drug at cost price (US$ 0.9 and 2.4 per child and adult treatment course, respectively)
Financing of ACTs Global fund expenditure on ACTs	GFATM, established in 2002, is now the largest funder of ACTs in countries, and have requested that countries apply for the most effective treatments to roll back malaria. The artemisinin Project is a program by Sanofi-Aventis, Amyris Biotechnologies, the Institute for OneWorld Health, and Jay Keasling, a researcher from the University of California, to combat malaria by producing artemisinin at low cost (Hamm, 2009)
Propagation of the plant *Artemisia annua*	Plans to have the plant *Artemisia annua* grow in other areas of the world outside Vietnam and China (Kenya, Tanzania and Madagascar) (Ro et al., 2006)

World Bank (2003) and WHO (2008).

Artemisinin- based combination therapies (ACTs)

Artemisinin itself has physical properties such as poor bioavailability that limit its effectiveness. Semi- synthetic synthetic derivatives and analogues of artemisinin, such as Artesunate, Artemether, Artelinic acid, Artenimol, and Artemotil, with more efficient bio-availabity have been developed. Artemisinin and its derivatives are fast-acting, but other drugs are often required to clear the body of all parasites and prevent recrudescence. For this reason, artemisinin is administered together with other antimalarial drugs, unrelated to the artemisinin family, in what is known as ACTs, which are the preferred treatment for malaria and are both effective and well tolerated in patients. The artemisinin derivative, Artemether, is typically administered, in simultaneous combination with lumefantrine (also known as benflumetol) to treat uncomplicated falciparum malaria. Lumefantrine has a half-life of about 3 to 6 days and prevents the disease from returning. Other examples of ACTs are artesunate-mefloquine, and artesunate-amodiaquine. ACTs are more than 90% efficient (Eline Korenromp et al., 2005; Bloland, 2001). Since 2001, 32 countries have adopted one of the aforementioned five combination therapies, several as first-line treatment and a few as second-line. A multi-artemisinin combination therapy is Artesunate-(Sulphadoxine-Pyrimethamine). The therapy is an initial administration of sulphadoxine-pyrimethamine combination with a subsequent administration of artesunate, approximately, 24hours after the initial administration (Elamin et al., 2005). Many others are in the process of policy change. WHO has provided continuous technical cooperation to ministries of health on all aspects of national treatment policy change monitoring the therapeutic efficacy of medicines, and updating and implementing ACT-based treatment policies and (Jambou et al., 2005; Grupper, 2005; Olumese, 2006). Information on how to access ACTs is given in Table 2.

CONCLUSION

Artemisinin, a sesquiterpene lactone, isolated from the plant *A. annua*, used as a drug, to treat multi-drug resistant strains of falciparum malaria, can be produced by a technique of synthetic microbiology, and also in the laboratory from basic organic reagents. In addition, artemisinin is curative of breast, ovary, liver, lung, pancreas and colon cancers. Artemisinin is a potent inhibitor of hemozoin formation activity of malaria parasite. Artemisinin have also been shown to inhibit the calcium transporter enzyme, thus posing toxicity to micro-organisms. Drug efficacy of artemisinin is optimized in ACTs.

ACKNOWLEDGEMENT

The author acknowledges the technical support given by Dr. Seb. Obasi and the resource contribution of Engr. Abraham Enyichukwu Obimba.

REFERENCES

Acton N, Roth RJ (1992). On the conversion of dihydroartemisinic acid into artemisinin. J. Org. Chem., 57: 3610-3614.

Basco LK (2004). Molecular Epidemiology of Malaria in Cameroon. XIX. Quality of Antimalarial Drugs Used for Self-medication. Am. J. Trop. Med. Hyg., 70(3): 245-250.

Bloland P (2001). Drug Resistance in Malaria. A Background Document for the WHO Global Strategy for Containment of Antimicrobial Resistance. Geneva: World Health Organization.

Bosman A, Mendis KN (2007). A major Transition in Malarial Treatment: The adoption and deployment of Artemisinin-based combination Therapies. Am. J. Trop. Med. Hyg., 77(6): 193-197.

Covello PS, Teoh KH, Polichuk DR, Reed DW, Nowak G (2007). Functional genomics and the biosynthesis of artemisinin. Phytochem., 6814 : 1864-1871.

Efferth T, Sauerbrey A, Olbrich A, Gebhart E, Rauch P, Weber HO, Hengstler JG, Halatsch ME, Volm M, Tew KD, Ross DD, Funk JO (2003). Molecular modes of action of artesunate in tumor cell lines. Mol. Pharmacol., 64: 382-394.

Elamin SB, Malik EM, Abdelgadir T, Khamiss AH, Mohammed MM, Ahmed ES, Adam I (2005). Artesunate plus sulfadoxine-pyrimethamine for treatment of uncomplicated Plasmodium falciparum malaria in Sudan. Malaria J., 4: 41.

Eline KJM, Nahlen B, Wardlaw T, Young M (2005). World Malaria Report: World Health Organization (WHO), Roll Back Malaria (RBM) and United Nations Children's Fund (UNICEF). Geneva: World Health Organization.

Firestone G (2006). Artemisinin Disrupts Estrogen Receptor-Alpha and Cell Growth.Carlifornia Breast cancer Research Program. http://www.cbcrp.org/research/PageGrant.asp?grant_id=4768

Firestone GL, Sundar SN (2009). Anticancer activities of artemisinin and its bioactive derivatives. Expert. Rev. Mol. Med., 11:e32.

Gao N, Budhraja A, Cheng S, Liu EH, Huang C, Chen J, Yang Z, Chen D, Zhang Z, Shi X (2011). Interruption of the MEK/ERK signaling cascade promotes dihydroartemisinin-induced apoptosis *in vitro* and *in vivo*. Apoptosis. 16(5): 511-523.

Grupper M (2005). Meeting on the Production of Artemisinin and ACTs. Arusha, Tanzania: DFID Health Resource Centre, Roll Back Malaria, World Health Organization.

Hamm S (2009). Crative Capitalism' versus Malaria. Business Week. 083.

Jambou R, Legrand E, Niang M, Khim N, Lim P, Volney B, Ekala MT, Bouchier C, Esterre P, Fandeur T, Mercereau-Puijalon O (2005). Resistance of *Plasmodium falciparum* field isolates to *in-vitro* artemether and point mutations of the SERCA-type PfATPase6. Lancet, 366: 1960-1963.

Jansen FH (2006). The herbal tea approach for artemesinin as a therapy for malaria? Trans R Soc Trop. Med. Hyg., 100(3): 285-286.

Lefevre G, Looareesuwan S, Treeprasertsuk S (2001). A clinical and pharmacokinetic trial of six doses of artemether-lumefantrine for multidrug-resistant *Plasmodium falciparum* malaria in Thailand. Am. J. Trop. Med. Hyg., 64(5-6): 247-256.

Li J, Zhou B (2010). Biological Actions of Artemisinin: Insights from Medicinal Chemistry Studies. Molecule, 15(3): 1378-1397.

Lu JJ, Meng LH, Cai YJ, Chen Q, Tong LJ, Lin LP, Ding J (2008). Dihydroartemisinin induces apoptosis in HL-60 leukemia cells dependent of iron and p38 mitogen-activated protein kinase activation but independent of reactive oxygen species. Cancer Biol. Ther., 7: 1017-1023.

Martin VJ, Yoshikuni Y Keasling JD (2001). The *in vivo* synthesis of plant sesquiterpenes by *Escherichia coli*. Biotech. Bioeng., 7: 497-503.

Miller LH, Baruch DI, Marsh K, Doumbo OK (2002). The pathogenic basis of malaria. Nature 415: 673-679.

Mutabingwa TK, Anthony D, Heller A (2005). Amodiaquine alone, amodiaquine+sulfadoxine-pyrimethamine, amodiaquine+artesunate, and artemether-lumefantrine for outpatient treatment of malaria in Tanzanian children: a four-arm randomised effectiveness trial. Lancet 365(9469): 1474-1480.

Ohgami Y, Elstad CA, Chung E, Shirachi DY, Quock RM, Lai HC (2010). Effect of Hyperbaric Oxygen on the Anticancer Effect of

Artemisinin on Molt-4 Human Leukemia Cells. Intl. J. Cancer Res. Treatment. 30(11): 4467-4470.

Olumese P (2006). Guidelines for the Treatment of Malaria. Geneva: World Health Organization.

Parker MH, Northrop J, Elias J, Ploypradith S, Xie P, Shapiro S, Theresa A (1999). Orally Active, Hydrolytically Stable, Semisynthetic, Antimalarial Trioxanes in the Artemisinin Family. J. Med. Chem., 42 (2): 300-304.

Ramacher M, Umansky V, Efferth T (2009). Effect of artesunate on immune cells in ret-transgenic mouse melanoma model. Anti-Cancer Drugs. 20(10): 910-917.

Ro DK, Paradise EM, Ouellet M, Fisher KJ, Newman KL, Ndungu JM, Ho KA, Eachus RA, Ham TS, Kirby J, Chang MC, Withers ST, Shiba Y, Sarpong R, Keasling JD (2006). Production of the antimalarial drug precursor artemisinic acid in engineered yeast. Nature 440: 940-943.

Rowen RJ (2009). Artemisinin: From Malaria to Cancer Treatment. Wikipedia encyclopaedia. http://en.wikipedia.org/wiki/Artemisinin. (3-12-2011).

Sarpong R, Keasling JD (2006). Production of the antimalarial drug precursor artemisinic acid in engineered yeast Nature. 440: 940-943.

Schmid G, Hofheinz W. (1983). Total Synthesis of qinghaosu J. Am. Chem. Soc., 105(3): 624-625.

Sutherland CJ, Ord R, Dunyo S, Jawara M, Drakeley CJ, Alexander N, Coleman R, Pinder M, Walraven G, Targett GA (2005). Reduction of malaria transmission to Anopheles mosquitoes with a six-dose regimen of co-artemether. PLoS Med., 2: e92.

Vugt MV, Wilairatana P, Gemperli B (1999). Efficacy of six doses of artemether-lumefantrine (benflumetol) in multidrug-resistant Plasmodium falciparum malaria. Am. J. Trop. Med. Hyg., 60(6): 936-942.

Wikipedia (2011). Isopentenyl pyrophosphate. http://en.wikipedia.org/wiki/Isopentenyl_pyrophosphate. (3-12-2011).

World Bank (2003). Report of the Expert Consultation on the Procurement & Financing of Antimalarial Drugs . Washington D.C.

World Health Organization. (2001a). The use of antimalarial drugs. Report of a WHO Informal Consultation. Geneva, World Health Organization. (WHO/CDS/RBM/2001.33).

World Health Organization. (2001b). Antimalarial drug combination therapy: Report of WHO technical consultation . Geneva, World Health Organization (WHO/CDS/RBM/2001.35).

World Health Organization. (2003). Procurement, quality and sourcing project: access to artemisinin-based combination antimalarial drugs of acceptable quality. Geneva, World Health Organization.

World Health Organization (2008). WHO ultimatum on artemisinin monotherapy is showing results. http://www.bmj.com/cgi/content/full/332/7551/1176-b. (3-12-2011).

16

Characterization of antioxidant and antimicrobial compounds of cinnamon and ginger essential oils

G. S. El-Baroty[1], H. H. Abd El-Baky[1], R. S. Farag[2] and M. A. Saleh[3]

[1]Department of Biochemistry, Faculty of Agriculture, Cairo University, Cairo, Egypt.
[2]Department of Plant Biochemistry, National Research Centre, Dokki, Cairo, Egypt.
[3]Department of Chemistry, Texas Southern University, Houston, Texas, USA.

Essential oils obtained from the bark of *Cinnamomum zeylanicum* (cinnamon) and the rhizomes of *Zingiber officinale* (ginger) were characterized by analytical TLC and GC/MS, and their antimicrobial and antioxidant compounds were detected by TLC-bio-autography assays. Essential oil of cinnamon bark (CEO) was found to be a unique aromatic monoterpene-rich natural source, with *trans*-cinnamaldehyde (45.62%) as the major constituents. Ginger oil (GEO) was characterized by high content of sesquiterpene hydrocarbons, including β-sesquiphellandrene (27.16%), caryophyllene (15.29%), zingiberene (13.97%), α-farnesene (10.52%) and *ar*-curcumin (6.62%). CEO and GEO oils showed significant inhibitory activity against selected strains of bacteria and pathogenic fungi, with MIC values ranging from 20 to 120 μg/ml depending upon the microbial species. Cinnamaldehyde (CA) and eugenol in cinnamon bark oil and β-sesquiphellandrene, caryophyllene and zingiberene in ginger rhizome oil were identified as the most active antibacterial components, with the aid of bioautography on TLC and GC-MS. Also, both oil exhibited appreciable *in vitro* antioxidant activity as assessed by 2, 2'-diphenyl-1-picrylhydrazyl (DPPH) radical scavenging and β-carotene bleaching methods, compared to α-tocopherol, BHT and BHA. Guided isolation through TLC-autography using 0.05% DPPH and β-carotene/linoleic acid as a detection reagent led to identified CA and eugenol as main active antioxidant compounds in CEO. The significant antimicrobial and antioxidant activities of both oils suggest that it could serve as a source of compounds with preservative phenomenon.

Key words: Antimicrobial, bioautographic assay, antioxidant, essential oils, ginger, cinnamon.

INTRODUCTION

The oxidative stress (OS), induces by reactive oxygen species (ROS), can be described as a dynamic imbalance between the amounts of free radicals generated in the body and levels of antioxidants to quench and or/scavenge them and protect the body against their deleterious effects (Shirwaikar et al., 2006). Excessive amounts of ROS may be harmful because they can initiated biomolecular oxidations which lead to cell injury and death, and create oxidative stress which results numerous diseases and disorders such as aging, cancer, atherosclerosis, cirrhosis and cataracts (Halliwell and Gutteridge, 2000). On other hand, the spread of drug resistant pathogens is one of the most threats to successful treatment of microbial diseases. In addition, the consumption of food contaminated with food-borne microorganisms can pose a serious threat to human health. The existence of microorganisms causes spoilage and results in reduction of the quality and quantity of possessed food (Anwar et al., 2009). Therefore, there has been a growing considerable interest to identify new sources of safe and inexpensive antioxidant and antimicrobial potential of natural origin (Abdel-Baky and El Baroty, 2008; Anwer et al., 2009).

Ginger (*Zingiber officinale*, Zingiberaceae) and cinnamon (*Cinnamomum zeylanicum*, Lauraceae) are widely been consumed as spices and food preservation. They

---

*Corresponding author. E-mail: abdelbakyh@hotmail.com.

Abbreviation: TLC, Thin layer chromatography.

are added to food products in the form of essential oils and various extracts (Yu et al., 2007). Also, both spices have been employed as a folk remedy to treat of several diseases, disorders and ailments (Geiger, 2005; Senhaji et al., 2007). Since long time, cinnamon and ginger have been used to treat dyspepsia, gastritis, blood circulation disturbance and inflammatory diseases in many countries (Wang et al., 2009). Also, they show potential antipyretic, antiallergenic, analgesic, antitussive (Gurdip et al., 2008) and chemopreventive activities (Sabulal et al., 2007). This potential activity was believed to be attributed to the major compounds in oils such as cinnamaldehyde and zingiberene, and their activity could be multiple (Ali et al., 2005; Singh et al., 2008; Anwer et al., 2009). However, cinnamon and ginger are locally named karfa and zingabil in several Arabic countries such as Egypt, and are used as common beverages like tea (in tea-bags form) among many people in particular in winter season, due to their protective effect and curative remedy for numerous disorders. Therefore, the aim of this study was to characterize the chemical constituents, and antimicrobial and antioxidant properties of essential oils obtained from two spices, viz. ginger (Z. officinale) and cinnamon (Cinnamomum zeylanicum). These beneficial characteristics could increase food safety and shelf life of fatty-rich foods and processed food products.

MATERIALS AND METHODS

Essential oil distillation

The bark of C. zeylanicum and rhizome of Z. officinale were purchased from the local spices store, Egypt. About 100 g of each spice were subjected to hydro-distillation for 3 h using a Clevenger-type apparatus. The obtained essential oil was dried over anhydrous Na_2SO_4, filtered and stored at −10°C in a sealed vial until use.

Determination of total phenols

The content of total phenols in the plant essential oils were calculated using the Folin-Ciocalteau reagent method as described by Singleton and Rossi (1965). Eugenol as the reference standard was used for preparation of calibration curve.

Gas chromatography/mass spectrometry (GC-MS) analysis

The analysis of the essential oils were performed using GC/MS system consisted of a HP 5890 series II gas chromatograph, HP 5972 mass detector and Agilent 6890 series auto-sampler (Agilent Technologies, USA). A Supelco MDN-5S capillary column (30 m × 0.25 mm i.d., 0.5 μm film thickness) was used with helium as the carrier gas, at a flow rate of 1 ml/min. GC oven temperature was programmed at an initial temperature of 40°C for 5 min, then heated up to 140°C at 5°C/min and held at 140°C for 5 min, then heated to 280°C at 10°C/min and held for 5 additional minutes. Injector and detector temperatures were 250°C. Diluted sample (1/100, v/v in heptane) of 1.0 μl were injected automatically. Mass spectrometry was run in the electron impact mode (EI) at 70 eV. The components were identified based on the comparison of their GC retention times,

interpretation of their mass spectra and confirmed by mass spectral library search using the National Institute of Standards and Technology (NIST) database (Massada, 1976; Adams, 2007).

Antioxidant activity

DPPH scavenging assay

The ability of the essential oil to scavenge DPPH radical was assessed as described by Tagashira and Ohtake (1998). Briefly, different concentrations of tested oil (ranged 5 - 200 μg) in 1 ml of ethanol were added to 25 ml of methanolic DPPH (100 mmol/L^{-1}) solution. The mixtures were incubated in the dark at 27 ± 1°C, then the absorbance was measured at 517 nm for 90 min, at 15 min intervals, against a blank (pure methanol). BHT, BHA and α-tocopherol (2 – 40 μg/ml) were used as reference standards. The radical scavenging activity of the each oil was calculated from a calibration curve. All tests were run in triplicate and averaged. The oil concentration providing 50% inhibition (IC_{50}) was calculated from a graph representing the inhibition percentage against oil concentration.

β-Carotene-linoleic acid bleaching

The ability of the oils to prevent the bleaching of β-carotene-linoleic acid was assessed as described by Abd El Baky and El Baroty (2008). An aliquot, β-carotene (0.2 mg) in chloroform (2 ml), linoleic acid (30 μL) and Tween-20 (200 mg) were transferred into round-bottom flask. Once the solvent was evaporated, 250 ml ultra-pure water was added and the resulting mixture was stirred vigorously. Then, 1 ml of aliquot essential oil (containing 5 – 200 μg oil and 10 mg Tween-20) was added to 50 ml reagent mixture and tested samples were subjected to thermal auto-oxidation at 50°C. At intervals up to 300 min, the absorbances of the reaction mixture (4 ml) were measured at 470 nm against a blank (1% Tween-20 solution). All samples were done in triplicates. Antioxidant capacities of algal extracts were compared with those of BHT, BHA and α-tocopherol (at 2-100 μg ml^{-1}) and control. Inhibition of bleaching β-carotene (I %) was calculated as follows:

Inhibition percentage (%I) = (Abs $_{initial}$ −Abs $_{sample}$ / Abs $_{initial}$) x 100

TLC rapid antioxidant assay: TLC plates were used to detect the most active constituents in both essential oils based on spraying the separated compounds on TLC plates either with β-carotene/linoleic acid reagent as described by Abdel Baky and El Baroty (2008) or with 0.05 % DPPH radical in methanol (Jaime et al., 2005), to locate the antioxidant compounds. The protection against the bleaching β-carotene gave orange spots and scavenging DPPH radical gave pale yellow colored spots were considered positive results.

Antimicrobial assay

Preparation of bacterial cultures

Four species of Gram-positive bacteria (Bacillus subtilis ATCC 6633; Bacillus cereus ATCC 14579, Staphylococcus aureus ATCC 27840 and Micrococcus luteus ATCC 4698) and two Gram-negative bacteria (Klebsiella pneumoniae ATCC 13883 and Serratia marcescens ATCC 13880) were routinely used for the antimicrobial assay in our laboratory. These specific strains were recommended for antibacterial screening purpose (NCCLS, 1990). The bacteria were sub-cultured on nutrient agar at 37°C prior to overnight growth in nutrient broth. All overnight cultures were standardized using sterile saline to produce approximately 1.5×10^7 colony forming units (cfu) per ml.

Disc diffusion method

The antibacterial activity of the essential oil was carried out by the disc agar diffusion method. Brief, Mueller Hinton agar (MHA) plates were swabbed with the respective broth cultures of the organisms. Sterile filter paper discs (Whatman's No. 1, 6 mm in diameter) were impregnated with the appropriate equivalent amount of the essential oil dissolved in sterile dimethylsulphoxide (DMSO) at concentrations of 1 - 10 mg/ disc. Control discs impregnated with 10 ml of the solvent DMSO (negative control) and 2 mg/disc chloramphenicol (positive standard antibacterial drug) were used to determine the sensitivity of one strain in each experiment. The plates were incubated at 30°C for 24 h and the antimicrobial activity was evaluated by measuring the inhibition zones expressed millimeters (mm) of inhibition against the tested organism.

Minimal inhibitory concentration

The minimal inhibitory concentration (MIC) values determined for the bacterial strains, as described by Daw et al. (1994). The MIC was defined as the lowest concentration tested samples showing no visible bacterial growth after 24 h incubation period at 37ºC.

Thin layer chromatography (TLC) bioautographic assay

A TLC bioautographic assay was used to detect components in ginger and cinnamon oil as well as the most bio-active constituents (as antibacterial agent). A set of three plates (5 x 20 cm, silica gel G, 60F 254 Merck, Darmstadt, Germany) were used one plate for each bacterial strain and in each experiment, a 5 µl of the undiluted oil was applied to each plate. The plates were then developed with toluene-ethyl acetate (95:5, v/v). The dried TLC plates were then cut with a diamond into three strips. One of the strips was inspected under UV light (254 nm) and also by visualization with 1% vanillin-sulfuric acid reagent and then heated at 110 C for 3 min; the second was used for the bioautography assay, while the active constituents on the third strip were eluted with hexane. TLC bioautography was carried out using the previously identified bacteria (B. subtilis and K. pneumoniae) that induced highest effectiveness in the disc diffusion assay. Suspensions of the bacteria in Difco-nutrient broth (Augsburg, Germany) containing agar and 0.1% iodonitrotetrazolum chloride media individually distributed over the TLC plate (second) was then incubated at 37°C for 48 h. Inhibition zones were shown as clear areas against a pink background. TLC zones that showed inhibition activities of the third strip of the TLC plats were scraped from the plates and eluted with dichloromethane, filtrated concentrated by nitrogen to a final volume of 50 µl and analyzed by GC/MS as described above (Abdel Baky and El Baroty, 2008).

Antifungal assay

Antifungal activity was assayed as described Daw et al. (1994), based on the determined growth inhibition rates of the mycelia of different mold strains (Aspergillus niger, Penicillium notatum, Mucora heimalis and Fusarim oxysporum) in Potato Dextrose broth (PDB, Sigma Co) medium. Under aseptic conditions, one ml of spore suspension (5×10^6 cfu/ml) of each tested fungus was added to 50 ml PDB medium in 100 ml Erlenmeyer flask. Appropriate volumes of tested oils were added to produce concentrations ranging from 10 to 100 µg ml^{-1}. Amphotericin B (Sigma Co., St.

Louis, MA) was used as a reference antifungal drug. All the flaks were incubated at 27 ± 1°C in the dark for 5 days and then the mycelium was collected on GF/C filter papers (5.5 cm in diameter). The mycelium was washed several times with sterile distilled water and placed in a drying oven at 105°C for 24 h. The filter papers were dried to a constant weight and the level of inhibition, relative to the control flasks was calculated from the following formula:

Percentage of inhibition = (C-T)/C × 100;

where T = weight of mycelium from test flasks and C = weight of mycelium from control flasks.

The values of minimal inhibitory concentration (MIC) were determined for testes samples, in which no growth was occurred. Each test was conducted three times and fungi growth was determined after 6 days.

Statistical analysis

All data are expressed as mean values ± standard deviation (S.D). Statistical differences between experimental groups were assessed by analysis of variance (ANOVA), using the COSTAT software package (Cohort Software, CA, USA). The main values were compared with LSD test (P < 0.05).

RESULTS AND DISCUSSION

The yields (g/100g) and total phenolic content in essential oil of cinnamon (C. zeylanicum) and ginger (Z. officinale) are given in Table 1. The yields of cinnamon and ginger oils were found to be 0.96 and 0.85%, respectively. These levels were found to be similar to that found in the literature (Massada, 1976). Also, as shown in Table 1, cinnamon oil was characterized by relatively high amounts of phenolic content (18.2% of oil, expressed as eugenol equivalent). While, ginger oil had lower phenolic content (= 1.2% of oil). Our results are in good agreement with the findings of Massada (1976), who reported that the essential oil of cinnamon bark have lower amount of phenolic compounds than that in leaf oil (ranging from 80 to 87% of the oil, as eugenol).

Chemical composition of ginger and cinnamon essential oils are presented in Table 1. Twenty seven and thirty five compounds accounting for 98.58 and 99.42%, respectively of the oils were identified with the aid of TLC and GC-MS analytical methods and literature comparison. Cinnamon oil was characterized with high amounts of oxygen-containing monoterpenes (69.65% of the total oil). Of which, cinnamyl aldehyde (45.13%), cinnamyl alcohol (5.13%), eugenol (7.47%), methyl-eugenol (5.23%), ethyl-cinnamate (3.86%) and dihydro-eugenol (3.31%) were found to be main components of the CEO.

Furthermore, some interesting oxygenated monoterpenic, that is, 1, 8-cineol (1.01%), nerol (1.06%) and geranial (1.79%) were detected in a minor amounts. Ginger oil showed a great chemical homogeneity characterized by relatively high amounts of sesquiterpene hydrocarbon (92.17%), including β-sesquiphellandrene

Table 1. Qualitative and quantitative composition of ginger (rhizomes) and cinnamon (bark) essential oils.

	Relative area %	
Components	**Ginger**	**Cinnamon**
α-Thafone		0.37
α-pinene	0.1	1.12
Benzaldehyde	-	0.25
Heptanol	-	0.79
Sabinene	-	0.52
1-octen-3-ol	-	0.68
β-pinene	-	0.77
Myrcene	-	0.39
p-cymene	-	0.66
Limonene	5.08	1.48
β-phellandrene	0.12	0.37
1,8-cineole	0.63	1.01
γ-terpinene	Tr.	0.99
Octanol	Tr.	0.33
Linalool	Tr.	0.54
terpinen-4-ol	Tr.	0.38
α-terpineol	Tr.	0.51
trans-carveol	Tr.	0.51
Nerol	0.25	1.06
Neral	Tr.	1.16
Geraniol	Tr.	0.78
Geranial	0.23	1.79
neryl acetate	Tr.	0.89
Trans- Cinnamaldehyde	-	45.13
Cinnamyl alcohol	-	5.13
Eugenol	-	7.47
Dihyroeugenol	-	3.31
Ethylcis-cinnamate	-	3.86
t-Methyl cinnamate	-	2.19
Cinnamyl alcohol	-	8.21
Methyl eugenol	-	5.23
Isoeugenol	-	1.59
Cis-Caryophyllene	15.29	Tr.
t-Cinnamic acid	-	0.41
Cinnamyl actate	-	0.21
α-Caryphyllene	Tr.	Tr.
E-ethyl cinnamate	Tr.	0.73
G-epi-Caryophyllene	Tr.	-
γ-Curcumene	Tr.	-
Ar-Curcumene	6.62	-
α-Zingiberene	13.97	-
Apo Farnesal-2-dihydro	5.08	-
α-(Z) Bisabolene	7.84	-
α-(E,E) Farnesene	10.52	-
β-Bisabolene	3.34	-
β-Sesquiphelladrene	25.16	-
γ-Bisabolene (Z)	4.35	-
Total of identified compounds	98.58	99.42
Oil yield (g/100g)	0.96	0.85

[a] Identification based on retention time authentic sample and mass spectrum data. [b] Trace: relative area % is less than < 0.05%.

(25.16%), cis-caryophyllene (15.29%), zingiberene (13.97%), α-farnesene (10.52%), α- (7.84%) and β-bisabolene (3.34%) and other. Also, both oils were contained a minor amounts of (1.48 - 5.08%) limonene (unique monoterpene hydrocarbon). Several studies have shown that cinnamon and ginger essential oils are very complex mixtures of compounds and many variations have been found in the chemical composition (Singh et al., 2008; Felipe et al., 2008; Wang et al., 2009). For instance, Jham et al. (2005) reported cinnamaldehyde (75%) as main constituents in cinnamon, while zingiberene (ZB) and β-sesquiterpene were found as major main components in ginger essential oil, ranged from 10 to 60% (Wohlmuth et al., 2006; Felipe et al., 2008).

In general, a literature search revealed cinnamaldehyde , cinnamyl alcohol, eugenol, methyl-eugenol and ethyl-cinnamate and β-sesquiphellandrene, cis-caryophyllene and zingiberene are the main constituents of cinnamon and ginger essential oils, respectively (Kaul et al., 2003; Pauli, 2008; Singh et al., 2008; Wang et al., 2009). On the other hand, based on a quantitative analysis, the amounts of some main compounds calculated in our present results are out the range generally identified in other reports (Vernin and Parkanyi, 1994; Raina et al., 2001; Singh et al., 2007). For example, a relatively high amount of eugenol was found as predominant components (> 85% of the oil) in cinnamon leaf oil, whereas trans-cinnamaldehyde was not detected (Singh et al., 2007). Singh et al. (2008) identified geranial (25.9%) as the major constituent in ginger oil, but it was detected in trace amount (0.78%) in our study.

Such variations in the chemical composition of distilled oils is known to differ considerably not only due to the existence of different subspecies, but also might be attributed to the varied agroclimatic condition (climatic, seasonal, geographic) of the regions, stage of maturity, adaptive metabolism of plants, distillation conditions, the plant part analyzed and some other factors (Anwar et al., 2009; Abd El Baky and El Baroty, 2008; Singh et al., 2008; Wang et al., 2009).

Antioxidant activity

It is known that free radicals are involved in the process of lipid per-oxidation and play a cardinal role in numerous chronic diseases such as cancer and coronary heart disease (Halliwell and Gutteridge, 2000). Thus, the ability to scavenge free radicals is an important antioxidant property in order to minimize oxidative cellular damage. Since, in a series of *in vitro* tests the essential oils from spices and medicinal plants exhibited remarkable antioxidant activity (Abd El-Baky and El-Baroty, 2008; Anwar et al., 2009).

Rapid TLC-screening assay

Antioxidant property of CEO and GEO was tested with a

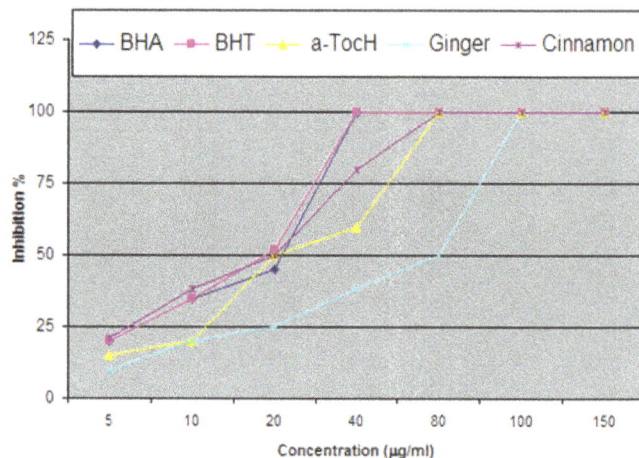

Figure 1. Effect of ginger and cinnamon essential oils on bleaching β-carotene/linoleic acid.

rapid and simple TLC screening based on decolorization of either DPPH radical (DPPH-TLC) or β-carotene/linoleic acid (C-TLC) reagent (Abd El-Baky et al., 2009). In both assays, bands of R_f = 0.56, 0.43 and 0.37 for cinnamon oil, corresponded to authentic volatile compounds of cinnamaldehyde, eugenol and methyl-eugenol exhibited remarkable antioxidant activity. Whereas, for ginger oil bands of R_f = 0.77 and 0.67 corresponded to sesquiphellandrene and caryophyllene showed a moderate antioxidant activity. Therefore, the most antioxidant activity in CEO appears to derive from phenolic components and other constituents are believed to contribute little effect.

β-carotene bleaching (BCB) in aqueous model system

The potency of the cinnamon (CEO) and ginger (GEO) essential oils on antioxidant activity (AA%) in emulsions, accompanied with coupled oxidation of β-carotene and linoleic acid was determined, by follow up the rate of β-carotene bleaching (Figure 1). GEO, CEO and α-TOC, BHT and BHA possessed an antioxidant activity with AA% values of 66.5, 82.3, 75.4, 74.4 and 81.2%, respectively. Hence, GEO (66.5%) showed a lower antioxidant activity than that shown by CEO (82.3%). Therefore, CEO exhibited an obvious antioxidant activity, by inhibiting the β-carotene bleaching due to retarding/inhibiting of linoleic acid hyderoperoxide-derived, which attack the chromophore-β-carotene. This revealed that the hyderoperoxide produced from linoleic acid auto-oxidation as free radicals will be neutralized by cinnamon oil. Thus, the degradation rate of β-carotene depends on the antioxidant activity of the oils. However, the order of antioxidant activity, expressed as the relative inhibition percentages (1%, of β-carotene oxidation), offered by

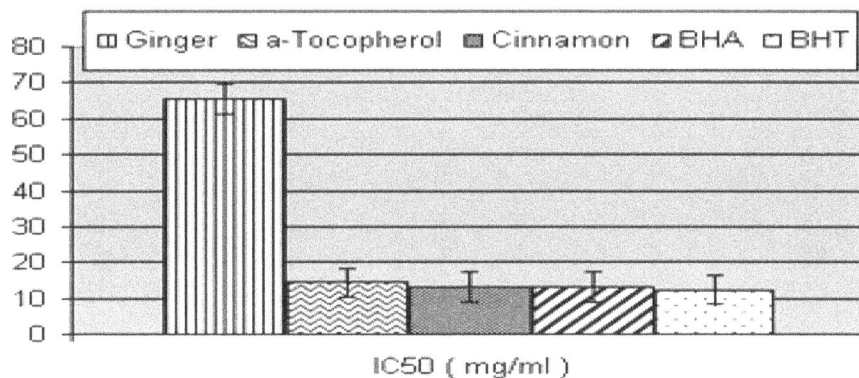

Figure 2. Scavenging activity of ginger and cinnamon essential oils on DPPH• radical.

essential oils and various commercial antioxidant were as follows: BHT = CEO > BHA > α-tocopherol > GEO. Thus, CEO had strong antioxidant capacity compared to synthetic antioxidants (BHT and BHA). These findings indicate that the antioxidant activity of CEO could be mainly attributed to its major compounds, which may be act as chain-breaking antioxidants (Farag et al., 1989 b, c; Abd El-Baky and El Baroty, 2008).

Free radical scavenging activity (FRSA)

In the DPPH assay the ability of CEO and GEO to act as hydrogen donors for transformation of DPPH into its reduced form DPPH-H was done in comparison with those of BHA, BHT and α-TOC. As shows in Figure (2), all tested samples exhibited good radical scavenging activity (FRSA) with varied degrees. The highest FRSA was shown by CEO, with IC_{50} of 13.1 µg/ml, compared to the values of 14.4, 12.2 and 13.1 µg/ml for α-TOC, BHT and BHA, respectively. GEO offered lower antioxidant activity (IC_{50} = 65.5 µg/ml) compared with the CEO. Thus, cinnamon oil had high potential DPPH radical scavenging activity and was similar to those of synthetic antioxidants. Overall, the protection of β-carotene from oxidation and radical scavenging activity of test samples increased in the order: GEO < α - TOC < BHA = CEO < BHT. Looking at the effects of cinnamon oil in different assays one would conclude that CEO contains relatively high amounts of phenolic compounds (18.2%, of the oil), their phenolic group plays an important role in antioxidant activity, which act as hydrogen donor. There are many reports emphasize that the positive correlation between volatile phenolic compounds in the essential and its antioxidant activity (Farag et al., 1989 [a]). On the other hand, the antioxidant activities observed in ginger oil could be due to the synergistic effect of two or more compounds present in it. However, Singh et al. (2008) identified some phenolic compounds in ginger oil such as shogaols, zingerone, gingerols and gengerdiols, as minor

component (< 2 % of oil). Herein, ginger oil consist of a very complex mixture of various classes of organic compounds (Table 1), which may produce either synergistic or antagonistic effects on the process of lipid oxidation or scavenging of radicals.

Antibacterial activity

The antibacterial activity of the essential oils cinnamon and ginger as well as chloramphenictol (antibiotic standard) against selected bacterial strains was assessed (Table 2). The results from the disc diffusion method revealed that both oils showed significant antibacterial activity toward all tested strains. The zone of inhibition was found to be 10 and 18 mm in diameter at doses of 1 and 5 mg/disc of CEO and GEO, respectively, for all tested bacterial strains (data not shown). However, this activity seemed to be lower than chloramphenicol (inhibition zone 14 -18 mm, at 2 mg/disc). Furthermore, the antibacterial activity of both oils quantitatively was assessed by determination of minimum inhibitory concentration. Cinnamon oil exhibited strong inhibitory action against all tested bacteria with MIC values ranged from 20 to 25 µg/ml), followed by ginger oil (MIC 90 to 120 µg/ml). However, the anti`bacterial activity of both essential oils was found to be concentrations depended. In general, antibacterial activity of cinnamon bark oil (MIC= 20 to 25 µg/ml) is comparable with the antibiotic standard, chloramphinicol (MIC= 18 µg/ml).

The essential oils of ginger and cinnamon essential oils revealed a high antibacterial activity against strains *B. subtilis*, *S. aureus* and *K. pneumoniae* as it was characterized by TLC-bioautotography and disc diffusion methods. For cinnamon essential oils, the most active compounds which induce large clear inhibition zones on TLC plate had R_f values of 0.56, 0.43 and 0.37 correspond to cinnamyl aldehyde, eugenol and methyleugenol as it was determined by GC/MS. Whereas, for

Table 2. Inhibition % and minimum inhibition concentration of ginger and cinnamon essential oils against the selected fungal strains.

Fungus strains	Ginger oil (µg/ml)						Cinnamon oil (µg/ml)						Amphotericin B
	10	25	50	75	100	MIC	10	25	50	75	100	MIC	MIC
A. niger	32	65	93	100	100	70	26	54	78	93	100	100	30
M. hemalis	34	62	90	100	100	75	27	58	80	95	100	100	30
F. oxysporum	36	60	93	100	100	75	24	53	75	92	100	100	30
R. stolonifer	35	60	90	100	100	75	26	57	82	96	100	100	25

Values represent the mean of three replicates and rebated three times MIC: Minimum inhibition concentration, values given as µg/ml for samples and for amphotericin B.

ginger oil, bands at R_f 0.77, 0.67 and 0.46 were found to correspond to sesqui-caryophellene and limonene.

Furthermore, those compounds were confirmed with GC-MS analysis. Thus, these findings emphasize the main compounds were mainly contributor to the antibacterial property of these oils. Our results also are comparable with the several investigations (Baratta et al., 1998; Senhaji et al., 2007; Ali et al., 2005). They found cinnamon and ginger essential oils exhibited an inhibitory effect against a wide range of pathogenic bacterial and fungi, and their effect were probably due to their main components in both oil.

Antifungal activity

The inhibitory effect of cinnamon (CEO) and ginger (GEO) essential oils on four fungal strains A. niger, P. notatum, M. heimalis and F. oxysporum were assessed. The results are presented in Table 2. CEO and GEO (in parentheses) at dilutions 10, 25, 50, 75 and 100 µg/ml inhibited the growth of the common spoilage fungus A. niger with 26 (32), 54 (65), 78 (93), 93 (100), 100 (100%), respectively. Thus, CEO and GEO completely inhibited (MIC=100%) the growth of A. niger at 75 and 100 µg/ml doses, respectively. Moreover, CEO and GEO oils showed similar inhibitory effect against P. notatum, M. heimalis and F. oxysporum. In general, on the bases of MIC values, CEO had stronger antifungal activity against tested fungi than that of GEO. However, antifungal activity of cinnamon and ginger essential oils is comparable with the standard drug, amphotericin B.

It appears that there is a relationship between the chemical constituents of oils and its antimicrobial activity. The cinnamon oil containing high amounts of phenolic compounds (18.2%), while ginger oil was rich in sesquiterpene hydrocarbons. Because both oils had a different chemical profiles, difference in antimicrobial activity could be expected. It has been reported that cinnamon (rich in eugenol and cinnamaldehyed) and ginger (rich in sesquiterpenes) essential oils possessed a wide spectrum of antimicrobial activity (Baratta et al.,

1998; Singh et al., 2005; Ali et al., 2005; Senhaji et al., 2007, Anwer, 2009). These results corroborated with the earlier reported data of Daw et al., (1994) and Farag et al. (1989b). They stated that the antimicrobial activity of volatile constituents was decreased in the decreasing order: phenols (highest active)> alcohols > aldehydes > ketones > ethers > hydrocarbons. Generally speaking, the extract of antimicrobial mechanism of essential oils has not been completely elucidated. However, it has been proposed that lipophilicity or hydrophobicity and chemical structure of essential oils or their main compounds such as the presence of functional polar groups and aromaticity could play an important role for the antimicrobial activity (Farag et al., 1989b; Daw et al., 1994), which enable them to partition between lipids of the bacterial or fungal cell membrane and mitochondria, disturbing the cell structures and rendering them more permeable, which will lead to cell death (Sikkema et al., 1994). Thus, as can be seen from Table 1, some of the major components present in cinnamon (CA and eugenol) and ginger oils can penetrate the membrane of the microorganisms and react with the membrane enzymes and proteins as well as phospholipids bilayer, which cause an impairment of microbial enzyme system and/or disturb genetic material functionality (Farag et al., 1989 b, c; Abd El-Baky and El-Baroty, 2008; Conner, 1993). Bang et al. (2000) reported that cinnamon oil contain high amount of cinnamaldehyde (CA), which inhibited the fungal-cell-well synthesizing systems through the reaction with sulfhydro groups present in active site of these enzymes. Therefore, the bioactivity of essential oils is dependent not only on the major compounds but also on the chemical structures of these compounds (Farag et al., 1989 b, c).

This study high light on the potential use of cinnamon and ginger essential oils in ethno-medicine as a preventer of cellular damage, and in food industries as preserver of foodstuffs against spoilage bacteria and fungi. Also, the both oils and bioactive components could be employed as natural food preservatives, preventing lipid peroxidation, which could cause food spoilage (at concentration levels 20 - 100 µg/ml), besides its traditional uses.

REFERENCES

Abd El-Baky HH, El Baz FK, El-Baroty GS (2009). Natural preservative ingredient from marine alga *Ulva lactuca* L. Int. J. Food Sci. Technol., 44: 1688-1695.

Abd El-Baky HH, El-Baroty GS (2008). Chemical and biological evaluation of the essential oil of Egyptian *Moldavian balm*. Int. J. Essential Oil Therap., 2: 76-81.

Adams RP (2007). Identification of Eessential Oils Components by Gas Chromatography/Quadruple Mass Spectroscopy, 4th edition. Allured Publishing Corporation, Carol Stream, Illinois, USA.

Ali SM, Khan AA, Ahmad I, Musaddiq M, Ahmed K, Polase H, Rao LV, Habibullah CM, Sechi LA, Ahmed N (2005). Antimicrobial activities of eugenol and cnnamaldehyde against human gastric pathogen *Helicobacter pylori*. 9doi: 10.1186/1476-0711-4-20. Ann. Clin. Microbiol. Antimicrob., 4: 20.

Anwar F, Ali M, Hussain AI, Shahid M (2009). Antioxidant and antimicrobial activities of essential oil and extracts of fennel (*Foeniculum vulgare* Mill.) seeds from Pakistan. Flav. Frag. J., 24: 170-176.

Bang KH, Lee DW, Park HM, Rhee YH (2000). Inhibition of fungal cell wall synthesizing enzymes by trans-cinnamaldeyyde. Biosci. Biotechnol. Biochem., 64: 1061-1063.

Baratta MT, Dorman HJ, Deans SG, Figueiredo AC, Barroso JG, Ruberto G (1998). Antimicrobial and antioxidant properties of some commercial essential oils. Flav. Frag. J., 13:235-244.

Conner DE (1993). Natural occurring compounds. In: Antimicrobial in food, Davidson P. M.; Branan A. L. (eds.). Marcel Dekker Inc., New York, pp. 441-468.

Daw ZY, EL-Baroty GS, Mahmoud AE (1994). Inhibition of *Aspergillus parasiticus* growth and aflatoxin production by some essential oils. Chem. Mikrobiol. Technol. Lebensm., 16(5/6): 129-135.

Farag RS, Badei AZM, Hewadi FM, EL-Baroty GS (1989[a]). Antioxidant activity of some spice essential oils on linoleic acid oxidation in aqueous media. Am. Oil. Chem. Soc., 66: 792-799.

Farag RS, Daw ZY, Hewadi FM, EL-Baroty GS (1989[c]). Antimicrobial activity of some Egyptian spice essential oils. J. Food Protection, 52: 665-667.

Farag, R.S.; Daw, Z. Y.; Abo-Raya, S. H. (1989[b]). Influence of some essential oils on *Aspergillus parasiticus* growth and aflatoxins production in a synthetic medium, J. food Sci., 54: 74-67.

Felipe CF, Kamyla SF, André L, José NSB, Manoel AN, Marta MF, Glauce SV (2008). Alterations in behavior and memory induced by the essential oil of *Zingiber officinale* Roscoe (ginger) in mice are cholinergic-dependent. J. Medicinal Plants Res., 2(7): 163-170.

Geiger JL (2005). The essential oil of ginger, *Zingiber officinale,* and anaesthesia. Int. J. Aromather., 15: 7–14.

Gurdip S, Kapoor IPS, Pratibha S, De Heluani CS, Marina PD, Cesar ANC (2008). Chemistry, antioxidant and antimicrobial investigations on essential oil and oleoresins of *Zingiber officinale*. Food Chemical Toxicol., 46(10): 3295-3302.

Halliwell B, Gutteridge JMC (2000). Free Radicals in Biology and Medicine. Oxford University Press, Oxford.

Jaime L, Mendiola JA, Herrero M, Soler-Rivas C, Santoyo S, Senorans FJ, Cifuentes A, Ibanez E (2005). Separation and characterization of antioxidants from *Spirulina platensis* microalga combining pressurized liquid extraction, TLC, and HPLC-DAD. Sep. Sci., 28: 2111–2119.

Jham GN, Onkar DD, Carolina MJ, Vânia MMV (2005). Identification of the major fungitoxic component of cinnamon bark oil. Fitopatol. Bras., 30(4): 404-407.

Kaul PN, Bhattacharya AK, Rao BRR, Syamasundar KV, Ramesh S (2003). Volatile constituents of essential oils isolated from different parts of cinnamon (*Cinnamomum zeylanicum* Blume). Journal of the Sci. Food Agric., 83: 53-55.

Massada Y (1976). Analysis of Essential Oils by Gas Chromatographyn and Mass Sepectrometry. Wiley, New York. USA.

NCCLS (1990). Performance for intimicrobial Disc susceptibility test, 4 th ed. Approved Standard. NCCLS Decument M2-A4. The National Committee for Clinical Laboratory Standards, Villanova PA.

Pauli A (2008). Relationship between lipophilicity and toxicity of essential oils. Int. J. Essential Oil Therapeut., 2: 60-68.

Raina VK, Srivastava SK, Aggraval KK, Ramesh S, Kumar S (2001). Essential oil composition of *Cinnamon zeylanicum* Blume leaves from little Andaman, India. Flav. Frag. J., 16: 374-376.

Sabulal B, Dan M, John JA, Kurup R, Purushothaman C, Varughese G (2007). Phenylbutanoid-rich rhizome oil of *Zingiber neesanum* from Western Ghats, Southern India. Flavour Fragrance J., 22(6): 521-524.

Senhaji O, Faid M, Ichraq K (2007). Inactivation of *Escherichia coli* O157:H7 by essential oil from *Cinnamomum zeylanicum*. Braz. J. Infect. Dis., 11(2): 234-236.

Shirwaikar A, Shirwaikar A, Kuppusamy R, Isaac SR (2006). *In Vitro* Antioxidant Studies on the Benzyl Tetra Isoquinoline Alkaloid Berberine. Biol. Pharm. Bull., 29(9): 1906-1910.

Sikkema J, De Bont JAM, Poolman B (1994). Interaction of cyclic hydrocarbons with biological membranes. J. Biol. Chem., 269: 8022-8028.

Singh G, Kapoor IS, Singh P, Heluani CS, Lampasona MP, Catalan CAN (2008). Chemistry, antioxidant and antimicrobial investigation on essential oil and oleoresine of *Zingiber officinale*. Food Chem. Toxicol., 46: 3295-3302.

Singh G, Maurya S, DeLampasona MP, Catalan CAN (2007). A comparison of chemical, antioxidant and antimicrobial studies of cinnamon leaf and bark volatile oils, oleoresins and their constituents. Food Chem. Toxicol., 45: 1650-1661.

Singleton VL, Rossi Jr. JA (1965). Colorimetry of Total Phenolics with Phosphomolybdic-Phosphotungstic Acid Reagents. Am. J. Enol. Vitic., 16(3): 144-158.

Tagashira M, Ohtake Y (1998). A new antioxidative 1, 3- benzodioxole from *Melissa officinalis*. Planta Med., 64: 555-558.

Vernin G, Parkanyi C (1994). Ginger oil (*Zingiber officinale* Roscoe). In Charalambous, G. (Ed.), Spices, Herbs and Edible Fungi. Elsevier Science B.V. pp. 579-594.

Wang R, Ruijiang W, Bao Y (2009). Extraction of essential oils from five cinnamon leaves and identification of their volatile compound compositions. Innovative Food Sci. Emerging Technol., 10: 289–292.

Wohlmuth H, Smith MK, Brooks LO, Myer SP, leach DN (2006). Essential oil composition of diploid and tetraploid clones of ginger (*Zingiber officinale* Roscose) grown in Australia, 54: 1414-1419.

Yu HS, Lee SY, Jang CG (2007). Involvement of 5-HT1A and GABAA receptors in the anxiolytic-like effects of *Cinnamomum cassia* in mice. Pharmacol. Biochem. Behav., 87: 164-170.

17

Purification of a mannose/glucose-specific lectin with antifungal activity from pepper seeds (*Capsicum annuum*)

Adenike Kuku*, Oludele Odekanyin, Kemi Adeniran, Mary Adewusi and Toyin Olonade

Department of Biochemistry, Obafemi Awolowo University, Ile-Ife, Nigeria.

A lectin was isolated and purified from the pepper seeds *Capsicum annuum*. The purification procedure involved anionic exchange chromatography on DEAE – Cellulose and QAE – Sephadex columns followed by gel filtration on Sephadex G–100. The heamagglutinating activity of the lectin towards human erythrocytes was sensitive to inhibition by D-mannose and D-glucose; and enhancement by $CaCl_2$ and $MgCl_2$. The lectin activity was enhanced at very high acidic pH, inhibited at high basic pH but stable at physiological pH range of 6- 8. The lectin was heat stable up to 30 °C. SDS-PAGE of the purified lectin revealed the presence of single band of 25 kDa. The lectin was capable of inhibiting the germination of spores and hyphal growth in the fungi *Aspergillus niger, Aspergillus flavus, Fuscarium solani* and *Fuscarium graminearum*.

Key words: Lectin, pepper, seeds, antifungal, glucose, mannose.

INTRODUCTION

Lectins are proteins that bind mono- and oligosaccharides specifically and reversibly but are devoid of catalytic activity (i.e. are not enzymes) and, in contrast to antibodies, are not products of an immune response (Sharon and Lis, 1989; Rudiger and Gabius, 2001). They are widely distributed in nature and can be found in almost all living organisms including plants, animals (vertebrates and invertebrates), algae, fungi, microorganisms and viruses (Goldstein, 1978; Loris, 2002). Most lectins that have been extensively studied are from plants and have been isolated from several parts such as the seeds, barks, leaves, pollen grains, roots, shoots etc. Over 500 different plant lectins have been isolated and characterrized and these lectins form a heterogeneous group of proteins due to the differences in structure, specificity and biological activities. Although their exact biological roles remain elusive, in many instances, lectins from plants and animals have been extensively exploited as biochemical tools in biotechnology and biomedical research (Van Driessche, 1988). In the last decade, substantial

progress has been made on the understanding of the roles of plant lectins; until recently, the role of most lectins was associated with their binding to foreign glycans in either recognition and/or defense-related phenomena (Petersen *et al.*, 2006; Sahly et al., 2008). Biochemical and molecular studies of numerous lectins demonstrated that only a limited number of carbohydrate-binding motifs evolved in plants and since the specificity of these binding motifs is primarily directed against foreign glycans, it is generally accepted now that many plant lectins are involved in the recognition and binding of glycans from foreign organisms, and accordingly play a role in plant defense (Pneumans and van Damme, 1995; Chen, 2008). Animal and insect studies with purified lectins and experiments with transgenic plants suggested that at least some lectins enhance the plant's resistance against herbivorous animals or phytophagous invertebrates (Carlini and Grossidesa, 2002). The ability of lectins to recognize specific carbohydrates makes them valuable tools for taxonomic studies and the isolation and purification of glycoconjugates (Van Leuven et al., 1993). Lectins extracted from plants may also function as lymphocyte polyclonal mitogens by binding to glycoconjugates on cell surface and thereby activating a series of events that result in cellular activation and proliferation (Sansford and Harris-H,

---

*Corresponding author. E-mail: adenikekuku@yahoo.com, akuku@oauife.edu.ng.

1990; Maennel et al., 1991; Singh et al., 2006; Huang et al., 2008). The biological importance of lectins has increased due to their potential for the purification, selection and cloning of subpopulations of cells involved in normal or pathological immune response (Cunnick et al., 1990; Tietz et al., 1991).

Over the past few years, evidence has accumulated to support the idea that when plants are stimulated by specific biotic or abiotic stimuli they respond through the expression of cytoplasmic and/or nuclear plant lectins. The location and the regulation of the expression of these lectins indicate that lectins are involved in specific endogenous protein–carbohydrate interactions. These novel findings led to the challenging idea that lectins might be involved in cellular regulation and signaling.

Although capsicum may cause heartburn for many individuals, it's most common oral use is to treat digestive complaints such as colic, gas, indigestion, and poor appetite. Chemicals in capsicum have been shown to increase not only the amount of acid the stomach produces, but also blood flow in the lining of the stomach and intestines. All these effects may improve digestion, but they may also irritate the stomach. The dried fruit is a powerful local stimulant with no narcotic effect. It has proved efficacious in dilating blood vessels and thus relieving chronic congestion of people addicted to drink. The pepper *Capsicum annuum* contains other active ingredients, including oily substances called oleoresins. One of the main oleoresins, capsaicin, is used topically as a counter-irritant, renowned for its extensive application in neuroscience research (Szolcsanyi and Bartho, 2001). Tropical capsaicin has been used to treat arthritis pain and it may also be useful for relieving pain from fibromyalgia and shingles. Some scientific evidence also support its topical use for itching associated with conditions such as psoriasis, but this use is less common (Mason et al., 2004; Kamo et al., 2008).

The fruit, raw or cooked is very hot and normally used as flavouring. The fruit can be dried and ground into a powder for use as flavoring. The seed can be dried, ground and used as pepper while the leaves can be cooked as a potherb.

This study aims at extracting and purifying a lectin from the seeds of dry pepper, *Capsicum annuum,* characterize the protein as well as investigate its antifungal activities.

MATERIALS AND METHODS

Crude extraction

Dried short pepper *Capsicum annuum* was purchased from a local market. The seeds were removed, weighed, and soaked in distilled water for 5 days before homogenization in distilled water, adjusted to pH 9. The homogenate was filtered through cheesecloth and allowed to stand at 4°C overnight. The suspension was centrifuged at 10,000 x g for 30 min and the resulting supernatant which constitutes the crude extract was lyophilized.

Protein concentration

The lyophilized powder was dissolved in 50 mM NH_4HCO_3 pH 9.2 (crude extract) and the protein concentration was determined by the method described by Gornall et al., 1949) using bovine serum albumin (BSA) as standard.

Purification of lectin

10 ml of the extract was applied to a column of DEAE- Cellulose (1.5 x 20 cm). After elution of unadsorbed proteins, the column was eluted sequentially with 200 mM, 300 mM and 500 mM NH_4HCO_3, pH 9.2. The fractions were tested for heamagglutinating activity and the active fractions were pooled and applied to a QAE -Sephadex column (1.5 x 20 cm) previously equilibrated with 10 mM Tris-HCl buffer, pH 7.2. After washing the column with the Tris-HCl buffer, the column was eluted with a linear concentration (0 - 0.1 M) gradient of NaCl in the Tris-HCl buffer. The fractions with hemagglutinating activity were pooled and dialysed and lyophilized and further purified on a Sephadex G-100 column previously equilibrated with 50 mM NH_4HCO_3, pH 9.2. The active peak represented the purified lectin.

Assay for lectin (hemagglutinating) activity

Agglutination of the red blood cells by the crude extract and the various fractions that were obtained during purification was estimated as described by Bing *et al. (*1967).

A serial two-fold dilution of the lectin solution in U-shaped microtitre plates (100 μl) was mixed with 50 μl of a 2% suspension of human erythrocytes in phosphate buffered saline, pH 7.2 at room temperature (the erythrocytes of human blood group A,B and O were fixed with 1% glutaraldehyde). The plate was left undisturbed for 1 h at room temperature in order to allow for agglutination of the erythrocytes to take place. The hemagglutination titre of the lectin expressed as the reciprocal of the highest dilution exhibiting visible agglutination of erythrocytes was reckoned as one hemagglutinating unit. Specific activity is the number of hemagglutination units per mg protein (Wang et al., 2000).

Blood group specificity

The blood group specificity of the lectin was established using red blood cells of different blood groups of the ABO system.

Test of hemagglutination inhibition by various carbohydrates

The hemagglutination inhibition tests to investigate inhibition of lectin-induced hemagglutinations by various carbohydrates were performed in a manner analogous to the hemagglutation test. Serial two-fold dilutions of sugar samples were prepared in phosphate buffer saline (0.2 M initial concentration). All the dilutions were mixed with an equal volume (50 μl) of the lectin solution of known hemagglutination units. The mixture was allowed to stand for 1 hr at room temperature and then mixed with 50 μl of a 2 % human erythrocyte suspension. The hemagglutination titres obtained were compared with a non-sugar containing blank. In this study, the sugars used were: glucose, mannose, cellobiose, galactose, maltose, arabinose, fructose, sucrose, lactose, raffinose, sorbitol, dulcitol and glucosamine-HCl. The minimum concentration of the sugar in the final reaction mixture which completely inhibited hemagglutination units of the lectin sample were calculated (Wang et al., 2000).

Estimation of subunit and native molecular weight

The purified lectin was subjected to sodium dodecyl sulfate-polyacrylamide gel electrophoresis (SDS-PAGE) for molecular weight determination in accordance with the procedure of Laemmli and Favre

(1970) using the following protein markers: α–lactabulmin(14,000), carbonic anhydrase (29,000) glyceraldehyde – 5-phosphate dehydrogenase (36,000), egg albumin (45,000) and bovine serum albumin (66,000). The protein bands were stained with Coomassie Brilliant Blue R, while the presence of covalently bound sugar in the lectin was detected by staining the gels with Periodic acid Schiff reagent (PAS staining) , as described in the Pharmacia Manual of Laboratory Techniques, revised edition (1983).

The native molecular weight was estimated under non-denaturing conditions by gel filtration on Bio gel P-300 column(1.5 x 100 cm) which had been calibrated with molecular weight markers: α–chymotrypsinogen (25,000, 3 mg/ml), thermolysin (37,500, 3mg/ml) ovine albumin (45,000, 3 mg/ml), and bovine serum albumin (66,000, 3mg/ml). One ml of each standard was applied to the column and ran separately using a 10 mM phosphate buffer, pH 7.2 as eluant at a flow rate of 10 ml/h. Fractions of 2.5 ml were collected and the elution was monitored for each protein at 280 nm. The void volume (V_0) of the column was determined using Ferritin (elution monitored at 620 nm).

Effect of temperature on hemagglutinating activity

The effect of temperature on the agglutinating activity of the lectin from *C. annuum* was determined by carrying out assay at different temperatures according to the method described by Patrick *et al.*, (2007). The purified lectin was incubated in a water bath for 30 min at various temperatutres: 10, 20, 30,40,50,60,70,80,90 and 100°C, and then cooled to 20°C. Hemagglutination assay was carried out as previously described.

Effect of pH on hemagglutinating activity

The effect of pH on the activity of the lectin from *C. annuum* was determined by incubating the lectin in the following buffers at different pH values: 0.2 M NaOAc buffer, pH 3 - 6, 0.2 M Tris-HCl buffer, pH 7 - 8, and 0.2 M Glycine NaOH buffer, pH 10 - 12, and assaying for hemagglutinating activity. The control values were the agglutination titre of the lectin in PBS, pH 7.2.

Effect of EDTA and divalent cations

The purified lectin was analysed for metal binding site by demetallizing with EDTA and then incubated in a water bath at 20°C for 30 min in the presence of chlorides of various metals such as KCl, NaCl, $CaCl_2$, $MgCl_2$, $MnCl_2$, $FeCl_2$, $FeCl_3$ and NH_4Cl, all at 25 mM, followed by hemagglutination assay.

The ouchterlony double diffusion experiment

1.5% (w/v) agar solution in PBS containing 0.01% (w/v) sodium azide was prepared. The solution was slowly heated until the agar had completely dissolved and poured into clean Petri dishes. A well was made at the centre of each Petri dish and eight other wells equidistant from the centre were made around it. 100 µl of the samples were dispensed at the centre wells and into the surrounding wells 100 µl of 10 mg/ml of dextrin, 100 mg/ml of dextrin, 10 mg/ml of inulin, 100 mg/ml of insulin, 10 mg/ml of glycogen, 100 mg/ml of glycogen and polysaccharide extract.

Assay for antifungal activity

The assay of the lectin for antifungal activity toward fungal species was carried out in 100 x 15 mm Petri plates containing 10 ml of potato dextrose agar (PDA) (Wang et al., 2004). At the centre of the plate was inoculated the tested fungal mycelia. After the mycelia colony had developed, sterile blank paper disks (0.625 cm in diameter) were placed at a distance of 0.5 cm away from the rim of the mycelia colony. An aliquot (15 µl) of the lectin was added to a disk while 15 µl of the buffer served as control. The plates were incubated at 25°C for 72 h until mycelia growth had enveloped peripheral disks containing the control and had formed crescents of inhibition around disks containing samples with antifungal activity. The zone sizes around each disk were measured. The organisms used for this test were *A. niger*, *Aspergillus flavus* and *Fuscarium spp.*

RESULTS

The phosphate buffered saline extract from *C. annuum* seeds agglutinated non-specifically the human red cells of the A, B and O blood groups. The soluble protein content and the specific activity of the crude lectin extract were 76 (mg/ml) and 2048 (HU/mg protein) respectively. For the purified lectin, the values were 6.5 (mg/ml) and 512 (HU/mg protein) respectively.

The hapten inhibition studies to define the sugar specificities of the crude extract (the phosphate buffered saline extract) of *C. annuum* seeds showed that Glucosamine-HCl, maltose, fructose, sucrose, arabinose, and cellobiose had no effect on the hemagglutinating activity. , dulcitol and sorbitol enhanced the activity of the lectin while galactose, lactose, rhamnose and raffinose slightly inhibited the activity of the lectin. The activity of the lectin was completely inhibited by mannose and glucose with minimum inhibitory concentration of 12.5 mM and 6.25 mM respectively (Table 1).

The elution profile of the ion exchange chromatography of the crude extract on DEAE-Cellulose column is as shown in Figure 1. Three protein peaks were obtained only one of which exhibited haemagglutination activity (D2), this was eluted with 200 mM NH_4HCO_3, pH 9.2. Peak D2 on QAE-Sephadex column was resolved into four protein peaks, with only Peak Q2 exhibiting haemagglutinating activity (Figure.2). Gel filtration of Peak Q2 on Sephadex G-100 column resulted in two peaks. CAL 1 and CAL 2. Lectin activity resided in CAL2 and constituted the homogenous preparation of the pepper seed lectin (Figure 3) which gave a distinct band in SDS- PAGE (data not shown).

The purified lectin sample was found to be heat stable up to 30°C, at incubation temperature of 30 to 40°C, a small decrease in the hemagglutinating activity of the lectin was observed whereas at 50 - 60°C, 50% of the activity of the lectin remained while at 65°C, the activity was completely lost (Table 2). The lectin activity was found to be stable at pH range of 6 - 8. At acidic pH, the activity of the lectin became indiscernible whereas at alkaline pH, the activity declined Table 3. The lectin activity was enhanced by both $CaCl_2$ and $MgCl_2.$

The PAS reaction revealed that the lectin was non glycosylated. The lectin when examined for possible interactions with some polysaccharides by Ouchterlony double diffusion experiment formed precipitin band with dextrin.

The lectin exhibited a strong inhibitory effect on growth

Table1. Sugar inhibition study of hemagglutinating activity.

(sugar in mmol/l)	200	100	50	25	12.5	6.25	3.12	1.56	0.78	PBS
Lactose	-	+	+	+	+	+	+	+	+	+
Glucose	-	-	-	-	-	-	+	+	+	+
Maltose	+	+	+	+	+	+	+	+	+	+
Sorbitol	+	+	+	+	+	+	+	+	+	+
Arabinose	+	+	+	+	+	+	+	+	+	+
Fructose	+	+	+	+	+	+	+	+	+	+
Sucrose	+	+	+	+	+	+	+	+	+	+
Glucosamine-HCl	+	+	+	+	+	+	+	+	+	+
Raffinose	-	+	+	+	+	+	+	+	+	+
Mannose	-	-	-	-	-	+	+	+	+	+
Dulcitol	+	+	+	+	+	+	+	+	+	+
Cellobiose	+	+	+	+	+	+	+	+	+	+
Galactose	-	-	+	+	+	+	+	+	+	+

Note: +, hemagglutinating activity; -, no hemagglutinating activity; PBS, phosphate-buffered saline.

Table 2. Effect of temperature on hemagglutinating activity of CAL.

Temperature (℃)	20	30	40	50	60	65	70	80	90
Hemagglutinating activity (number of units)	64	64	32	8	8	0	0	0	0

Table 3. Effect of pH on hemagglutinating activity of CAL.

pH	3.0	4.0	5.0	6.0	7.0	8.0	10.0	11.0	12.0
Hemagglutinating activity (number of units)	-	-	32	64	64	64	32	2	2

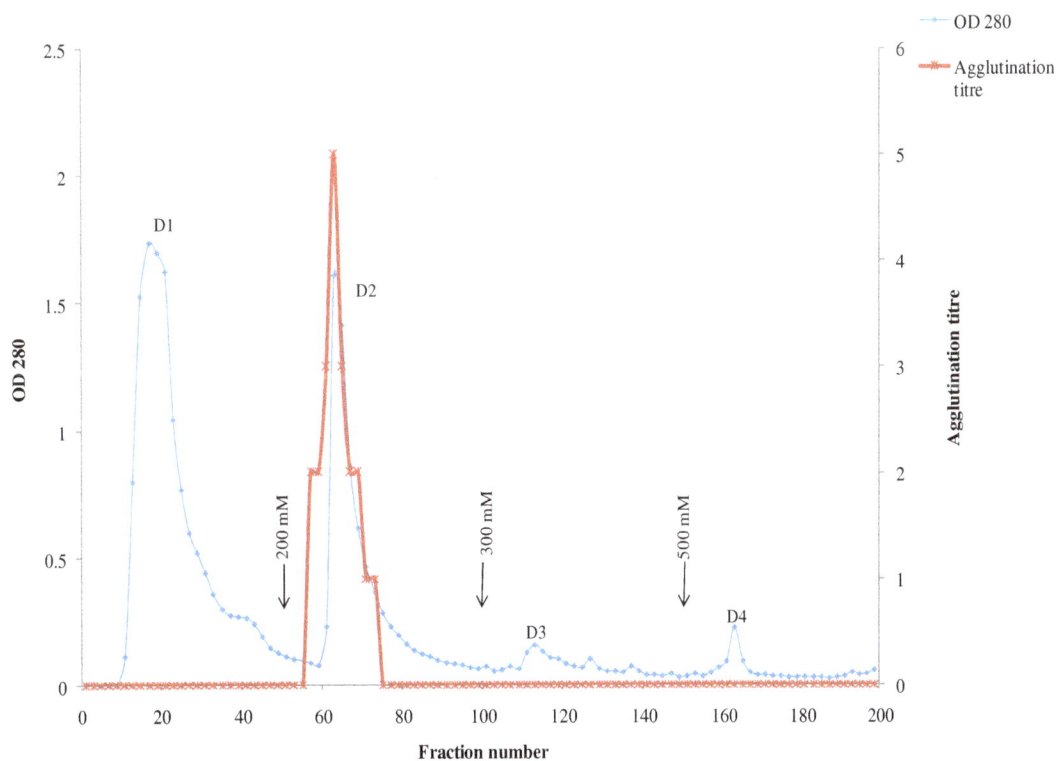

Figure 1. Ion exchange chromatography of *Capsicum annuum* extract on DEAE-Cellulose column.

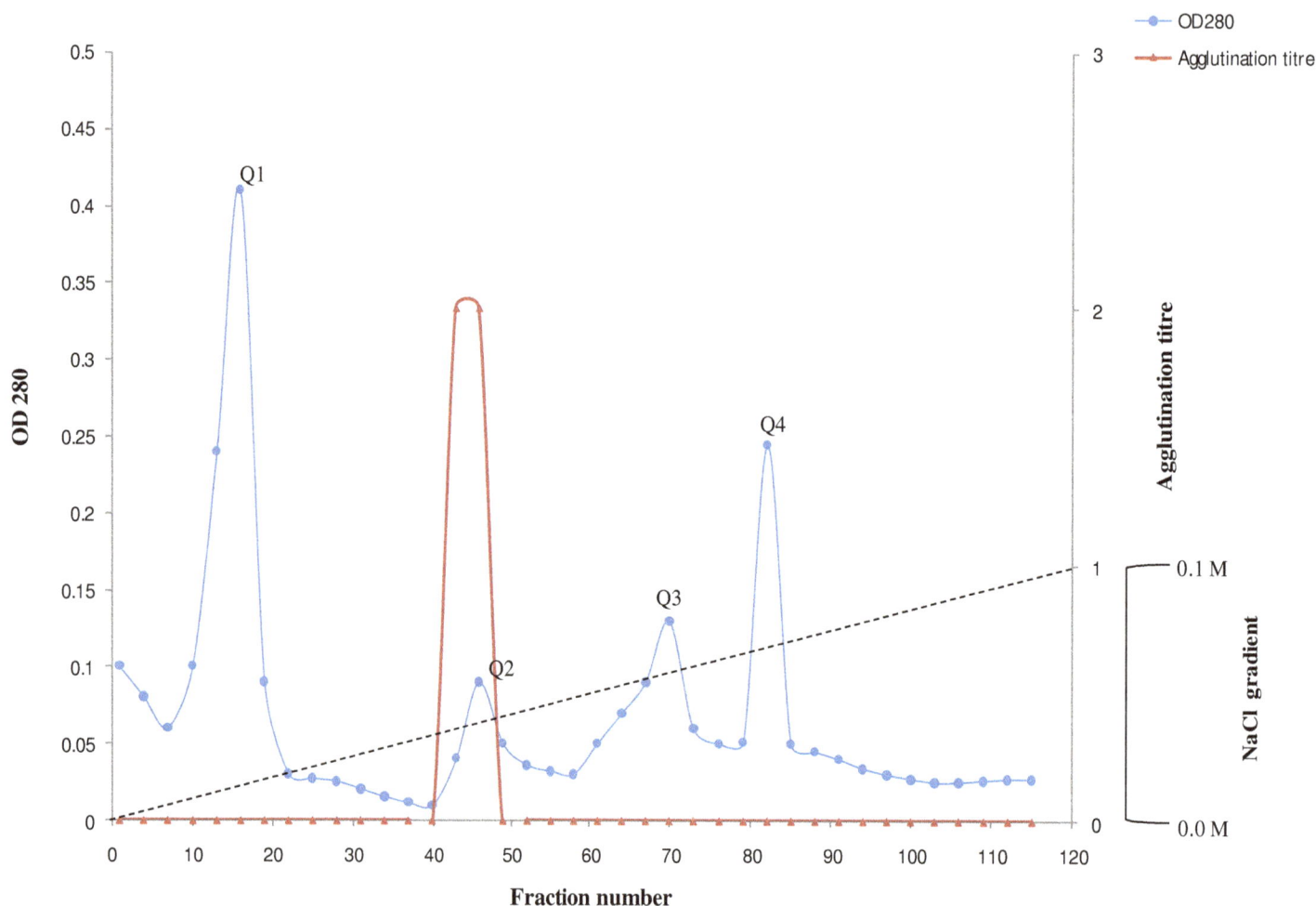

Figure 2: Ion exchange chromatography of Fraction D2 on QAE-Sephadex column.

Column size	1.5 x 20cm
Elution buffer	10mM Tris-HCl buffer pH 7.2
Volume of extract layered	5ml (46mg protein)
Fraction volume	2ml
Flow rate	24ml/h

Protein was eluted with gradient solution of 0 – 0.1M NaCl in Tris-HCl buffer.

Agglutination titre

Absorbance at 280 nm

and spore germination in the fungi, *A. flavus* and *Fuscarium graminearum* while its effect on the other fungal species was insignificant. Inhibition of hyphal growth was 55 ± 5% for *A .flavus* and 70 ± 5% for *F. graminearum* was 70 ± 5% at a dose of 1 mg/ml lectin. The widths of inhibition zone in the spore germination test in the two fungi at 200 µg lectin/ml were 3 ± 0.4 and 5 ± 0.4 mm respectively. (Mean ± SD, n = 3)

DISCUSSION

The data presented from this study showed that the extract of the seeds of *C. annuum* contained a measurable

amount of haemagglutinating protein (lectin). The lectin from *C. annuum* agglutinated red blood cells non-specifically which is typical of many lectins.

The thermostability and pH stability characteristics of lectins are known to differ from lectin to lectin (Patrick and Ngai, 2007) the haemagglutinating activity of this pepper seed lectin is thermostable and pH sensitive. This investigation showed that *C. annuum* was stable in the pH range 6 - 8. Lectins are known to be heat labile and their activity can be decreased by heat treatment (Leiner, 1994). The haemagglutinating activity of lectin from *C. annuum* was heat stable up to 30°C, beyond which the activity started declining, similar observation has been re-

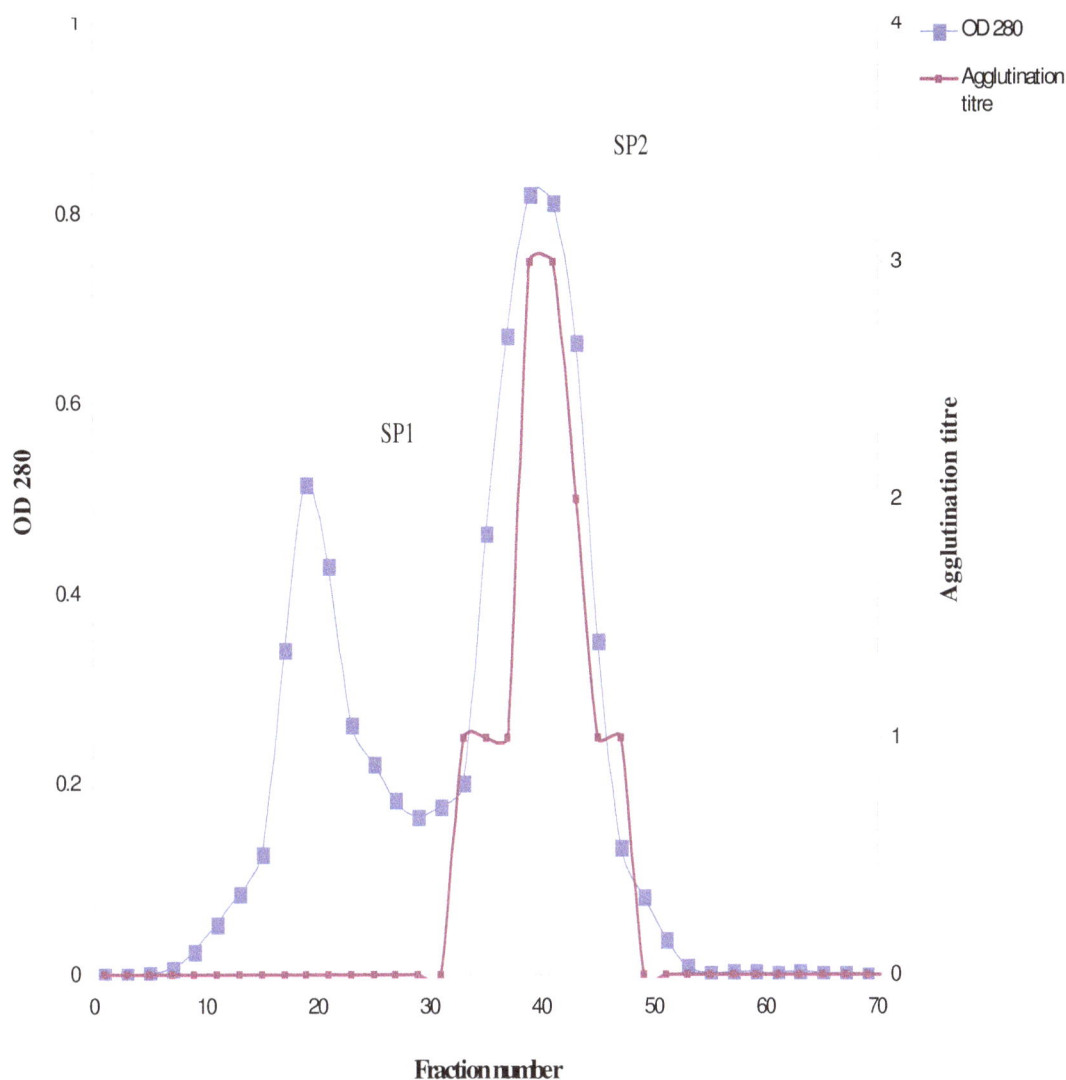

Figure 3: Gel Filtration of Fraction Q2 on Sephadex G-100

Column size	2.5 x 40cm
Elution buffer	50 mM NH_4HCO_3, pH 9.2
Volume of extract layered	10ml (46mg protein)
Fraction volume	2ml
Flow rate	24ml/hr

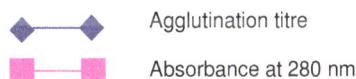

◆——◆ Agglutination titre

■——■ Absorbance at 280 nm

ported for many lectins. Ca^{2+} and Mg^{2+} showed ability to potentiate the activity of the pepper seed lectin which is consistent with the observation with Con A. Polyacylamide gel electrophoresis revealed that the purified lectin was homogenous and has a monomeric structure consisting of a single polypeptide chain, the molecular mass of the seed lectin is similar to that of Con A subunit. A few numbers of lectins with a single polypeptide chain have been reported; for instance, Utarabhand and Akkayanont (1995) reported that *Parkia speciosa* lectin has a single

polypeptide chain, also, the purified lectin from mycelia and fruiting bodies of *Ganoderma lucidum* appeared as a single band on SDS-PAGE (Kawagishi et al., 1997).

The Ouchterlony double-diffusion experiment revealed that there was interaction between the lectin and Dextrin among the polysaccharides tested; failure to form precipitin line with other polysaccharides could however be due to many factors such as the concentration of the protein as well as the molecular size of the polysaccharides. This could also be explained based on the theory that a lectin may either fail to precipitate a polysaccharide or form precipitin bands in agar gel because the lectin may not be specific for that polysaccharide.

There are only a few lectins known to possess antifungal activity such as the lectins from the seeds of *Phaseolus vulgaris* and *Pisum sativum*, from the pepper seed *Capsicum frutescens* and from the mushroom *Astragalus mongholicus* (Ye et al., 2001; Yan et al., 2005; Ngai and Ng, 2007and Sitohy et al., 2007). The lectin from *C. annuum* like the one from *Capsicum frutescens* (Ngai and Ng, 2007) possess antifungal and sugar binding characteristics that make them potentially exploitable and interesting lectins.

REFERENCES

Bing DH, Weyand JG, Satvitsky AB (1967). Hemagglutination with aldehyde-fixed erythrocytes for assay of antigens and antibodies. Proc. Soc. Exp. Biol. Med. 124(4): 1166-1170.

Carlini CR, Grossi-de-sa MF (2002). Plant toxic proteins with insecticidal properties. A review on their potentialities as bioinsecticides. Toxicon 40(11): 1515-1539.

Chen MS (2008). Inducible direct plant defense against insect herbivores: A Rev. Insect Sci. 15: 101-114.

Cunnick JE, Sakamoto K, Chapes S K, Fortner GW, Takemoto DJ (1990). Induction of tumor cytotoxic immune cells using a protein from the bitter melon (*Momordica charantia*) Cell Immunol. 126(2): 278-289.

Gornall AG, Bardawill CJ, David MM (1949). Determination of Serum Proteins by means of the Biuret Reaction. J. Bio. Chem. 177: 751-766.

Huang L, Adachi T, Shimizu Y, Goto Y, Toyama J, Tanaka H, Akashi R, Sawaguchi A, Iwata H, Haga T (2008). Characterization of lectin isolated from *Momordica charantia* seed as a B cell activator. Immunol. Lett. 121(2):148-56.

Kamo H, Honda K, Kitagawa J, Tsuboi Y, Kondo M, Taira M, Yamashita A, Katsuyama N, Masuda Y, Kato T, Iwata K (2008) .Topical capsaicin application causes cold hypersensitivity in awake monkeys. J. Oral Sci. 50: 175-179.

Kawagishi H, Mitsunaga S, Yamawaki M, Ido M, Shimada A, Kinoshita T, Murata T, Kimura A, Chiba S (1997). A lectin from mycelia of the fungus *Ganoderma lucidum*. Phytochem. 44:1-10.

Laemmli UK, Favre M (1993). Maturation of the head of bacteriophage T₄ . DNA packaging events. J. Mol. Biol. 80:573-599.

Liener IE (1994). Implication of antinutritional components in soybean foods. Crit. Rev. Food. Sci. Nutr. 34(1): 31-67.

Loris R(2002). Principles and structure of animal and plant lectins. Biochim. Biophys. Acta. 1572:198-208.

Mäennel DN, Becker H, Gundt A, Kist A, Franz H (1991). Induction of tumor necrosis factor expression by a lectin from *Viscum album*. Cancer Immunol. Immunother. 33(3): 177-182.

Mason L, Moore RA, Derry S, Edwards JE, McQuay HJ (2004). Systematic review of topical capsaicin for the treatment of chronic pain. BMJ: 328:991-998.

Ngai PHK, Ng TB (2007). A lectin with antifungal and mitogenic activities from red cluster pepper (*Capsicum frutescens*) seeds. Appl. Microbiol. Biotechnol. 74: 366-371.

Petersen KA, Matthiesen F, Agger T, Kongerslev L, Thiel S, Cornelissen K, Axelsen M (2006). Phase I safety, tolerability, and pharmacokinetic study of recombinant human mannan-binding lectin. Clin. Immunol. 5: 465–475.

Pneumans WJ, van Damme EJM (1995). Lectins as Plant Defense Proteins. Plant Physiol. 109: 347-352.

Rudiger H, Gabius HJ (2001). Plant lectins: occurrence, biochemistry, functions and applications. Glycoconj J. 18: 589-613

Sahly H, Keisary Y, Crouch E, Sharon N, Ofek I (2008). Recognition of bacterial surface polysaccharides by lectins of the innate immune system and its contrbution to defense against pulmonary pathogens. Infect. Immun. 76, 1322–1332

Sansford GL, Harris-Hooker S (1990). Stimulation of vascular cell prolixferation by beta-galactoside specific lectins. FASEB J. 4(11): 2912-2918.

Sharon N, Lis H (1989). Lectins as Cell Recognition Molecules. Sci. 246: 227-234.

Singh R, Subramanian S, Rhodes JM, Campbell BJ (2006). Peanut lectin stimulates proliferation of colon cancer cells by interaction with glycosylated CD44v6 isoforms and consequential activation of c-Met and MAPK: functional implications for disease-associated glycosylation changes. Glycobiol. 16(7): 594-601.

Sitohy M, Doheim M, Badr H (2007). Isolation and characterization of a lectin with antifungal activity from Egyptian *Pisum sativum* seeds. Food Chem. 104: 971-979.

Szolcsanyi J, Bartho L (2001). Capsaicin-sensitive afferents and their role in gastroprotection: an update. J. Physiol. Paris 95: 181-188.

Tietz HJ, Montag T, Volk HD, Brose E, Gantenberg R, Weichold FF, Hiepe T (1991). Activation of human CD4+ and CD8+ cells by Sarcocystis gigantean lectin. Parasitol. Res. 77(7): 577-580.

Utarabhand P, Akkayanont P(1995). Purification of a lectin from *Parkia javanica* beans. Phytochem. 38: 281-285.

Van Driesche E (1988). Structure and function of leguminosae lectins. In: Advances in Lectin Res. (1):73-135.

Van Leuven F, Torrekens S, Van Damme E, Peumans W, Van den Berghe H (1993) Mannose-specific lectins bind alpha-2-macroglobulin and an unknown protein from human plasma. Protein Sci. 2(2): 255–263.

Wang H, Gao J, Ng TB (2000). A new lectin with highly potent antihepatoma and antisarcoma activities from the oyster mushroom, *Pleurotus ostreatus* Biochem. Biophys. Res. Commun. 275: 810-816.

Yan Q, Jiang Z, Yang S, Deng W, Han L (2005). A novel homodimeric lectin from *Astragalus mongholicus* with antifungal activities. Arch. Biochem. Biophys. 442: 72-81.

Ye XY, Ng TB, Tsang PW, Wang J (2001). Isolation of a homodimeric lectin with antifungal and antiviral activities from red kidney bean (*Phaseolus vulgaris*) seeds. J. Protein Chem. 20: 367-375.

18

Investigation of antimicrobial and plasma coagulation property of some molluscan ink extracts: Gastropods and cephalopods

R. Vennila, R. K. Rajesh kumar*, S. Kanchana, M. Arumugam and T. Balasubramanian

Center of Advanced Study in Marine Biology, Annamalai University, Portonovo, Tamil Nadu, India.

The ink secretion of molluscan species was identified as one of the novel sources of bioactive compounds. Aqueous ink extracts of *Dollabella auricularia* inhibited the growth of Gram-positive and Gram-negative bacteria. In addition to *D. auricularia*, *Octopus vulgaris* and *Sepia aculeate* ink samples showed antifungal activity. The antimicrobial activities of the samples were not due to the presence of protease activity. All tested ink samples were not shown the property of agglutinating chicken erythrocytes. The *D. auricularia* ink fluid was haemotoxic which shows 100% lyses of chicken RBC with the minimum concentration of protein 4.4 µg/ml. In plasma coagulation assay *S. aculeate* ink showed procoagulant property and it coagulated chicken plasma within 180 s; all the remaining samples took more than 5 min for clot formation. Taken together, all these data suggest that, the presence of a number of factors in the ink secretion of mollusk and some of which are proteins in the range from 62 to 249 kDa which are all playing specific roles in the chemical defense mechanism of inking mollusk.

Key words: Anti-microbial activity, aqueous extract, molluscan ink, procoagulant, protease activity.

INTRODUCTION

In nature, animals are provided with their own protective response against their predators, likewise marine mollusks are protected by their shells, but many of them are not fully protected by shells. Chemical defenses are used extensively by both shelled and shell-less mollusks. Among the chemical defenses, a class of defense including sea hares, squid, octopus and cuttlefish, have a striking defensive behavior-releasing ink when attacked. The ink of cephalopods functions as anti predatory visual stimuli either as like distracting "smoke screens" or as decoys. Very few have proposed that the ink of cephalopods contain compounds that are capable of disrupting predator's chemical senses but evidences are not fully recorded (Caldwell, 2005). The defensive secretions of inking mollusks: sea hares and cephalopods

secretions contain millimolar levels of free amino acids (FAA) and ammonium, among the total FAA highest concentration found were taurine, aspartic acid, glutamic acid, alanine and lysine. Fishes and Crustaceans are the major predators of these mollusks and are having specific receptor systems for these FAA (Derby et al., 2007).

Most of the studies concerning antimicrobial activity includes specific compartments like egg masses, hemolymph or whole body extracts of mollusk (Haug et al., 2003). Mollusks not only exhibit the anti-microbial activity, it constitutes many classes of bioactive compounds which includes antitumor, antileukemic and antiviral activities have been reported world-wide (Pettit et al., 1987; Kamiya et al., 1989; Premanand et al., 1997; Rajaganapathy et al., 2000). The sea hare species Aplysia and Dollabella have been reported to contain some biologically active substances, including antibacterial compounds (Faulkner et al., 1973), haemagglutins (Melo et al., 2000), toxic compounds (Kato and Scheruer, 1974), cytotoxic compounds

*Corresponding author. E-mail: rk.rajeshkumar@yahoo.co.in.

(Yamazaki et al., 1990) and substances for chemical defenses (Yamamura et al., 1977). Most of these substances are derived from their algal diets of the sea hares (Kinnel, 1977). The presence of antimicrobial activity has been reported in the digestive gland, albumin gland, egg masses and purple fluid of the Nudibranch (Minale and Riccio, 1976; Kamiya et al., 1989; Yamazaki, 1993). In case of cephalopods, the antimicrobial activity has been reported in the mucous and cuttle bone of the giant snail (Iguchi, 1982; Rajaganapathi, 2001).Other than antimicrobial activity, a novel agglutinin which is responsible for hemagglutination was isolated from the sea hare *A. kurodai*, *A. juliana*, *A. dactylomela*. Apart from ink as a possible first line of defense, sea hares possess a toxic opaline-gland secretion (Ando, 1952) and it has a broad spectrum of algal-derived toxins in the skin and digestive gland (Carefoot, 1987).

The bioactive compounds involved in sensory disruption and phagomimicry include free amino acids (FAA) and ammonium, which are extraordinarily concentrated in ink and opaline of the sea hares (Kicklighter et al., 2005) and various simple amines and paralyzing proteins were found in the cephalopods (Walker and Masuda, 1990; Cariello and Zantli, 1977). In the past few decades, mining of bioactive compounds from marine sources are considered promising because of its rich species diversity. So the present study focuses the antibacterial, antifungal, protease, hamagglutination and plasma coagulation activity of sea hare, octopus, cuttlefish and squid ink extracts.

MATERIALS AND METHODS

Collection of ink samples

Squid (*Loligo duvalucelii*), octopus (*Octopus vulgaris*) and cuttlefish (*Sepia aculeate*) were collected from annankoil landing centre near Portonovo, ink glands were removed and extracted with water. The sea hare (*Dollabella auricularia*) specimens were collected from the region of Gulf of Mannar (Thondi). The ink fluid was obtained by disturbing the animals and extracted with water. All aqueous ink samples were centrifuged at 15,000 g for 15 min and the supernatant was taken and stored in -20°C for further use.

Estimation of protein concentration

Protein concentration was determined by the method of Lowry et al. (1951) using bovine serum albumin (BSA) as a standard. The protein concentration of aqueous extracts of sea hare, squid, octopus, cuttlefish ink samples were 44, 108, 144 and 420 µg/ml respectively.

Microorganisms and inoculum preparation

The microorganisms used in the study were molds (*Fusarium* sp and *Aspergillus fumigatus*) and two strains of Gram positive bacteria *Pseudomonas aeruginosa* and *Staphylococcus aureus*; five strains of Gram-negative bacteria *Vibrio cholerae*, *Salmonella*

paratyphi, *Shigella boydii*, *Shigella dysenteriae*, *Klebsiella pneumoniae*. All microorganisms were clinical isolates, obtained from the Department of Microbiology, Annamalai University, Annamalai Nagar, TamilNadu, India.

Nutrient broth and Sabouraud Dextrose Agar (SDA) were used for growing and diluting the microorganism suspensions. Bacterial strains were inoculated and grown to exponential phase in nutrient broth at 37°C for 18 h and adjusted to a final density of 108 CFU/ml by diluting fresh cultures by comparing with McFarland density. *Fusarium* sp and *A. fumigatus* were aseptically inoculated on Petri plates containing sterile SDA medium. Petri plates were incubated at 28°C for 48 h and the colonies were aseptically sub-cultured on SDA slants. The mold colonies from SDA slants was suspended in sterilized saline and compared with McFarland solution. The final concentration was adjusted to 2×10^7 cells/ml.

Microbial sensitivity test

Inhibition of bacterial growth by the ink samples was determined as described by Bauer et al. (1966). Sterile swabs were immersed in the microbial suspensions (108 cells/ml) and evenly applied to Petri dishes containing Mueller Hinton agar. Sterile whatman No 1 filter paper discs (6 mm in diameter) were fully incubated with 30 µl of the ink samples and placed over the agar in the plates. Erythromycin disc (Himedia, India) and chloramphenicol (Himedia, India) were used as positive control the plates were incubated overnight at 37°C and then examined for zone of growth inhibition around each disc.

Growth inhibition of Mold strains by the ink samples was determined as described by Roberts and Selitrennikoff 1990. Briefly, agar assay plates were prepared by autoclaving potato dextrose agar (PDA). Sterile swabs were immersed in the microbial suspensions and evenly applied to Petri dishes containing PDA. Sterile whatman No 1 filter paper discs (6 mm in diameter) were fully imbibed with 30 µl of the ink samples and placed over the agar surface of the plates. Nystatin (Himedia, India) was used as positive control. Plates were incubated at 37°C for 48 to 72 h and examined as described by the antibacterial assay.

Protease assay

Zymographic method was used to assay the protease activity of the samples. Casein, gelatin were used as substrate and the method was adapted from Heussen and Dowdle (1980). Briefly, 2 mg/ml of casein and gelatin (Himedia, India) was incorporated as a substrate in the 10% of resolving gel with a 5% stacking gel without substrate. Ink samples were mixed with the non-reducing sample buffer and loaded in the gel. The gel was run at 20 mA at 4°C. After electrophoresis, the gel was washed twice with Triton X-100 to remove the SDS for 20 min, then incubated in incubation buffer containing 20 mM Tris-HCl, 0.4 mM calcium chloride pH 7.4 at 37°C for 16 h and stained with Coomassie blue. The clear area in the gel indicates the region of enzyme activity.

Coagulation assay

The effect of sea hare, octopus, cuttlefish and squid ink upon coagulation was accessed using the recalcification time assay (Hougie, 1963) adopted for the SpectraMaxPro microplate reader. In a final volume of 150 µl, 50 µl of citrated chicken plasma was incubated with different amount of ink samples in 90 µl of 20 mM Tris–HCl buffer, pH 7.4. After 5 min at 37°C, 10 µl of 150 mM CaCl₂ was added and clot formation was monitored at 37°C for 20 min in the Spectra Max system at 650 nm. To access calcium independent coagulation activity, EDTA was added instead of CaCl₂, to a final

Investigation of antimicrobial and plasma coagulation property of some molluscan ink extracts...

101

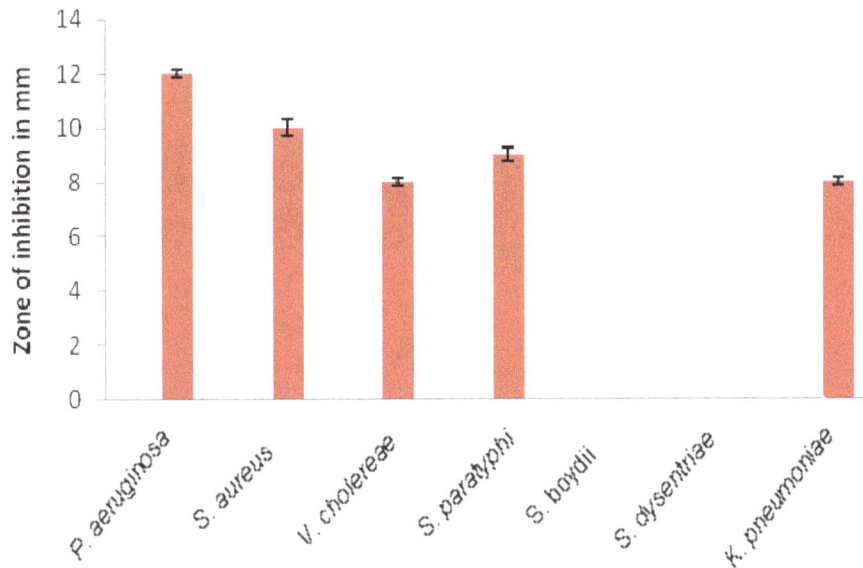

Figure 1. Antibacterial activity of sea hare ink against *P. aeruginosa*, *S.* aereus, *V. cholereae*, *S. paratyphi*, *S. boydii*, *S.* dysenteriae, *K. pneumoniae*.

concentration of 10 mM.

Erythrocyte agglutination assays

The hemagglutinating activity was assayed according to vasconcelos et al. (1994). Briefly 1: 2 serial dilutions of ink in Tris-Cl buffer pH 7.4 was mixed in small glass tubes with 0.25 ml of a 2% suspension of erythrocytes. The extent of agglutination was monitored visually, after the tubes had been left at 37°C for 30 min and subsequently at room temperature for a further 30 min. The results were reported as the number of hemagglutination units (HU) per mg of fluid protein able to induce visible erythrocyte agglutination. One HU was defined as the minimum protein concentration required producing visible agglutination.

Hemolytic assay

Hemolytic activity was assayed on washed chicken erythrocytes as described earlier by Garnier et al. (1995). To 1 ml samples containing various concentration ink protein in 150 mM NaCl, 200 µl of resuspended 2% erythrocytes was added and kept for 30 min at room temperature. The suspensions were centrifuged for 5 min at 3000 rpm. The absorbance of the supernatant was measured at 540 nm to released hemoglobin. A negative control (erythrocyte suspension in 150 mM NaCl) and a positive control erythrocyte suspension in distilled water were prepared to enable the calculation of percentage hemolysis; all assays were carried out in triplicate.

SDS-Polyacrylamide gel electrophoresis

Electrophoresis of the crude ink was carried out by the method of Laemmli (1970) on a 1-mm vertical gel consisted of 5% stacking gel mix, and main running gel mix of 12.0% acrylamide. Ink samples containing 2% SDS and 1% 2-mercaptoethanol were incubated at 100°C for 10 min. A few sucrose crystals were dissolved in the samples before being applied (30 µl) to the gel. Electrophoresis

was carried out at 20-mA constant current for 60 min and protein bands were visualized by staining in Coomasie brilliant blue. Standard molecular weight markers from BANGALORE GENEI size ranging from 29 to 205 kDa were used to determine the molecular weight of individual proteins.

Statistical analysis

Results were expressed as mean ± SD (n-4). One way ANOVA followed by Duncans multiple range test was used to analyze data, using SPSS windows version 11.5 with $p < 0.05$ were considered statistically significant.

RESULTS

Antibacterial activity

Among the four ink samples tested for antibacterial activity against two Gram positive bacteria *P. aeruginosa*, *S. aureus* and five Gram negative bacteria *V. cholerae*, *S. paratyphi*, *S. boydii*, *S. desenteriae*, *K. pneumoniae*. Sea hare ink extract (1.32 µg) showed maximum activity against *P. aeruginosa*, *S. aureus* with growth inhibition of 12 and 10 mm respectively. Similar range of inhibition zone was recorded against *V. cholerae*, *S. paratyphi*, *K. pneumoniae* in which the growth of inhibition was found to be 8, 9 and 8 mm respectively (Figure 1). There was no anti-bacterial activity in the ink extracts of squid, octopus, and cuttlefish against the test organisms. Data were reported as the mean ± SD, which was carried out in duplicate. All strains were sensitive to the control erythromycin (15 mcg/disc) except *S. boydii* and chloramphenicol (30 mcg/disc) were resistant to *P. aeruginosa* and *S. dysenteriae*.

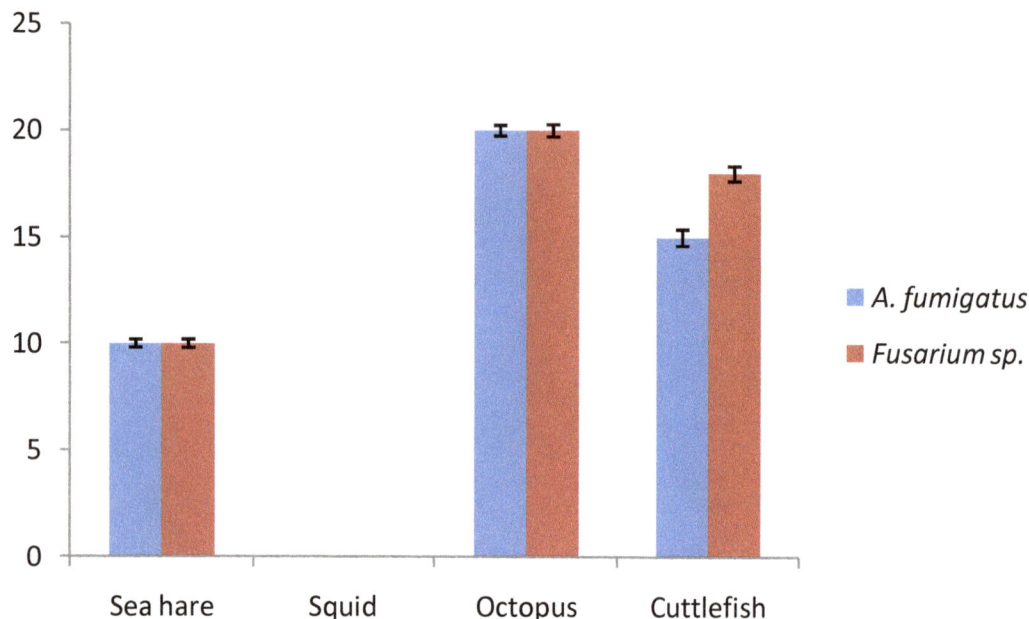

Figure 2. Antifungal activity of sea hare, squid, octopus, and cuttlefish ink against *A. fumigatus* and *Fusarium* spp.

Antifungal activity

The results of antifungal activity of four ink extracts were shown in Figure 2. In the total of four ink samples tested against two fungal strains, the maximum growth inhibition was exhibited by octopus ink with the inhibition range of 20 mm against *A. fumigatus* and *Fusarium* sp and it was followed by cuttlefish with the maximum inhibition zone of 15 and 18 mm against *A. fumigatus* and *Fusarium* sp. The minimum growth inhibition was recorded by sea hare ink against *Fusarium* sp with the growth inhibition zone of 10 mm. Both strains were resistant to squid ink.

Data were reported as the mean ± SD which was carried out in duplicate. The antifungal controls Nystatin inhibited the growth of both Fusarium and *A. fumigatus*.

Protease activity

Protease activity from the four ink sample was analyzed using gelatin and casein as substrate in zymographic method. Protease activity was observed in squid ink in both the substrate zymography. Gelatin and Casein zymograms revealed common protease band with the molecular range from 79 to 249 kDa (Figure 3). The remaining ink samples did not show any protease activity in our experimental condition.

Hemagglutination and hemolytic activity

Molluscan ink extracts did not show hemagglutination

activity on the chicken RBC. The hemolytic property of the ink extracts were tested by using chicken RBC. Among the four inks extracts tested sea hare ink exhibited hemolytic activity. Lyses of erythrocytes by sea hare ink were dose dependent, 2.1 µg of ink protein produced 50% hemolysis and 4.4 µg produced 100% hemolysis shown in Figure 4. Remaining ink samples of squid, octopus and cuttlefishes did not having the hemolytic property.

Plasma coagulation assay

The effect of ink samples on blood coagulation was assessed by the plasma coagulation assay. To analyze the effect of ink samples upon clotting, citrated chicken plasma was incubated with ink samples prior to the induction of coagulation by calcium. From Figure 5, it is clear that the cuttlefish ink showing potent procoagulant effect is capable of shortening the clotting time of human plasma. At the same time, control plasma and other ink samples took more than 5 min to initiate coagulation, after the addition of calcium, plasma incubated with cuttlefish which took around 180 s to start coagulation.

SDS-PAGE analysis

The electrophoretic profile of the ink samples showed the presence of small to high molecular weight protein, upon these some were distinct (Figure 6). Sea hare ink sample has bands ranging from 84 to 237 kDa, octopus has

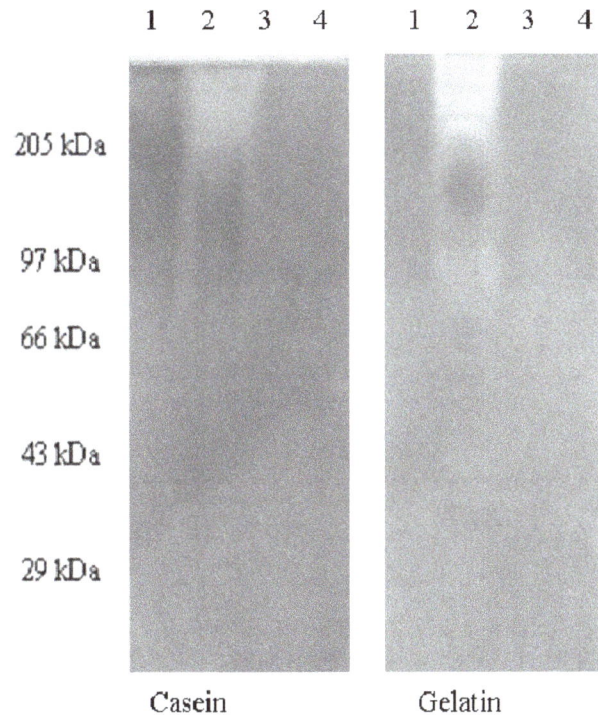

Figure 3. Protease activity: Caesinolytic, gelatinolytic activities of the ink samples were determined using the technique of substrate SDS-PAGE 10%. Number on the left indicate the molecular weight markers. Lane, (1) Sea hare (2) Squid (3) Octopus (4) Cuttlefish. Clear area in the gel indicates the region of protease enzyme activity.

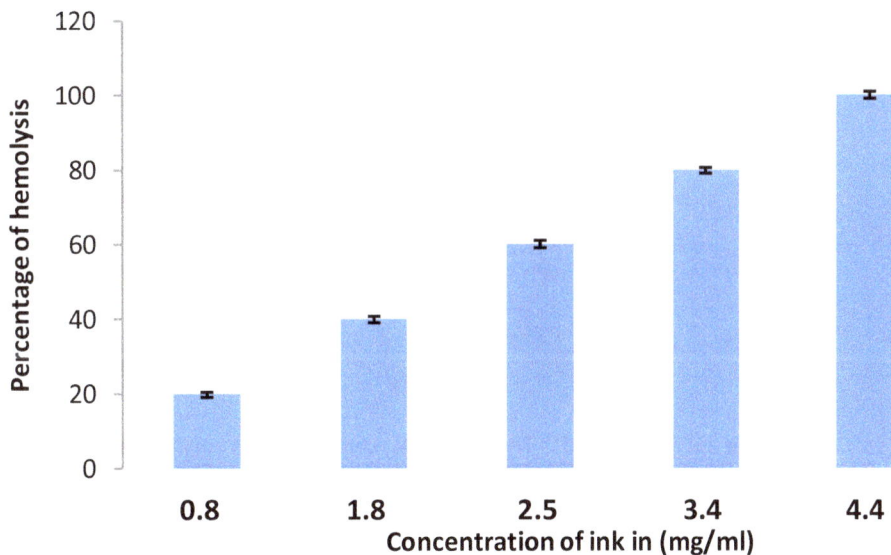

Figure 4. Hemolytic activity of sea hare ink on chicken blood erythrocytes. chicken blood erythrocytes were incubated with increasing concentration of ink sample for 30 min. Release of hemoglobin was determined by measuring the absorbance at 540 nm.

prominent bands from 82 to 248 kDa, squid has bands from 62 to 240 and the cuttlefish having 94 to 240 kDa.

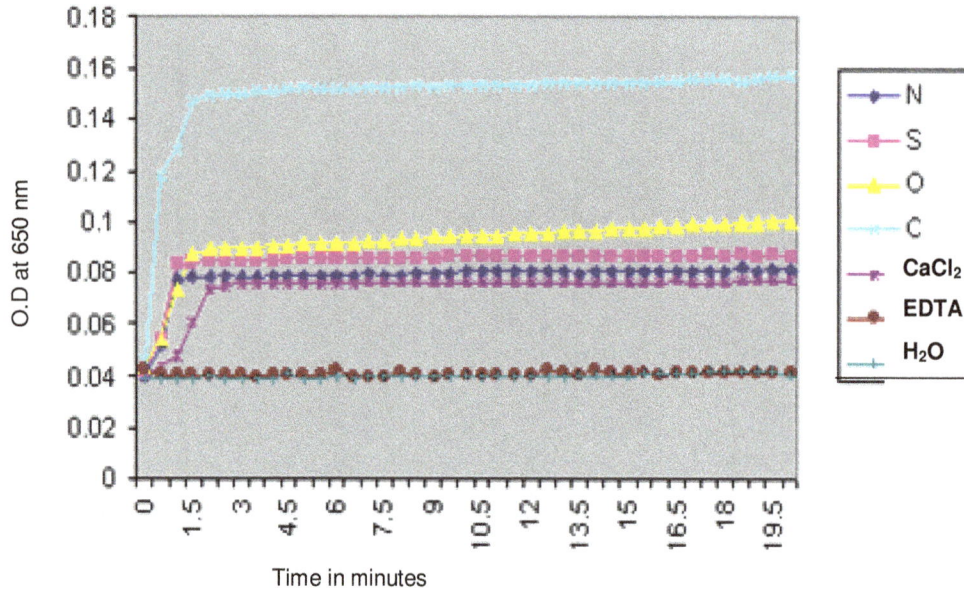

Figure 5. Plasma coagulation assay: The effect of ink sample in the blood coagulation of chicken plasma was monitored at 650nm in SpectraMax system at 650 nm at 37°C. In the experiment plasma incubated with either sea hare,(♦) octopus,(▲) squid (■)cuttlefish (*) ink was added prior to the addition of $CaCl_2$.(x) Plasma incubated with calcium act as control reaction.(●) plasma incubated with EDTA instead of $CaCl_2$. Each values represents mean ± SD of four independent experiments (*P < 0.05).

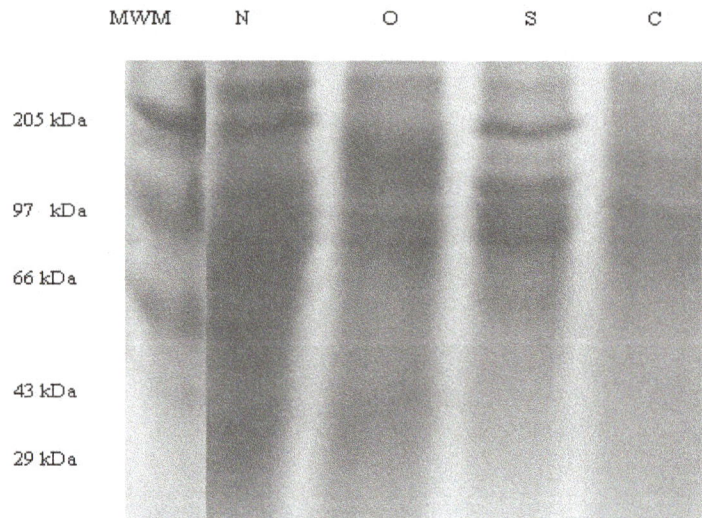

Figure 6. SDS-PAGE: The four ink samples were subjected to electrophoresis in 10% gel. Lane, (1) Molecular weight marker (2) Sea hare (3) Octopus (4) Squid (5) Cuttlefish.

DISCUSSION

Marine mollusks are protecting themselves from predators through their unique way, one of them is releasing ink when disturbed. This ink secretion contains a rich array of chemical secretions to escape from predators. The chemical composition of the ink of all inking mollusk will not be the same. In order to explore the components and its effect on various living systems, we have accessed antimicrobial, protease, hemagglutination, hemolytic, and coagulation assay of the ink samples.

Both Gram positive bacteria as well as Gram negative bacteria showed susceptibility towards the ink extract of sea hare, which showed the zone of growth inhibition ranging from 9 to 12 mm. The inhibition zone for positive control erythromycin and chloramphenicol was ranging from 15 to 35 mm and the discrepancies between the results could be due to aqueous extracts of test samples might have lower concentration of antibacterial compounds. Kamiya et al. (1984) isolated aplysianin-E, an antibacterial glycoprotein from nudibranch Aplysia. Yamazaki et al. (1990) have reported the antibacterial activity of the purple fluid of *Aplysia kurodai*. An antibacterial peptide Dolabellanin-A, was identified and characterized from albumin gland of sea hare, *D. auricularia* (Kisugi et al., 1992).

The results from the present work revealed the strongest antifungal activity of octopus ink with the inhibition zone of 20 mm against *Fusarium* sp and *A. fumigatus* respectively. Cuttlefish ink shows the inhibition zone of 18 and 15 mm against *Fusarium* sp and *A. fumigatus* respectively and minimum activity found in the sea hare ink against *Fusarium* sp. The highest activity in octopus probably may be due to the presence of potential antifungal compound. This result supports the previous work done by the Lane (1962) who reported the antibiotic effects of the fluid from the ink sac of the cephalopods. Iijima et al. (1995) successfully isolated the compound Aplysianin-E from *Aplysia* sp, which inhibit the growth of yeast species- *S. cerevisiae*, *Schizosaccharomyces* sp. and *Candida albicans*. The presence of anti-fungal activity in mollusca has been reported in egg mass of the sea hare *A. kurodai* which inhibited the growth of *C. albicans* (Kisugi et al., 1989b). A potential polysaccharide with potent antifungal activity was extracted from the cuttle bone of *S. aculeata* and Brevimana (Shanmugam et al., 2008).

To determine whether the anti-microbial activity was due to protease activity in the sample, we have conducted the protease zymography analysis. Protease are considered antimicrobial proteins because they are involved in the regulatory production of antimicrobial peptides (Aranishi and Nakane, 1997a,b). Zymography analysis revealed the fact that, anti-microbial property of the ink samples were not primarily due to the protease activity indicating that proteases were not responsible for the activity. Notably squid ink having protease activity which was active on broad range of substrates like casein and gelatin but it did not exhibited other activities.

None of the ink samples showed hamagglutination activity against chicken erythrocytes. A different glycoprotein is responsible for agglutination of erythrocytes. These ink samples may not contain agglutinin proteins to agglutinate chicken erythrocytes. Marine opisthobranch mollusks are able to incorporate and accumulate terpenoid toxin from their algal dietary sources (Wagele et al., 2005). Sea hare ink showed hemolytic activity (Figure 4), this activity possibly may contain terpenoid like toxic compound, which may cause

lyses of chicken RBC. The eunicellin based diterpenes isolated from a Japanese *lipophyton* species showed ichthyotoxic and hemolytic activities (Miyamoto et al., 1994).

Test results of plasma coagulation assay showed the presence of blood clotting factors in cuttlefish ink, which shorten the blood clotting time of chicken blood after the addition of $CaCl_2$, indicating that cuttlefish ink has effect on blood clotting. The result emphasized that the cuttlefish ink having compounds which is calcium dependant procoagulant. This is the first time finding that cuttlefish ink having strongest procoagulant effect which takes only 180 s to clot chicken blood whereas other samples took more than 5 min to clot (Figure 5). Procoagulant activity may be due to presence of compounds which are calcium dependant prothrombin activator (Guerrero et al., 1992). The remaining samples showed only moderate clotting effect which is equivalent to positive control. SDS polyacrylamide gel electrophoresis of aqueous extracts of ink samples (Figure 6) showed the presence of proteins with the molecular weight ranging from 62 to 249 kDa. These proteins may be responsible for various biological activities of the ink samples.

From this study, it is clear that molluscan ink sample contains a large number of compounds with various biological and physiochemical properties. These compounds might be one of the factors which are playing a crucial role in the defensive mechanism of the inking mollusk. The ink samples are having properties like antimicrobial, hemolytic, procoagulant etc. These results give additional support that ink secretions are toxic to lower organisms and source of biologically important compounds for biomedical research.

REFERENCES

Ando Y (1952). Toxicity of Tethys kurodai. Kagaku (Tokyo), 22: 87-88.
Aranishi F, Nakane M (1997a). Epidermal proteinases in the European eel. Physiol. Zool., 70: 563-570.
Aranishi F, Nakane M (1997b). Epidermal proteinases of the Japanese eel. Fish Physiol. Biochem., 16:471-478.
Bauer AW, Kirby WMM, Sherris JC, Turck M (1966). Antibiotic susceptibility testing by a standardized single disc method. Am. J. Clin. Pathol., 45: 93-495.
Caldwell RL (2005). An observation of inking behavior protecting adult Octopus bocki from predation by Green Turtle (Chelonia mydas) hatchlings. Pac. Sci., 59: 69-72.
Carefoot TH (1987). Aplysia: its biology and ecology. Oceanog. Mar. Biol. Ann. Rev. 25, 167–284.
Faulkner DJ, Stallard MO (1973). 7-chloro-3, 7-dimethyl-1, 4, 6-tribuano-1-octen-3-01, A novel monoterpene alcohol from Aplysia californica. Tetrahedron Lett., 14: 1171-1175.
Garnier P, Goudey-perriere F, Breton P, Dewulf C, Petec F, Perriere C (1995). Enzymatic properties of the stonefish (Synanceia verrucosa Bloch and Schneider, 1801) venom and purification of a lethal, hypotensive and cytolytic factor. Toxicol. 33:143-155.
Guerrero B, Arocha-Pinango CL (1992). Activation of human prothrombin by the venom of Lonomia achelous (Cramer) caterpillars. Thromb Res., 66: 169-178.
Haug T, Stensverg K, Olsen O, Sandsdalen E, Styrovld OB (2003). Antibacterial activities in the various tissue of the horse mussel

Modiolus. J. Invertebr. Pathol., 85: 112-119.

Heussen C, Dowdle EB (1980). Electrophoretic analysis of plasminogen in polyacrylamide gels containing sodium dodecyl sulfate and copolymerized substrates. Anal. Biochem., 102: 196-202.

Hougie C (1963). Fundamentals of Blood Coagulation and Clinical Medicine. McGraw-Hill, New York, pp. 25-48.

Iguchi SMM, Aikawa T, Matsumoto JJ (1982). Antibacterial activity of snail mucus mucin. Comp. Biochem. Physiol., 72: 571-574.

Iijima RJ, Kisugi J, Yamazaki M (1995). Antifungal activity of Aplysianin E, a cytotoxic protein of Sea hare (Aplysia kurodai) eggs. Develop. Comp. Immuno., 19: 13-19.

Kamiya H, Muramoto K, Ogata K (1984). Antibacterial activity in the egg mass of a sea hare. Experientia, 40: 947-949.

Kamiya H, Muramoto K, Goto R, Sakai M, Endo Y, Yamazaki M (1989 a). Purification and characterization of an antibacterial and antineoplastic protein secretion of a sea hare, Aplysia juliana. Toxicon, 27: 1269-1277.

Kamiya H, Muramoto K, Goto R, Yamazaki M (1989 b). Characterization of the antibacterial and antineoplastic glcoproteins in a seahare Aplysia Juliana. Nippon Scusan Gkkaishi, 54:773-777.

Kato Y, Scheruer PJ (1974). Aplysiatoxin and debronoaplysiatoxin, constituents of the marine mollusk Stylocheilus iongicauda (Quoy and Gaimard,1824). J. Chem. Soc. 96 (7): 2245–2246.

Kicklighter CE, Shabani SP, Johnson M, Derby CD (2005). Sea hares use novel antipredatory chemical defenses. Curr. Biol., 15: 549-554.

Kinnel R, Duggan AJ, Eisner T, Melnwals J, Miura U (1977). Panacene: an aromatic bromoallene from a sea hare (Aplysia kurodai). Tetrahedron Lett., 18: 3913-3916.

Kisugi J, Ohye H, Kamiya H, Yamazaki M (1989 b). Biopolymers from marine invertebrates. Mode of action of an antibacterial glycoprotein Aplysianin E, from eggs of a sea hare, Aplysiakurodai. Chem. Pharma. Bull., 37(10):2773-2776.

Kisugi J, Ohye H, Kamiya H, Yamazaki M (1992). Biopolymers from marine invertebrates: XIII.Characterization of an antibacterial protein, Dollabellami-A from albumin gland of the sea hare, Dollabella auricularia. Chem. Pharma. Bull., 40(6): 1537-1539.

Lane FW (1962). Economic.In: Kingdom of the octopus, the worlds of science (ecology) pyramid publication, New York, pp. 181-201.

Laemmli UK (1970). Cleavage of structural protein during the assembly of the head of bacteriophage T4. Nature, 227:680-685.

Lowry OH, Rosebrough NJ, Farr AL, Randall RJ (1951). Protein measurement with the Folin phenol reagent. J. Biol. Chem., 193: 265–275.

Minale L, Riccio R (1976). Constituents of the digestive gland of the molluscs of the genus Aplysia –I.Novel diterpenes from Aplysia Depilans .Tetrahedon Lett., 31: 2711-2714.

Miyamoto T, Yamada K, Ikeda N, Komori T, Higuchi R (1994). Bioactive terpenoids from octocorallia,I. Bioactive diterpenoids:Litophynols A and B from the mucus of the soft coral Litophyton sp. J. Nat. Prod., 57: 1212-1219.

Premanand T, Rajaganapathi J, Pattersson Edward JK (1997). Antibacterial activity of marine mollusk from portonovo region. Indian J. Mar. Sci., 26: 206-208.

Rajaganapathi J (2001). Antimicrobial activities of marine mollusk and purification of anti-HIV protein, Ph.d thesis, India.

Roberts WK, Selitrennikoff CP (1990). Zeamantin, an antifungal protein from maize with membrane-permeablizing activity. J. Gen. Microbiol., 136: 1771-1778.

Shanmugam A, Mahalakshmi TS, Barwin V (2008). Antimicrobial activity of Polysaccharides isolated from the cuttle bone of Sepia aculeate and Sepia brevimana: An approach to selected antimicrobial activity for human pathogenic microorganism. J. fish. aquat. sci., 3 (5): 268-274.

Vasconcelos IM, Trentin A, Guimaraes JA, Carlini CR (1994). Purification and physicochemical characterization of soyatoxin,a novel toxic protein isolated from soyabeans (glycine max). Arch. Biochem. Biophys., 312: 357-366.

Wagele H, Klussmann-Kolb A (2005). Opisthobranchia (Mollusca,Gastropoda)–more than just slimy slugs. Shell reduction and its implications on defense and foraging. Front. Zool., 2: 3.

Walker MJA, Masuda VL (1990). Toxins from marine invertebrates. In: "Marine toxin (Origin, Structure and molecular Pharmacology")" (S.Hall and G.Strichartz eds.,) American chemical society, Washington DC, pp. 113-332.

Yamamura S, Teraday Y (1977). Isoaplysin-20, A natural bromine-containing diterpene, from Aplysia kurodai. Tetrahedron Lett., 18: 2171-2172.

Yamazaki M, Kimura K, Kisugi J, Muramoto K, Kamiya H (1990). Bacteriostatic and cytolytic activity of purple fluid from the Sea hare. Dev. Comp. Immunol., 14: 379-383.

Yamazaki M (1993). Antitumor and antimicrobial glycoprotein from sea hares. Comp. Biochem. Physiol., 105: 141-146.

19

Anti-plasmodial activity of aqueous root extract of *Acacia nilotica*

Alli L. A.[1]*, Adesokan A. A.[2], Salawu O. A.[3], Akanji M. A.[2] and Tijani A. Y.[3]

[1]Department of Medical Biochemistry, College of Health Sciences, University of Abuja, Nigeria.
[2]Department of Biochemistry, Faculty of Sciences, University of Ilorin, Nigeria.
[3]Department of Pharmacology and Toxicology, National Institute for Pharmaceutical Research and Development (NIPRD), Abuja, Nigeria.

Acacia nilotica, of family *Fabaceae,* is a thorny tree commonly used in Northern Nigeria for the treatment of cough, diabetes and malaria. Aqueous root extract of *A. nilotica* was analyzed for antiplasmodial activity in mice. Acute toxicity of the extract was studied using Organization for Economic Cooperation and Development (OECD) guideline 423. Suppressive activity, curative and prophylactic effect was studied in chloroquine-sensitive *Plasmodium berghei berghei* NK 65 infected mice. Five groups, of five mice in each group were used. Group 1 or control, was administered with 10ml distilled water/kg body weight; groups 2, 3 and 4 were administered with 100, 200, and 400mg extract/kg body weight, respectively, while group 5 was administered with 5mg chloroquine/kg body weight. The doses were administered orally. All doses of the extract produced significant, dose-dependent, chemo suppressive activity against the parasite in the suppressive, curative and prophylactic tests. This is comparable to the group treated with chloroquine. The extract also prolonged the mean survival time of treated mice compared to the untreated group. The oral median lethal dose (LD$_{50}$) of the extract in mice was 5000mg/kg body weight. The results of this study showed that the aqueous root extract of *Acacia nilotica* is safe and has anti plasmodial activity.

Key words: *Acacia nilotica*, antimalarial, *Plasmodium berghei berghei,* medicinal plant.

INTRODUCTION

Malaria remains one of the most dreaded human parasitic diseases in the tropics and subtropics, especially the African and Asian developing/under developed nations, because it is still a major cause of mortality in children (< 5 years) (WHO, 2008). Mortality, currently estimated at about 781,000 people per year (WHO, 2010), is attributed to resistance of the parasite to commonly used antimalarial drugs. In addition to its direct health impact, malaria imposes a huge economic burden on afflicted individuals and nations, through high health care cost, missed days at work or school, and reduced economic output and productivity (Sachs and Malaney, 2002).

Despite the success recorded with the Artemisinin Combination herapy (ACT), most malaria endemic

Combination Therapy (ACT), most malaria endemic communities still rely on traditional herbal medicines, which are often more affordable and available (Etkin, 2003). In view of the problems associated with antimalarial drug resistance and the use of substandard ACT's, researchers are now focusing on other alternatives, including investigation of medicinal plants known to have antiplasmodial activity (Ajaiyeoba et al., 2006; Etkin, 1997). In Africa, up to 80 per cent of the population still rely on herbal medicine to treat malaria and other diseases (Agbedahunsi, 2000), because of their affordability and accessibility. One of such popularly used medicinal plants is *Acacia nilotica,* a scented thorny tree commonly found and used in Northern Nigeria as a traditional herbal remedy against malaria (Etkin, 1997). The fruits and root of the plant was reported to have antitubercular (Oladosu et al., 2007) and antidiabetic activities (Dalziel, 1997), while the bark is used in treatment of cough, diarrhea and as an aphrodisiac (Van Wyk, 2000).

*Corresponding author. E-mail: adewalealli@gmail.com.

With this view, the present study was executed to analyse the antiplasmodial activity of the aqueous root extract of *Acacia nilotica* in *Plasmodium berghei berghei* infected mice in order to provide scientific evidence for its continuous use in ethno therapeutic management of malaria.

MATERIALS AND METHODS

Plant materials

A. nilotica roots were collected at Chaza village, Suleja, Niger State, Nigeria. It was identified and authenticated by Mrs. Grace Ugbabe, a taxonomist at the Department of Medicinal Plant Research and Traditional Medicine (MPR & TM) of National Institute of Pharmaceutical Research and Development (NIPRD), Abuja, Nigeria. A voucher specimen (NIPRD/H/6401) was prepared and deposited at the NIPRD herbarium for future reference. The root samples were cleaned, air-dried and pounded into fine powder using mortar and pestle. The powder was stored in a dry air-tight container.

Extract preparation

400 g of powdered root was macerated in 1L of distilled water for 24 h. The mixture was filtered using muslin cloth, followed by Whatman filter paper (NO. 1) and freeze-dried using AMSCO/FINN-AQUA GT2 Freeze dryer (Germany). Aliquot portion of this crude extract were weighed and dissolved in distilled water for preparation of appropriate doses on each day of the experiment.

Phytochemical screening

The extract was screened for phytochemical constituents using standard procedures as described by Evans (2005).

Animals

Both sexes of Wistar albino mice having body weight of 18 to 22 g, obtained from Animal Facility center, NIPRD, Abuja, were used as test animals for the study after receiving approval from NIPRD animal ethics committee on use of laboratory animals. They were housed in standard cages and maintained under standard laboratory conditions in accordance with the "NIH guideline for the care and use of Laboratory animals" (NIH Publication No. 85; rev. 1985).

Chemicals

The standard chloroquine used for the study was obtained from Sigma –Aldrich (C 6628-25G) representative in Nigeria (Zayo-sigma International ltd, Jos, Nigeria).

Acute toxicity test

The safety of the extract was assessed by determining its median lethal dose (LD_{50}) using the OECD Guideline 423 (2001).The extracts were administered at a stepwise doses of 300, 2000 and 5000 mg/kg orally to three groups of mice, comprising three females. The mice were observed for signs of toxicity after treatment for the first four (critical) hours, then over a period of 24 h, thereafter daily for 7days. Mortality occurring at a particular dose will indicate either to continue administration of subsequent higher dose or to estimate the LD_{50} by comparing the mortality to a fixed LD_{50} cut-off values provided in the guideline.

Rodent parasite

Chloroquine sensitive rodent *Plasmodium berghei berghei* NK 65 was obtained from National Institute for Medical Research (NIMR), Lagos, Nigeria and maintained alive in mice by continuous intraperitoneal passage in mice after every five days. The reinfected mice were kept at the Animal facility Center of NIPRD where the study was carried out. A standard inoculum of 1×10^7 of parasitized erythrocytes from a donor mouse in volumes of 0.2 ml was used to infect the experimental animals intra-peritoneally.

Antiplasmodial studies

Test on early malaria infection (4-day suppressive Test)

The Peter's 4-day suppressive test against chloroquine sensitive *Plasmodium berghei berghei* (NK 65) infection in mice was employed (Peters, 1965). Twenty five albino mice of both sexes were inoculated as described above. They were randomly grouped, having five mice in each group and administered extract daily for four (4) consecutive days. Treatment started immediately after the mice were infected with the parasite. Group 1 that served as control was administered with 10ml/kg body weight of distilled water. Groups 2, 3 and 4 were orally administered with 100, 200 and 400 mg extract/kg body weight daily respectively, while group 5 was administered with 5 mg chloroquine /kg body weight orally daily. On the fifth day (D_5), blood was collected from the tail of each mouse and spread on a microscope slide to make a thin film. The blood films were stained with Giemsa and examined microscopically following Cheesbrough (2004). The parasite count was recorded and the suppression of parasitemia was expressed as per cent for each dose, by comparing the parasitemia in the control group with the treated one.

Average suppression = APC – APT/APC X 100.
APC = Average parasitemia in the control.
APT = Average parasitemia in the test group.

Test on established infection (Rane test)

Evaluation of the curative potential of *A. nilotica* root extract against established infection was carried out as described by Ryley and Peters (1970). Twenty five mice were all inoculated as described above, and left untreated until the fourth day (D_4) post inoculation. The mice were weighed and randomized into five groups of five mice each. Group 1 was administered with 10ml/kg of distilled water; groups 2, 3 and 4 received graded extract doses of 100, 200 and 400 mg extract/kg body weight/day orally respectively, while group 5 was administered with 5 mg chloroquine /kg body weight /day orally for four days (D_4-D_7). On Day-7 each mouse was tail-bled and a thin blood film was made on a microscope slide. The films were stained with Giemsa stain and examined microscopically to monitor the parasitemia level. The mean survival time of the mice in each treatment group was monitored for 30 days (Saidu et al., 2000; Adzu and Salawu, 2009).

Repository test

The prophylactic activity of the extract was tested using the residual infection procedure described by Peters (1965). Twenty-five mice of

Table 1. Phytochemical constituent of aqueous root extract of *A. nilotica.*

Phytochemical	Tannin	Saponin	Flavonoid	Terpene	Sterol	Phenol	Alkaloid	Anthraquinone
Qualitative	++	++	+	+	+	+ +	++	+
Quantitative (%)	27.0	9.8	0.5	0.1	0.1	34.5	23.3	4.7

++ = moderately present, + = slightly present.

both sexes were weighed and randomized into five groups of five mice each. Group 1 was administered with 10ml/kg distilled water, group 2, 3 and 4 were administered with 100, 200 and 400 mg extract /kg body weight orally respectively, while group 5 was administered with 5mg chloroquine/kg body weight orally daily. Treatment continued daily for four days (D_1-D_4) and mice were all infected with the parasite on the fifth day (D_5). Thin blood films were prepared from each mouse 72hours (D_7) post treatment and mean parasitemia in each group determined microscopically. The mice were reweighed on seventh day and the differences between the pre- and post-treatment body weight recorded.

Statistical analysis

Graph pad prism version 5.02 was used to analyze the data obtained and these were expressed as mean ± standard error of mean. The differences between means were compared using one-way analysis of variance (ANOVA), followed by Dunnet's test. $p < 0.05$ was considered significant.

RESULTS

Phytochemical tests

The aqueous root extract of *A. nilotica* comprised of tannins, saponins, flavonoids, terpenes, sterols, phenols, alkaloids and anthraquinones (Table 1).

Acute toxicity test

The oral median lethal dose (LD_{50}) of the extract was estimated to be 5000 mg/kg in mice. There were no remarkable behavioral changes in the extract-administered mice (reaction to food supply, contact and noise), however activity was reduced in all the extract-administered groups within the first four hours. No mortality occurred within observation period of a week.

Evaluation of antiplasmodial activity

Test on early malaria infection (4-day suppressive test)

The administration of extract resulted in a significant dose-dependent decrease in parasite counts. The average parasite, percentage chemo suppression recorded was 68.8, 78.5 and 79.5% at 100, 200 and 400 mg extract/kg body weight, respectively, while administration

of 5 mg chloroquine/kg body weight resulted into complete chemo suppression (Table 2).

Test on established infection (Curative test)

The administration of extract also resulted in significant and dose dependent decrease in parasite counts in the treated groups when compared to the control group (Table 3). The mean parasite count was 10, 7 and 6, at the doses of 100, 200 and 400 mg extract/ kg body weight, respectively, as compared with the mean parasite count of 44 in the control group. Chloroquine administration of 5 mg/kg chloroquine reduced the mean parasite density to 3. The dose of extract administered also affected the survival period of the mice. Mortality started in the control group from seventh day after extract administration, and completed on eleventh day (mean survival time was 9 days after extract administration). Mice administered with100 and 200 mg extract/kg body weight survived for 17 and 21days respectively, but those administered with 400 mg/kg survived for 18 days only. Chloroquine administered mice had longest survival of 28 days after administration (Table 3).

Test on residual infection (Repository test)

The *Plasmodium* count also reduced significantly with increase in the dose of extract when compared with control. The mean parasite counts at 100, 200 and 400 mg extract /kg body weight were 19.2, 12.8 and 10.0, compared with 26.4 for the control group. The mean parasite count for chloroquine administered group was 2.8. Significant reduction in body weight of the mice in the control and the mice administered with 100 and 400 mg/kg of the extract was observed (Table 4).

DISCUSSION

The results obtained from the present study showed that the aqueous root extract of *A. nilotica* possess significant suppressive effect against early *Plasmodium* infection, curative effect against established infection and prophy-lactic effect against residual infection in *P. berghei berghei* infected mice.

Survival of mice, after oral administration of 2500 mg/kg body weight of the extract, up to 7 days, indicates

Table 2. Suppressive activity of aqueous root extract of *Acacia nilotica* in *P. berghei berghei* infected mice.

Treatment	Dose (mg/kg) p. o.	Mean parasitaemia count D_5	Inhibition (%)
Control	-	26.5 ± 1.04	-
Extract	100	8.25 ± 0.48*	68.8
	200	5.5 ± 0.80*	78.5
	400	5.25 ± 1.11*	79.5
Chloroquine	5	0*	100

D_5 = Day five, *significantly different from the control at $p < 0.05$.

Table 3. Curative effect of aqueous root extract of *A. nilotica in P. berghei berghei* infected mice.

Treatment	Dose Mg/kg, p.o	Mean parasitemia count		Survival time (Days)
		Pre- (D_3)	Post- (D_7) - treatment	
Control	-	18.0 ± 0.73	44.0 ± 0.48	9 ± 0.19
Extract	100	16.0 ± 0.63	10.0 ± 0.58***	17 ± 0.48
	200	16.0 ± 0.80	7.0 ± 0.58***	21 ± 0.14
	400	17.0 ± 0.58	6.0 ± 0.68***	18 ± 0.46
Chloroquine	5	14.0 ± 0.82	3.0 ± 0.37***	28 ± 0.58

D_3 = Day three, D_7 = Day seven, *** significantly different at $p < 0.001$.

Table 4. Prophylactic effect of aqueous root extract of *A. nilotica in P. berghei berghei* infected mice.

Treatment	Dose (mg/kg, p.o)	Mean parasitemia count D_7	Body weights (g)	
			D_1	D_7
Control	—	26.4 ± 1.0	18.6 ± 0.68	15.5 ± 0.50*
Extract	100	19.2 ± 0.86*	18.2 ± 0.66	16.0 ± 0.98*
	200	12.8 ± 0.37**	19.2 ± 0.86	19.0 ± 0.01
	400	10.0 ± 0.71**	22.0 ± 0.68	18.5 ± 0.50*
Chloroquine	5	2.8 ± 0.37***	18.8 ± 0.67	18.3 ± 0.33

D_1 = Day one, D_7 = Day seven, *, ** and *** = significantly different at $P < 0.05$, 0.01 and 0.001, respectively.

that the estimated oral median lethal dose (LD_{50}) of the extract at 5000 mg/kg body weight (OECD, 2001) is non-toxic. This suggests that acute oral administration of the extract is safe, and also explains the reason why the root portion of the plant is widely used in traditional treatment of malaria.

Although rodent models do not produce exactly the same signs and symptoms observed in the human plasmodial infection but they have been reported (Pedroni et al., 2006; Pierrot et al., 2003) to produce disease features similar to those of human plasmodial infection, when infected with *P. berghei berghei* (Thomas et al., 1998). Moreover, several studies (Calvalho et al., 1991;

Agbedahunsi, 2000; Adzu and Salawu 2009) have employed *P. berghei berghei* in predicting treatment outcome of suspected antimalarial agents, because of its high sensitivity to chloroquine, making it appropriate for this study. Substances that reduce parasite multiplication (anti plasmodial effect) in the host were considered to possess antimalarial activity (Ryley and Peters, 1970).

The 4 day suppressive test is a standard test commonly used for antimalarial screening (Peters, 1965). The extract produced significant dose related chemo suppression in all the treated groups with the highest chemo suppression (79.5%) observed in the group treated with 400 mg extract/kg. The closeness of the chemo-suppression value of 78.5 and 79.5% in 200 and 400 mg/kg body weight administered group respectively, and the higher survival time in the former group suggests that the 200 mg extract/kg dose may be the optimal therapeutic dose in mice. The higher doses of extract may not possess significantly more beneficial antiplasmodial effect. The aqueous root extract also demonstrated significant dose related reduction in parasite count in both established (curative) and residual (repository) infection, comparable to the effect of chloroquine, which in this study was used as standard control drug.

The reduction of parasite count in the curative test is similar to the values recorded for reduction in parasite count in the suppressive test, but lower than the mean parasite count in the repository test. This may probably be due to rapid parasite clearance by the extract in early and established infection, as against a situation where the extract was initially administered for days (Prophylactic) before inoculation with parasite. The high parasite count in the repository test may be attributed to rapid metabolism of administered extract (before inoculation) to inactive products (Dahanukar et al., 2000).

The significant reduction in body weight in the group administered with 400 mg/kg body weight as well as the control group may be due to combined effect of plasmadial infection (Thomas et al., 1998) and possible catabolic effect of high dose of the extract on stored lipids.

These observations showed that the extract is active against the malaria parasite used in this study and is consistent with the ethnomedicinal use of A. nilotica roots, as anti malaria in Northern part of Nigeria (Etkin, 1997).

The mechanism of anti plasmodial action of this extract has not been elucidated, however, anti plasmodial effects of natural plant products have been attributed to some of their active phytochemical components (Ayoola et al., 2008; Sofowora, 1980). Some of these phytochemicals such as terpenes and flavonoids (detected in A. nilotica) were reported to have antiplasmodial activity (Phillipson and Wright, 1990; Christensen and Kharazmi, 2001; Go, 2003). Earlier studies by Etkin (1997), reported the oxidant generation potential of A. nilotica extract, based on the ability of the extract to increase conversion of reduced glutathione (GSH) to oxidized glutathione (GSSG). Increased oxidation has also been shown to create an intracellular environment that is unfavourable to plasmodial growth (Borris and Schaeffer 1992; Levander and Ager, 1993). The mechanism of action of artemisinin, which depends on oxidant action for its potent antimalarial activity, validates this (Etkin, 2003). However, lack of oxidizing action in some plants does not rule out anti plasmodial activity since they may be active through other biochemical mechanisms.

The anti plasmodial effect of aqueous root extract of A. nilotica may therefore be due to the phytochemical components (alkaloids, flavonoids and terpenes) or the oxidant generation potential or a combination of these mechanisms.

It can therefore be concluded that aqueous root extract of A. nilotica possess good potential as antimalarial phytomedicine and there is a scientific basis for its continuous use in traditional medicine for the management of malaria.

REFERENCES

Adzu B, Salawu OA (2009). Screening Diospyros mespiliformis extract for antimalarial potency. Int. J. Biol. Chem. Sci., 3(2): 271-276.

Agbedahunsi JM (2000). Screening of crude drugs for the treatment of malaria in Nigeria, Phytomedicine in malaria and sexually transmitted diseases: Challenges for the new millennium. Drug Research and Production Unit, Faculty of pharmacy, Obafemi Awolowo University, Ile Ife, Nigeria, pp. 13-22.

Ajaiyeoba EO, Abiodun OO, Falade MO, Ogbole NO, Ashidi JS, Happi CT, Akinboye DO (2006). In vitro cytotoxicity studies of 20 plants used in Nigerian antimalarial ethno medicine. Phytomedicine, 13: 295-298.

Ayoola GA, Coker HAB, Adesegun SA, Adepoju-Bello AA, Obaweya K, Ezennia EC, Atangbayila TO (2008). Phytochemical screening and antioxidant activities of some selected medicinal plants used for malaria therapy in southwestern Nigeria. Trop. J. Pharm. Res., 7(3): 1019-1024.

Borris RP, Schaeffer JM (1992). Antiparasitic agents from plants. Phytochemical Resources for medicine and Agriculture. New York: Plenum, pp.117-158.

Calvalho LH, Brandao MGL, Santos-Filho D, Lopes JLC, Krettli AU (1991). Antimalarial activity of crude extracts from Brazilian plants studied in vivo in plasmodium berghei berghei infected mice and in vitro against Plasmodium falciparum in culture. Br. J. Med. Biol. Res., 24: 1113-1123.

Cheesbrough M (2004). District Laboratory Practice in Tropical Countries. 2nd ed. Cambridge Univ. Press, pp. 239-258.

Christensen SB, Kharazmi A (2001). Antimalarial natural products: isolation, characterization and biological properties. In Bioactive compounds from natural sources: Isolation, Characterization and biological properties, Tringali C (ed). Taylor and Francis: London.

Dahanukar SA, Kulkarni FA, Rege NN (2000). Pharmacology of medicinal plants and natural products. Indian J. Pharmacol., 32: 1081-118.

Dalziel JM (1997). Useful plants of West Africa. Revised 2nd ed. Vol IV, M-R. Royal Botanical Gardens, England, pp. 138-139.

Etkin NL (1997). Antimalarial plants used by Hausa in Northern Nigeria. Trop. Doct., 27: 12-16.

Etkin NL (2003). The co-evolution of people, plants, and parasites: biological and cultural adaptation to malaria. Proc. Nutr. Soc., 62: 311-317.

Evans WC (2005). Trease and Evans Pharmacognosy, (14th ed), WB Saunders Company Limited, London, pp. 357-358.

Go ML (2003). Novel antiplasmodial agents. Med. Plant Rev., 23: 456-487.

Levander OA, Ager AL (1993). Malaria parasites and oxidant nutrients. Parasitology, 107: S95-S106.

OECD 423 (2001). Oral Toxicity Study in Rodents. OECD guideline for the testing of chemicals, 423: 1-8.

Oladosu P, Samuel BB, Okhale SE, Ibrahim K, Okogun JI (2007). Antitubercular activity of the dried fruits of Acacia nilotica. J. Phytomed. Therapeut., 12: 76-79.

Pedroni HC, Bettoni CC, Spalding SM, Costa TD (2006). Plasmodium berghei: Development of an irreversible experimental malaria model in wistar rats. Exp. Parasitol., 113: 193-196.

Peters W (1965). Drug resistance in plasmodium berghei. Vinka and Lips. Exp. Parasitol., 17: 80-89.

Phillipson JD, Wright CW (1990). Can ethno pharmacology contribute to the development of antimalarial agents? J. Ethno. Pharmacol., 32: 155-165.

Pierrot C, Adam E, Laffite S, Godin C, Dive D, Capron M, Khalife J (2003). Age related susceptibility and resistance to plasmodium berghei in mice and rats. Exp. Parasitol., 104: 81-85.

Ryley JF, Peters W (1970). The anti malarial activity of some quinolone esters. Ann. Trop. Med. Parasitol., 64: 209-222.

Sachs J, Malaney P (2002). The economic and social burden of malaria. Nature, 415: 680-685.

Saidu K, Onah J, Orisadipe A, Olusola A, Wambebe C, Gamaniel K (2000). Antiplasmodial, analgesic and anti inflammatory activities of the aqueous stem bark of *Erythrina senegalensis*. J. Ethnopharmacol., 71: 275-280.

Sofowora A (1980). The present status of knowledge of the plants used in traditional medicine in West Africa: A medical approach and a chemical evaluation. J. Ethno. Pharmacol., 2: 109-118.

Thomas AM, Van Der Wel AM, Thomas AW, Janse CJ, Waters AP (1998). Transfection system for animal models of malaria. Parasitol. Today, 14: 248-249.

Van Wyk P (2000). Field Guide to trees of Southern Africa. Struik, Cape Town, 2: 25-27.

World Health Organization (WHO) (2008). World Malaria Report, pp. 7-10.

World Health Organization (WHO) (2010). World Malaria Report, pp. 13-15.

20

In-vitro assessment of antioxidant potential and phenolic capacity of *Temnocalyx obovatus* leaves

P. Dzomba*, E. Togarepi and C. Mahamadi

Chemistry Department, Faculty of Science Education, P. Bag 1020, Bindura, Zimbabwe.

Temnocalyx obovatus is widely found in many areas in Zimbabwe, Nigeria and Zambia where it is used to treat a variety of ailments. Phenolic compounds in *T. obovatus* assessed by Folin-Ciocalteu method varied from 1.18 to 2.89 mg tannic acid g^{-1}. Acetone extract showed the greatest flavonoids, flavonols and proanthocyanidins content 5.12, 4.13 and 3.07 mg catechin g^{-1} respectively. 2, 2-diphenyl-1-picrylhydrazyl radical (DPPH⁻) scavenging effect, Ferric reducing ability and egg lipid peroxidation inhibition assays were adopted to evaluate antioxidant activity. Acetone extracts exhibited the greatest antioxidant activity for all the assays, followed by methanol extracts. Hexane extracts showed the weakest activity. Correlation studies showed that antiradical activity is explained more by flavonols and proanthocyanidins (73%) and flavonoids (71%) and weakly by phenolic contents (43%). The results revealed significant phenolic capacity and antioxidant potential of *T. obovatus* to warrant its use as a source of antioxidants. It can be added to foods, such as, meat and soups for enhancement of nutritional content and promotion of health.

Key words: Antioxidant activity, phenolics, *T. obovatus*.

INTRODUCTION

Researches in traditional food and medicinal plants have increased previously (Prasad et al., 2011, 2010; Miliauskas, 2006). This is as a result of the need to find new sources of natural antioxidants which are believed to be safer than their synthetic counterparts. Synthetic antioxidants are cheap and very efficient however they have been implicated in the etiology of cancers such that some countries are now banning or enforcing restrictions to their use (Bergfeld et al., 2005; Wangensteen et al., 2004). Tert-butyl-hydroquinone (TBHQ) a synthetic antioxidant widely used to prevent rancidity in oils and lipid based foods is banned in Japan and certain European countries (Shahidi and Wanasundara, 1997). Since the report by Chipault et al. (1956) on antioxidant activity of 72 different spices, many researches reports the possibility of using plant extracts as potent antioxidants to prevent food rancidification and diseases as a result of oxidative stress. Rosemary (*Rosmarinus officinalis*), sage (*Salvia officinalis*) and oregano

(*Origanum vulgare*) were found to be effective sources of antioxidants resulting in their application in nutraceutical and pharmaceutical industry (Miliauskas, 2006). In Zimbabwe, there are many unstudied traditional food and medicinal plants which can be sources of the increasingly sort natural antioxidants. The advantage of these plants is that they have been used for several years as either medicines to treat ailments or as food sources therefore placing a plus sign to their safety concerns. *Temnocalyx obovatus* (Figure 1) is an example of such plant. The plant is widely found in many areas in Zimbabwe, Nigeria and Zambia. It falls under the family Rubiaceae. It is an under shrub, sometimes in clumps, it is 2 to 3 ft. high, with 3-angled slightly pubescent stems; flowers greenish with darker apex, solitary or few of them are found together in the axils. In many African societies, its leaves are fused to make a particular kind of tea. It is taken as a medication or merely as a beverage. Its leaves are used to treat a variety of ailments such as, boosting the immune system, abdominal pain, including menstrual pain, backache and chest pains, strengthening bones, building stamina, coughs and flu, whooping cough, muscular toning, oedema, constipation, ulcers, asthma, loss of appetite and hypertension. *T. obovatus* is used to

*Corresponding author. E-mail: pdzomba@gmail.com or pdzomba@buse.ac.zw.

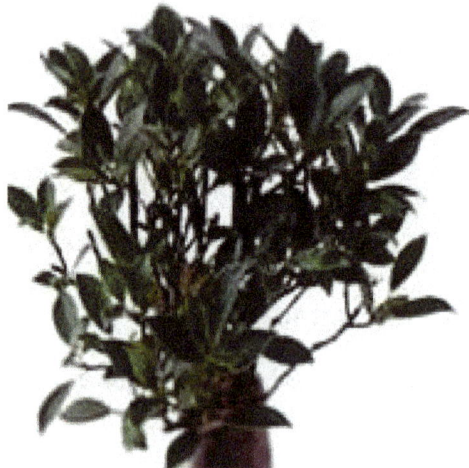

Figure 1. Scientific name: *Temnocalyx obovatus* (family Rubiaceae).

treat diarrhoea in chickens and stomach disorders in turkeys, goats and cows (Mahamadi et al., 2011). It is also used as an antidote for poisoning which includes snakebites (Mahamadi et al., 2011). These properties are akin to the presence of polyphenols (Maestri et al., 2006), thus this study sought to investigate the antioxidant potential and phenolic capacity of *T. obovatus*.

MATERIALS AND METHODS

Plant material

The leaves were collected in April, June and July 2010 from Mashonaland East in Chivhu, Zimbabwe. The plants were identified by their characteristic leaves and validated by a taxonomist at Harare Botanical Garden specimen 2010/2011 and was deposited in the Chemistry Department (Natural Product Section) of Bindura University for future reference.

Sample preparation

Plant leaves were air-dried at room temperature for three weeks to obtain a constant mass. The dried leaves were later ground two times into powder using a wooden mortar and pestle, followed by sieving through a laboratory king test sieve of 0.75 µm. The fine material which passed through the sieve was collected. The remaining residues were then discarded. A quantity of 10 g of the ground material was extracted continuously with cold organic solvents 100 ml; acetone, methanol, ethanol, hexane, petroleum ether and diethyl ether (Merck Co. Germany) for 5 h on a shaker at room temperature followed by filtration through Whatman no. 1 filter paper. The residues were re-extracted under the same treatment and the filtrates combined. The extracts were then centrifuged at 1536 × g for 20 min at 20°C. The supernatants were taken into 100 ml flasks and then evaporated in a Bucchi rotary evaporator at 40°C. The extracts obtained after evaporation were weighed to determine the yield and re-suspended in 100 ml of each solvent and stored in a deep freeze before use.

Determination of total phenolics

Total phenolic compounds in plant extracts were determined by Folin-Ciocalteu method as reported by Wolfe et al. (2003) with minor modifications. For the preparation of the calibration curve, 1 ml aliquots of 0.1, 2.0, 4.0 and 6.0 mg/L tannic acid solutions in each respective solvent: methanol, ethanol, petroleum ether, hexane, diethyl ether and acetone were mixed with 5 ml of Folin-Ciocalteu reagent (diluted ten-fold) and 4 ml of sodium carbonate solution (75 g/L). The absorbance was read after 30 min at 20°C and at 725 nm and the calibration curves were constructed. A volume of 1 ml of each plant extract (0.1 mg/ml) was mixed with the same reagents as described previously, and after 30 min the absorbance was measured for the determination of total plant phenolics. All determinations were performed in triplicate. Total content of phenolic compounds in plant extracts in tannic acid equivalents (TAE) was calculated by the following formula:

$$T = \frac{c \times v}{m}$$

where; T is total content of phenolic compounds in mg/g plant extract, in TAE; C is the concentration of tannic acid established from the calibration curve in mg/L; V is the volume of extract in ml; and m is the weight of plant solvent extract in gram.

Determination of total flavonoid content

The method of Ordon et al. (2006) was employed with slight modifications. This was done by adding 0.5 ml of 2% $AlCl_3$ ethanol solution to 0.5 ml plant sample (0.1 mg/ml). Absorbance of the mixture was measured after one h at 425 nm. Total flavonoids content was evaluated as mg/g quercetin equivalents by a calibration method of 0, 0.5, 1.0, 1.5 and 2.0 mg/ml quercetin.

Determination of total flavonols

The amount of flavonols was evaluated using the method of Kumaran and Karunakaran (2007). A volume of 2.0 ml of 2% ethanolic $AlCl_3$ and 3 ml (50 g/L) sodium acetate solutions was mixed with 2.0 ml of the sample extract of concentration 0.1 mg/ml. The absorbance was measured at 440 nm after standing for 2 to 5 h at 20°C. Total flavonols was estimated as mg/g of quercetin equivalent using a calibration method of 0, 0.5, 1.0, 1.5 and 2.0 mg/ml quercetin.

Determination of total proanthocyanidins

The total proanthocyanidin compounds of the samples were estimated using UV-spectrometry as reported by Sun and Ho (2005) by adding 0.5 ml of 0.1 mg/ml of the extract solution to 3 ml of 4% vanillin methanol solution and 1.5 ml hydrocloric acid, and the mixture was to stand for fifteen minutes. The absorbance was measured at 500 nm and the results expressed as catechin equivalents using a calibration method of 0, 0.5, 1.0 1.5 and 2.0 mg/ml catechin.

Antioxidant activity determination

Antioxidant test systems differ significantly such that the results of a single assay can give just a limited assessment of the antioxidant properties of a sample (Dejian et al., 2005; Gianni et al., 2005). As such, in the present research, total antioxidant activity was

Table 1. Total phenolic, flavonoids, flavonols and proanthocyanidins content of the different solvents.

Sample	Solvent	Average ± SD			
		TP	TFD	TF	TPR
Powdered leaves	Methanol	2.89 ± 0.03	2.08 ± 0.01	3.84 ± 0.02	2.25 ± 0.01
	Ethanol	1.82 ± 0.01	1.00 ± 0.01	1.45 ± 0.01	1.93 ± 0.01
	Acetone	1.67 ± 0.01	5.12 ± 0.01	4.13 ± 0.01	3.07 ± 0.01
	Hexane	1.46 ± 0.02	0.86 ± 0.02	0.25 ± 0.03	1.68 ± 0.01
	Petroleum ether	1.31 ± 0.01	1.46 ± 0.01	0.90 ± 0.01	1.87 ± 0.01
	Diethyl ether	1.18 ± 0.01	0.91 ± 0.01	0.87 ± 0.01	1.69 ± 0.02

DW, Dry weight; TP, total phenols (mg tannic acid g^{-1} DW); TFD, total flavonoids (mg quercetin g^{-1} DW); TF, total flavonols (mg quercetin g^{-1} DW); TPR, total proanthocyanidins (mg catechin g^{-1} DW).

evaluated through three assays, DPPH˙ scavenging activity, the ferric reducing ability of plasma (FRAP) and inhibition of egg lipid peroxidation.

DPPH˙ radical scavenging assay

The DPPH˙ radical scavenging activity was evaluated according to a slightly modified method described by Pothitirat et al. (2009) and Masuda et al. (2007). The reagent (1 ml of $1×10^{-3}$ molL^{-1}) DPPH˙ solution in methanol was mixed with 1 ml of plant extract, butylated hydroxytoluene (BHT), ascorbic acid and catechin [standard antioxidants (Sigma Chemical Co. St Louis, USA)] of different concentrations. The reaction mixture was incubated in the dark for 30 min and there after the optical density was recorded at 517 nm. For the control, 1 ml of DPPH˙ solution in methanol was mixed with 1 ml of each solvent without extract and optical density of solution was recorded after 30 min. The decrease in optical density of DPPH˙ on addition of test samples in relation to the control was used to calculate the antioxidant capacity as percentage of inhibition (% I) of DPPH radical:

$$\% \ I = \frac{Ac - As}{Ac} × 100$$

where; A_s is the absorbance with extract/standards after 30 min and A_c is the absorbance without the extract after 30 min. Each assay was carried out in triplicate.

Total antioxidant power (FRAP)

This was done as reported by Benzie and Strain (1996) with slight modifications. Fresh working solutions consisting of 25 ml acetate buffer, 3.1 g sodium acetate, 16 ml acetic acid, and pH 3.6 were used for this analysis. A volume of 2.5 ml of 2, 4, 6-tripydal-s-triazine solution in 40 ml HCl (10 Mm) and 20 Mm FeCl$_3$.6H$_2$O solution were mixed at 37°C. Extracts, catechin and ascorbic acid of different concentrations were allowed to react with the mixture for 30 min in the dark and absorbance was measured at 563 nm. Total antioxidant power to reduce Fe(III) to Fe(II) was determined by the change in absorbance which was then calculated and related to absorbance change of an Fe(II) standard solution.

Inhibition of lipid peroxidation

The assessment was performed following a method reported by Zhang et al. (1996). An equal volume 2 ml of egg yolk was added to 0.1 mol/dm^3 phosphate buffer solution (PBS) (pH 7, 45). The

mixture was stirred magnetically for 10 min and then diluted with 24 ml of phosphate buffer solution. The homogenized yolk (1 ml), extract, ascorbic acid, catechin (0.5 ml) of different concentrations, PBS 1 ml and $25 × 10^{-3}$ mol dm^{-3} (1 ml) iron sulphate were mixed and shaken at 37°C for 15 min. The reaction was stopped by the addition of trichloroacetic acid and the mixture was centrifuged. Then 1 ml of 8 g/dm^3 thiobarbituric acid was added to 3 ml of the supernatant. The solution was heated at 10°C for 10 min and then absorbance was measured at 523 nm. Percentage lipid peroxidation inhibition was calculated as follows.

Statistical analysis

All analyses were performed in triplicate and data reported as mean ± standard deviation (SD). The data was subjected to analysis of variance (ANOVA) ($p < 0.05$). Results were processed by Excel and SPSS Version 16.0 (SPSS Inc., Chicago, IL, USA). Least significant difference (LSD) tests and T test was applied to separate the means and to compare antioxidant activity of extracts and that of standards respectively.

RESULTS AND DISCUSSION

Total phenolic content

The concentration of phenolic compounds in *T. obovatus* varied in different extracts ranging from 1.18 to 2.89 mg tannic acid g^{-1} dry weight and they were in the order methanol > ethanol > acetone > hexane > petroleum ether > diethyl ether (Table 1). The results revealed that methanol and ethanol were better compared to other solvents in extracting phenolic compounds (ANOVA and LSD test analysis $p < 0.05$). This is because they have higher polarity and favourable solubilities for phenolic compounds from plants (Kequan and Liangh, 2006). The less polar solvents such as petroleum ether, diethyl ether and hexane revealed less capability of extracting phenolic compounds. Stecher et al. (2003) observed that low-polarity solvents yield more lipophilic components, while alcoholic solvents give a larger spectrum of apolar and polar material. In comparison to the food taken daily in diets, total phenolic compounds in *T. obovatus* was lower than that obtained from tomatoes (2.29 to 5 mg

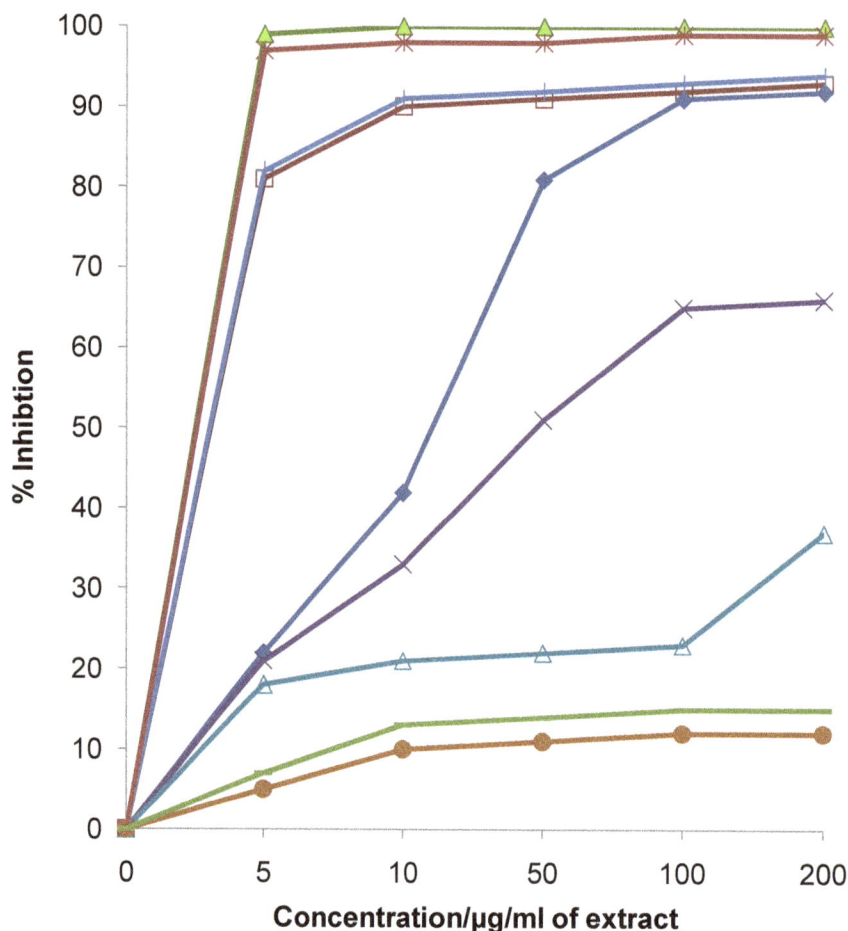

Figure 2. DPPH radical scavenging assay.

gallic g^{-1}) (Wolfe et al., 2003) but higher than that found in carrot (1.52 mg gallic acid g^{-1}) (Kequan and Liangli, 2006) and onion (2.5 mg gallic acid g^{-1}) (Kahkonen et al., 1999).

Total flavonoids and flavonols content

Flavonoids and flavonols exhibit a wide spectrum of biological and chemical activities including antiradical activities. Because of this, all extracts were assayed for total flavonoids and flavonols content. Acetone extracts showed the greatest yield for both flavonoids and flavonols (5.12 and 4.13 mg quercetin g^{-1} respectively). The least yield was obtained with hexane (0.84 mg quercetin g^{-1} for flavonoids and 0.27 mg querceting^{-1} for flavonols) (Table 1).

Total proanthocyanidins content

Among the tested solvents, acetone was the most efficient solvent in extracting proanthocyanidins (3.07 mg

catechin g^{-1}) followed by methanol (2.25 mg catechin g^{-1}) and then ethanol (1.94 mg catechin g^{-1}) (Table 1). The results disagree with the results obtained by Lapornik et al. (2005) that described methanol and ethanol as the best extractors of anthocyanins from red and black current. In the studies of Zhao et al. (2006), Kequan and Liangli (2004) and Tabart et al. (2007), similar results were obtained as reported in this study. Acetone (80%) showed the highest extraction capacity for (+) catechin, caffeic, vanillic and coumaric acid from barley. Kequan and Liangli (2004) found out that 50% acetone exhibited superior extraction efficiency of anthocyanins from wheat based foods.

ANTIOXIDANT ACTIVITY DETERMINATION

DPPH scavenging assay

The DPPH antiradical activity of different solvents shown in Figure 2 generally show that the percentage inhibition was concentration dependent. All extracts exhibited antioxidant activity with acetone showing the

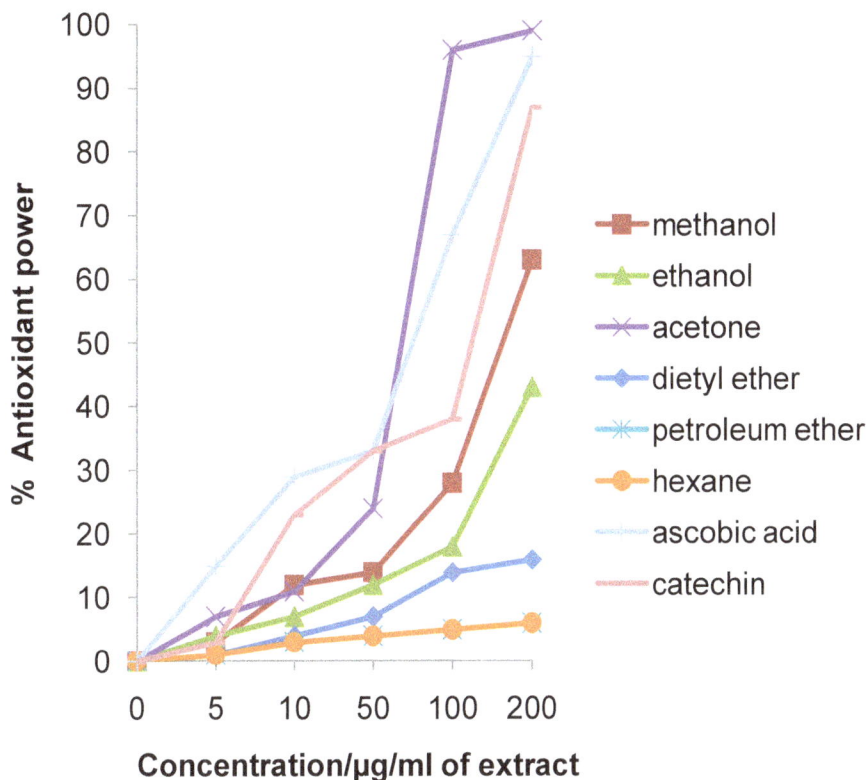

Figure 3. Total antioxidant power *(FRAP)*.

greatest activity profile just above that of ascorbic acid. It should be noted that the reaction of acetone extract and DPPH· radical was very rapid in all replicas and was completed within 0.5 to 1 min. Methanol extracts were second with activity slightly below that of standard antioxidant BHT. At a concentration of 10 µg/ml, the scavenging activity of ascorbic acid, methanol, and acetone extracts were 99.6, 89.7 and 100% respectively. Hexane extracts showed the weakest radical scavenging activity just like catechin. At 10 µg/ml the percentage inhibition was 10.4 for hexane extracts and 12.8% for catechin. The concentration of antioxidant activity required to decrease the initial DPPH· concentration by 50% (IC_{50}) is a parameter widely used to measure antioxidant activity. The lower the IC_{50} value the higher is the antioxidant activity. The antioxidant activity was in the following order: acetone IC_{50}, < 5, methanol < 5, ethanol, 15, diethyl ether 30, petroleum ether > 200 and hexane > 200 µg/ml. Significant difference was observed in the results, though ANOVA analysis showed that p < 0.05 at concentrations of 5, 10 and 50 µg/ml.

FRAP assay

In the present study, acetone extract exhibited the greatest reducing power followed by methanol. However, the results were lower than those of ascorbic acid and

catechin at concentration below 50 µg/ml. Above 50 µg/ml, acetone extract showed better antioxidant activity than catechin and ascorbic acid. This may indicate a possibility of competitive kinetics (Figure 3). Diethyl ether, petroleum ether and hexane extracts were poor reducing agents. The results were compared to those reported by Zhao et al. (2006). The highest reducing power was found in acetone extracts as compared to ethanol and methanol using barley as the sample. When the test was performed with plasma in the absence of Fe(III) added to the reaction mixture, it was observed that no color developed. This indicated that there was no detectable free Fe(II) in plasma, and that, there was no detectable agent in normal plasma that reacts directly with 2, 4, 6-tripydal-s-triazine (TPTZ) to form the blue chromogen. Monitoring complete reagent, that is reagent containing TPTZ and Fe(III) but with no sample addition, it also showed that no color developed.

Inhibition of lipid peroxidation

This assay makes use of the ability of egg yolk lipids to undergo a fast non enzymatic oxidation in the presence of iron sulphate (Watson et al., 2006). The results for lipid peroxidation shown in Figure 4 revealed that, acetone extract was the best egg lipid peroxidation inhibitor followed by methanol and then ethanol extracts.

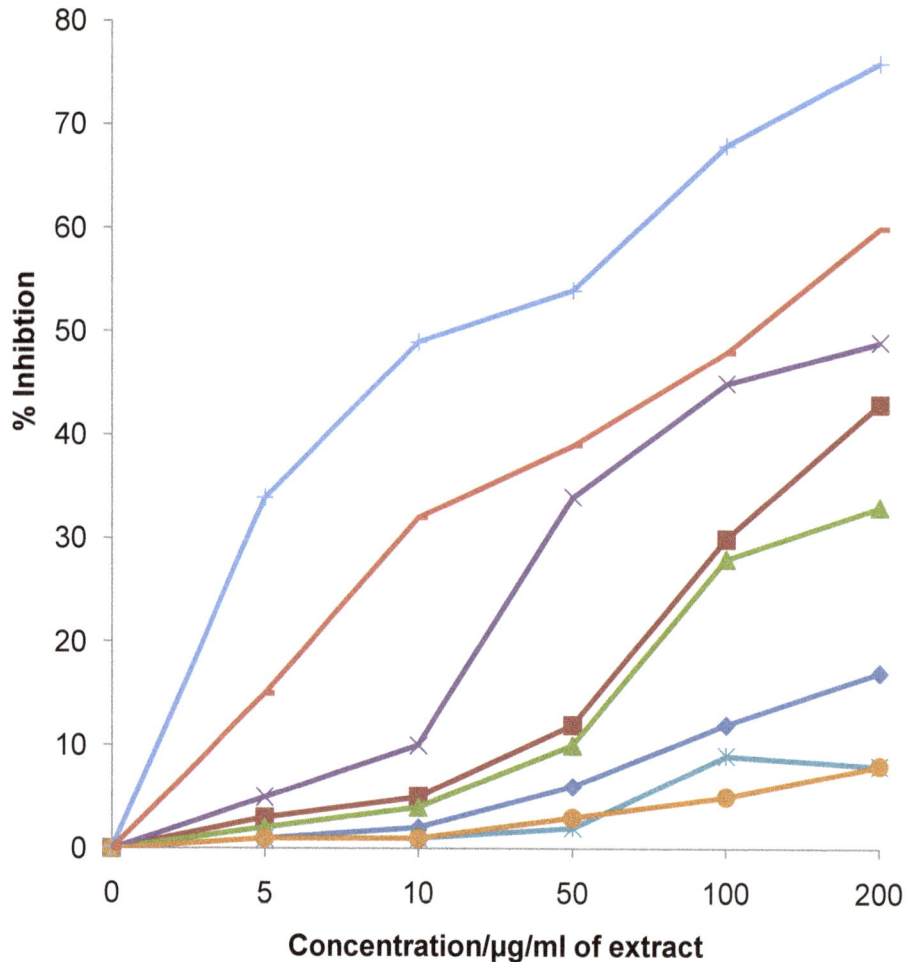

Figure 4. Inhibition of lipid peroxidation.

Compared to ascorbic acid and catechin, acetone was significantly inferior [t-test $p < 0.05$ at concentrations, 5; 10 and 50 ($\mu g/ml$)]. The less polar solvent extracts (diethyl ether, petroleum ether and hexane) were observed with poor lipid peroxidation inhibitors even at concentrations above 200 $\mu g/ml$. Lipid peroxidation inhibition of the extracts was also concentration dependent.

Relationship between yield, phenolic, flavonoids, flavonols and proanthocyanidins with antioxidant activity

This study's analysis showed that there was good correlation between yields ($R^2 = 0.901$), flavonols ($R^2 = 0.729$), proanthocyanidins ($R^2 = 0.729$), flavonoids ($R^2 = 0.708$) and antioxidant activity, but weak correlation in phenolic compounds ($R^2 = 0,426$). Similar results were reported by Chung et al. (1999). These results suggested that the antioxidant capacity of extracts was largely due to the contribution of flavonoids, flavonols and proanthocyanidins.

Conclusion

The results indicate that extraction solvents have a significant impact on antioxidant activity as well as selectivity for different polyphenols. Basing the employed models for antioxidant activity test, acetone proved to be the best solvent for extracting polyphenols from *T. obovatus*. The antioxidant activity of *T. obovatus* can be explained significantly in terms of flavonols, proanthocyanidins and flavonoids. *T. obovatus* consists of significant antioxidant activity and some amounts of flavonoid, flavonols and proanthocyanidins compounds to warrant its use as a source of natural antioxidants which can be used to promote health and delay of food rancidification. *T. obovatus* can also be used as alternative medicine for treatment of ailments therefore authenticating its use in traditional medicines.

ACKNOWLEDGEMENTS

The authors would like to express sincere gratitude to Professor M. F. Zaranyika and Mr .Dotito (University of Zimbabwe), Mr. Makahamadze and Mr. Mapfaka (Bindura University) for their kind supports.

REFERENCES

Benzie IFF, Strain JJ (1996). The ferric reducing ability of plasma as a measure of antioxidant power: the FRAP assay. Anal. Biochem., 239: 70-76.

Bergfeld WF, Belsito DV, Marks JGJ, Andersen FA (2005). Safety of ingredients used in cosmetics. J. Am. Acad. Dermatol., 52: 125-132.

Chipault JR, Mizuno GR, Lundberg WO (1956). The antioxidant properties of spices in Foods. Food Technol., 10: 209-210.

Chung HYT, Soung DY, Kye IS, No JK, Baek BS (1999). Peroxynitrite-scavenging activity of green tea tannin. J. Agric. Food Chem.. 46: 4484-4486.

Gianni S, Silvia M, Mariavittoria M, Martina S, Stefano M, Matteo R (2005). Comparative evaluation of 11 essential oils of different origin as functional antioxidants, antiradicals and antimicrobials in foods. Food Chem., 91: 621-632.

Kahkonen MP, Hopia AI, Vuorela HJ, Rauha JP, Pihlaja K, Kujala TS (1999). Antioxidant activity of plant extracts containing phenolic compounds. J. Agric. Food Chem., 47: 3954-3962.

Kequan Z, Liangli Y (2006). Total phenolic contents and antioxidant properties of commonly consumed vegetables grown in Colorado. LWT – Food Sci. Technol., 39: 1155-1162.

Kequan Z, Liangli Y (2004). Effects of extraction solvents on wheat bran antioxidant activity estimation. LWT – Food Sci. Technol., 37(7): 717-721.

Kumaran A, Karunakaran RJ (2007). In vitro antioxidant activities of methanol extracts of phyllanthus species from India. Lebens-Wiss Tech., 40: 344-352.

Lapornik B, Prosek M, Wondra GA (2005). Comparison of extracts prepared from plant by products using different solvents and extraction time. J. Food Eng., 77(2): 214-222.

Maestri DM, Nepote V, Lamarque AL, Zygadlo JA (2006). Natural products as antioxidants. Res. signpost., 37: 105-135.

Mahamadi C, Togarepi E, Dzomba P (2011). Extraction of phenolic compounds from Temnocalyx obovatus. A. J. Biotech., 10(54): 11245-11248.

Masuda T, Yonemori S, Oyama Y, Takeda Y, Tanaka T, Andoh T (2007). Evaluation of the antioxidant activity of environmental plants: activity of leaf extracts from seashore plants. J. Agric. Food Chem., 47: 1749-1754.

Miliauskas G (2006). Screening, isolation and evaluation of antioxidative compounds from Geranium macrorrhizum, Potentilla fruticosa and Rhaponticum carthamoides. Europian Food Res. Technol., 218: 253-261.

Ordon EAA, Gomez JD, Vattuone MA, Isia M (2006). Antioxidant activities of Sechium edule Jacq Swart extracts. Food Chem., 97: 452-458

Prasad KN, Fouad AH, Yang B, Kong KW, Ramannan RN, Azrina A, Amin I (2011). Response surface optimization for the extraction of phenolic compounds and antioxidant capacities from Mangifera pajang Kosterm. peels. Food Chem., 128: 1121-1127

Prasad KN, Chew LY, Khoo HE, Kong KW, Azlan A, Amin I (2010). Antioxidant capacities of peel, pulp and seed fractions of Canarium odontophyllum Miq. fruit. J. Biomed. Biotech., pp. 1-8.

Pothitirat W, Chomnawang M T, Supabphol R, Gritsanapan W (2009). Comparison of bioactive compounds content, free radical scavenging and anti-acne inducing bacteria activities of extracts from the Mangosteen fruit rind at two stages of maturity. Fitoterapia, 80: 442-447.

Shahidi F, Wanasundara UN (1997). Measurement of lipid oxidation and evaluation of antioxidant activity, in natural antioxidants, chemistry, health effects, and applications. AOCS Press. Champaign, pp. 379-396.

Stecher G, Huck CW, Stoggl WM, Bonn GK (2003). Phytoanalysis: a challenge in phytomics. Trends Anal. Chem., 22: 1.

Sun T, Ho C (2005). Antioxidant activities of buckwheat extracts. Food Chem., 90: 743-749.

Tabart J, Kevers C, Sipel A, Pincemail J, Defraigne JO, Dommes J (2007). Optimisation of extraction of phenolics and antioxidants from black currant leaves and buds and of stability during storage. Food Chem., 3: 1268-1275.

Wangensteen H, Samuelsen AB, Malterud KE (2004). Antioxidant activity in extracts from coriander. Food Chem., 88: 293-297.

Watson J, Arnold M, Ho YS, O` Dell T (2006). Age-dependent modulation of Hippocampal long term potentiation by antioxidant enzymes. J. Neurosci. Res., 84: 1564-1574.

Wolfe K, Wu X, Liu RH (2003). Antioxidant activity of apple peels. J. Agric. Food Chem., 51: 609-614.

Zhang EX, Yu LJ, Zhou YL, Xiao X (1996). Studies on the peroxidation of polyunsaturated fatty acid from lipoprotein induced by iron and the evaluation of the anti-oxidative activity of some natural products. Acta Biochem. Biophys. Sin., 28: 218-222.

Zhao H, Dong J, Lu J, Chen J, Li Y, Shan L, Lin Y, Fan W, Gu G (2006). Effects of extraction solvent mixtures on antioxidant activity evaluation and their extraction capacity and selectivity for free phenolic compounds in barley (Hordeum vulgare L.). J. Agric. Food Chem., 54(19): 7277-7286.

21

Variation in antioxidant and aroma compounds at different altitude: A study on tea (*Camellia sinensis* L. Kuntze) clones of Darjeeling and Assam, India

Sudeshna Bhattacharya and Swati Sen-Mandi*

BOSE INSTITUTE, Division of Plant Biology, MC, 93/1 APC Road, Kolkata – 700 009, India.

Plants at high altitude are subject to enhanced oxidative stress due to high UV fluence (resulting from air rarefaction) compared to places at low altitude. For survival, plants have developed specific cell protective compounds viz. the flavonoids. Flavonoid derivatives (viz. flavonoid glycoside) may also serve as precursor of aroma producing compounds and are thus relevant in studies on plant quality under varying UV fluence. This study was conducted with an aim to understanding the effect of geographic location viz. altitude on aroma compounds in tea leaf, focusing on the internationally reputed Darjeeling tea. Darjeeling grown tea clones (compared with the same clones growing in Assam) are found to have higher; (a) accumulation of flavonoids and flavonoid glycosides that are known to function as UV screens and antioxidants with flavonoid glycosides, additionally serving as aroma precursors, (b) activity of phenylalanine ammonia lyase for flavonoid biosynthesis, (c) activity of β-D glucosidase that releases aroma conferring aglycons from flavonoid glycosides, (d) accumulation of aglycons viz. linalool that is known to cause aroma in tea. In all the cases, a varietal difference (manifested in respective clones) was observed. The understanding developed from the study should help not only for plant survival in the face of global climate change but also for aroma enhancement in tea plants cultivated at non-conventional sites.

Key words: UV radiation, reactive oxygen species, flavonoid glycoside, aroma, tea, high altitude.

INTRODUCTION

Plants at high altitude under naturally prevailing high UV fluence are subject to enhanced oxidative stress (Lesser, 1996; Balakrishnan et al., 2005). To combat such stress, plants have evolved effective cell protective mechanisms that retard cell damaging processes thus enabling plants to survive on earth. In this context, a group of effective antioxidants, viz. the flavonoids specifically present in plants (Stapleton and Walbot, 1994) are particularly relevant. These compounds maintain antioxidant potential in cells due to the phenol-quinone tautomerism in the side chain; the flavonoid group of compounds serves as electron acceptors from reactive oxygen species (ROS)

mediated oxidized macromolecules, thereby protecting cells against UV caused ROS mediated damaging effect (Kirsch, 2001; Rebeiro et al., 2002). Accumulating in plant epidermis and showing absorption for UVA and UVB (Cockell and Knowland, 1999) by virtue of π →π* transition in core nucleus make flavonoids good contenders for sun screening protection in plant cells. Robberecht and Caldwell (1978) demonstrated that flavonoids block up to 95 to 98% transmittance of incoming UV radiation into plant cells. Derivatives of flavonoids, viz. flavonoid glycosides are also involved in conferring aroma compounds to various extents under variation in environment (Carrao-Panizi and Bordington, 2000). In view of the on going, study of plants growing at high altitude and at low altitude (under natural UV radiation-high and low respectively) seems a worthwhile proposition for generating information of interest particularly in the face of a global climate change. In this context, tea clones cultivated under similar tea cultivation

*Corresponding author. E-mail: swatism@bosemain.boseinst.ac.in, Senmandi.swati@gmail.com.

practices in Darjeeling and clones of the same varieties cultivated in Assam, both places at the same latitude (-27°N), ensures comparison in data between the two locations (Cabrera et al., 1995) on altitudinal variation in cell protection and quality of plants.

UV fluence is higher in the subtropical regions (Turunen and Latola, 2005); during the months of April to July, when the sun shifts to the Northern hemisphere, highest UV fluence is recorded within 15 to 35°N latitude (http//teanewsdarjeeling.blogspot.com/2010/04/rain-cheer for teaindustry-plantars-html), that encompasses many of the developing nations in northern Africa and southern parts of Asia including India. During this period, tea plants of Darjeeling and Assam produce the first flush (that is, first yearly burst) of leaves that produces best tea each year. Of the cultivation sites at these two places at different altitude, tea leaf of Darjeeling, India, is internationally reported for flavor/aroma quality (Lachman et al., 2003). For an in depth understanding towards developing strategies for value addition in tea plants cultivated at other sites, a comparison of experimental data between clones of different varieties of tea plants growing in tea cultivation sites of Darjeeling at ~4500 ft msl and of Assam at ~350 ft msl, where UV fluence presents single major variation in environmental factor, is presented here.

Plants growing in same location, that is, under equal UV fluence may exhibit variation in the degree of cell damage actually incurred; this is due to their variation in varietal/genetic make-up that determines the extent of genetically conferred flavonoid mediated defense against UVB radiation (Mazza et al., 2000). Reports that genetic block in the synthesis of flavonoids (that is, phenolic UV absorbing sunscreens) in phenylpropanoid mutants of *Arabidopsis* (Kliebenstein et al., 2002) and susceptibility of such plants to UV radiation (Li et al., 1993; Lois and Buchanan, 1994; Landry et al., 1995; Ryan et al., 2002) provide evidence to suggest a genetic effect as the basic cause for plant protection against natural UV radiation. Survival/occurrence of different plant groups at different altitudinal levels exemplifies such a phenomenon (Kreft et al., 2002). Constitutive levels the basic genetically controlled UV absorbing compounds viz. flavonoids and the readiness of plants to accumulate/enhance these in plants under enhanced UV radiation have been correlated with UV-B tolerance in several studies (Murali and Teramura, 1986). Such reports indicate epigenetic up-regulation of enzymes in the biosynthetic pathway for synthesis of flavonoids. Accumulation of flavonoids (in *Pisum sativum* leaf) only within hours of UV induction (Strid and Porra, 1992; He et al., 1994) provide further evidence for UV effect superimposed on the basic genetic attribute for flavonoid production and thereby establishes the existence of a relationship between increased UVB radiation and enhancement of genetically attributed flavonoid synthesis level in plant cells. Induction of enhanced flavonoid group of compounds in response to enhanced UV fluence may thus be seen as a prophylactic induction of reactionary biosynthesis of the flavonoid group of compounds (Strid and Porra, 1992). Phenylalanine ammonia lyase (PAL) and other enzymes involved in the biosynthetic pathway for phenolic compounds viz. flavonoids is also reported to be up-regulated by enhancement of UV (Logeman et al., 2000; Kubasek et al., 1992). This and other more direct studies (Strid and Porra, 1992; He et al., 1994) indicate an UV up-regulation effect on biosynthesis of flavonoids. Studies on effect of UV on the biosynthetic pathway involving the supply pathways from primary metabolism and also the final steps for flavonoid secondary product formation indicates an enhancing effect of UV on most of the enzymes involved in flavonoid production (Logeman et al., 2000).

In leaf of a number of plant species, the major flavonoids are found as derivatives in the form of flavonoid glycosides. These compounds exist as flavonoids linked by 1-2 and/or 1-6 glycoside bonds with sugar rings and exhibit a number of biological activities particularly conferring antioxidant potential (Rebeiro et al., 2002). Antioxidant potential of flavonoid glycosides have been reported in black berry, blue berry and red wine grape (Cho et al., 2004) and several other plants. In tea leaf, flavonoid glycosides is added to antioxidant potential, such compounds also contribute towards better quality in tea (Goswami and Barbora, 1994); the author suggests that the tasters' score for strength could be due to presence of higher amounts of flavonoid glycosides in the tasted tea. Das et al. (1994) also demonstrated the presence of flavonoid glycosides in Indian tea clones. In Chinese tea clones, Li et al. (2005) have reported glycosides with monoterpene alcohols and aryl alcohols as aglycons that on enzymatic hydrolysis, release aglycons (Conesa et al., 2002) such as linalool and geraniol that confer aroma in black tea, oolong tea and green tea (Sakata et al., 1995; Ogawa et al., 1995). Other derivatives of flavonoids viz. methylated flavonoid di- and tri glycosides (Franski et al., 2002) acetylated flavonol glycosides (Shahat et al., 2003) have also been reported in different plant species.

In different plants, the aglycon moiety is known to confer typical flavour. In soybean, flavonoid glycosides on cleavage at the glycosidic bonds by the enzyme β-D glucosidase, releases non reducing β-D glucose, and the terminal aglycone that have been reported to confer flavour, and also antioxidant potential in plants (Carrao-Panizzi and Bordington, 2000). Expression of the gene for β-D-glucosidase, the enzyme reported to split flavonoid glycoside, has also been reported to be enhanced (up-regulated) under abiotic stress (Spano et al., 2005) including UV radiation.

MATERIALS AND METHODS

Plant materials

Sampling scheme selection of leaves from high and low altitude tea gardens were randomly selected, each following the scheme simple random sampling without replacement (SRSWOR). Young leaves were collected from tea plants/clones of genotypes T78, AV2 and CP1 growing in conventional tea cultivation sites viz. Ging tea estate, Darjeeling, (at high altitude ~4500 ft msl) and Tocklai experimental station of tea research association (TRA), Tocklai, Assam (at low altitude ~ 350 ft msl). Both these places are at ~27°N latitude where variation in UV radiation at the respective altitudes represents the major variable environmental factor. From both these cultivation sites, leaves from clones of different varieties were collected for experimentation each year during the 1st flush (April to June) that provides the best tea of fresh and strong flavour (http//teanewsdarjeeling.blogspot.com/2010/04/rain-cheer for teaindustry-plantars-html).

Method

Flavonoid analysis

Total flavonoid in young leaf of clones originating from different varieties growing both at high and at low altitude was estimated by high performance liquid chromatography (Figure 1 and Table 1a) according to the method of Moriguchi et al. (2001). Experimental sample (young leaf) was extracted in 1 ml of a (1:1) (v/v) mixture of dimethyl sulphoxide (DMSO) and methanol; debris was removed by centrifugation at 6000 rpm for 3 min. The supernatant was diluted with distilled water and aliquots were injected into the chromategraphic system consisting of waters 501 pump, an automatic sampler, a Hypersil ODS reverse phase column (Hewlett Packard, $125 \times \phi$ 4 mm r.d.), and UV diode array detector (waters, detector 486). The elution schedule consisted of an initial 2 min of 20% methanol in 10 mM phosphoric acid followed by a gradient with increasing concentration of methanol from 20 to 100% in 55 min at the flow rate of 1 ml/min. The detector was set to measure spectra from 220 to 400 nm since the conjugated π systems of flavonoids afford good UV absorption; the eluent was monitored at 285 nm, that is, within the UV range of wavelength coinciding with absorption maxima (λ max) of flavonoids (that matches with UVB absorption). Rutin (quercetin-3-rutinoside) (Santa Cruz Biotechnology) was used as standard (0.01 mg/ml).

Flavonoid glycoside analysis

Flavonoid glucoside was specifically assayed (Poole and Poole, 1994) by thin layer chromatography (TLC). Methanol: water (1:1) extracts (in aliquots) were spotted with micro-capillary tube on silica gel coated plates (Figure 2). The silica plate (stationary phase) was placed in chloroform: acetone: methanol (20:6:5) that provided the mobile phase for the TLC run of the chemical components of the leaf extracts. Constituents of leaf were observed by specific (for flavonoid glycosides) color development using aqueous solution of 1% $FeCl_3$ and $K_3 Fe (CN)_6$.

Assay of rutin (specific flavanoid glycoside)

Rutin related assay of tea clones were done according to the modified method of Atanassova and Bagdassarian (2009). 500 mg of tea leaves are extracted in 50 ml of 80% methanol. With that, 2 ml distilled water and 5 ml ammonium molybdate were added. The mixture was diluted to 50 ml by adding distilled water. The standard rutin solution was prepared by dissolving 0.02 g of rutin in 50 ml of 80% methanol. Then, 2 ml of this standard rutin solution extract was considered comparable with sample material (tea clones) extract as mentioned. The absorbance of the sample extract and also the rutin

preparation were determined at 360 nm. The percent rutin content (%) of the samples was determined according to the following calculations and as shown in Table 1b.

Calculations:

Calculations are based on averaging results from analyses of triplicate samples.

The rutin content (R) % in the sample is calculated as follows:

$$(R) \% = \frac{A_{sample} \times C \times 50 \times 100}{A_{standard} \times W \times 2}$$

Where A_{sample} = absorbance of the sample at 360 nm, $A_{standard}$ = absorbance of the standard solution at 360 nm, C= concentration of standard solution of rutin in gm/ml, W = weight of the sample in gm, 2 ml = volume of the sample taken.

Assay for phenylalanine ammonia lyase (PAL)) (EC number 4.3.1.24)

200 mg tissue were homogenized at 4°C in a pre-cooled mortar and pestle with sea sand and 150 mg of poly vinyl pyrrolidone (PVP) in 3 ml of 0.1 M borate buffer (pH 8.8) containing 50 mM β-mercapto ethanol according to Saunders and McClure (1974). The homogenate was centrifuged at 18,200 g for 30 min at 4°C. Supernatant (1 ml) containing the enzyme phenylalanine ammonia lyase (PAL) was added to 0.5 ml of 50 mM L-phenylalanine (substrate) for enzyme assay. PAL activity was assessed by monitoring the increase in A_{290} against a control without phenylalanine over a period of 4 h at 1 h intervals. The rate of appearance of trans-cinnamic acid was taken as a measure of enzyme activity using an increase of 0.01 $A_{290} \equiv 3.09$ nmol of trans-cinnamic acid formed. The PAL activity is expressed in P_{kat} (pmol trans- cinnamic acid) formed per second per mg total protein (Figure 3) (total protein in leaf extract was assessed according to the method of Bradford (1976).

Total UV absorbing compounds analysis

200 mg of each sample were placed in 1.4 ml of 99:1 methanol: HCl and allowed to extract for 48h at -20°C. Absorbance of extract was read spectrophotometrically at 305 nm for determination of total UV absorbing compounds (Mazza et al., 2000) (Figure 4).

Antioxidant assay

The antioxidant potential of leaf extracts was determined as Ribeiro et al. (2002) on the basis of scavenging activity of the stable 2, 2'-diphenyl-1 picrylhydrazyl (DPPH) free radical (Figure 5). Aqueous extract (0.1 ml) of experimental leaf was added to 3 ml of a 0.004% methanolic solution of DPPH. Absorbance at 517 nm was determined after 30 min, and the percent inhibition activity was calculated as [(Ao-Ae) / Ao] x 100 (where Ao = absorption without extract, Ae= absorption with extract).

β-D glucosidase (EC number 3.2.1.21) enzyme assay

A method, modified over that of Matsuura et al. (1989) and Jiang and Li (1999) was used. Experimental leaf tissue was extracted in buffer (50 mM sodium acetate buffer pH 5.0 containing 1 mM ethylene diamine tetra acetic acid (EDTA), NaCl, $MgSO_4$, 1 mM

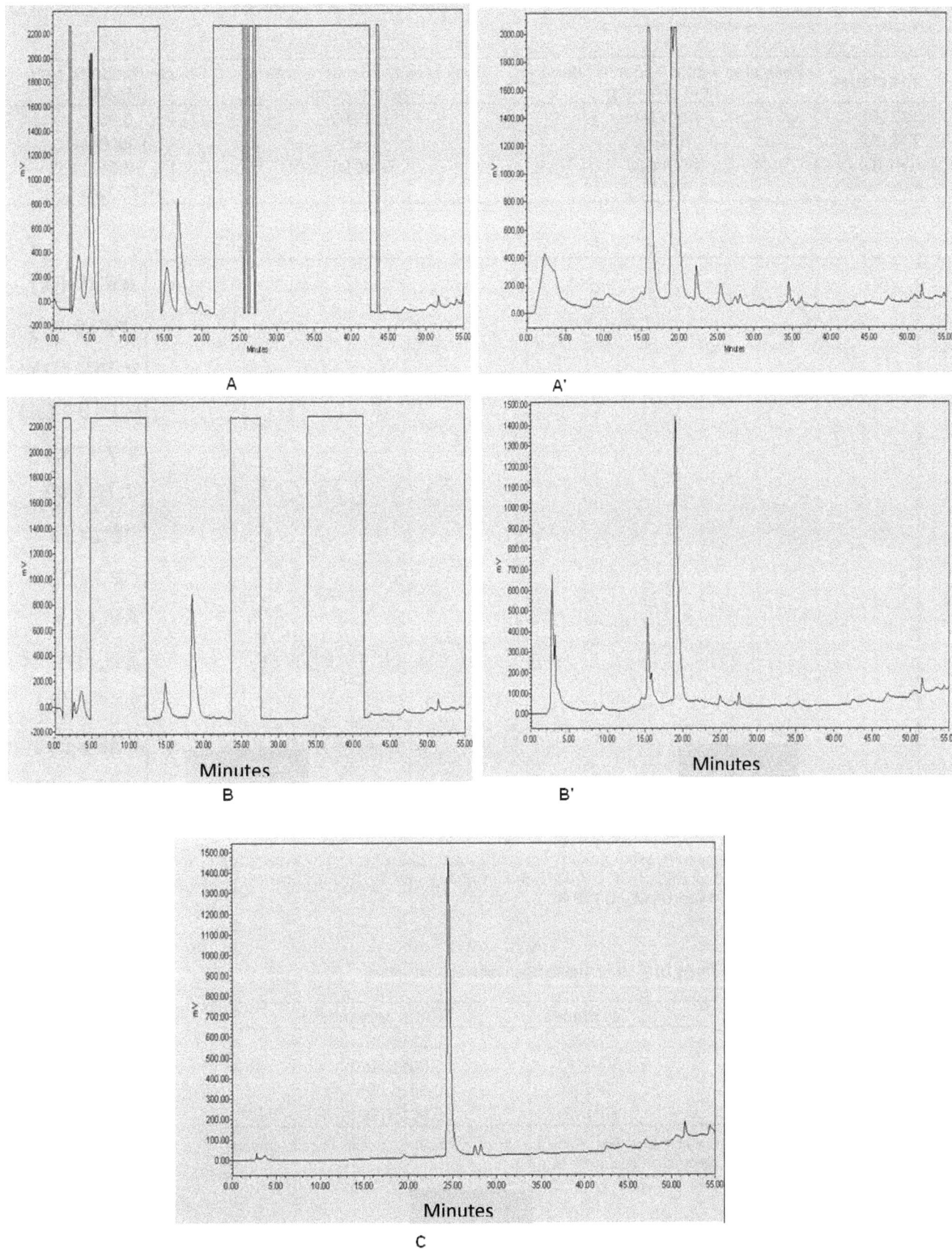

Figure 1. Flavonoid analysis by HPLC scan recorded at 285nm using DMSO: MeOH solvent system at 0-55min retention time in hypersil ODS2 column A = T78(D), A' = T78(A), B = CP1(D), B' = CP1(A), C = standard rutin.

Table 1a. Quantitative estimation for total flavonoids and flavonoid glycosides taken from HPLC scan, eluant taken at 285nm by UV diode array detector (waters 486) (Figure 1).

Tea clones	Peak area within 0-55 min retention time (mV-min)	Peak area at 25 min retention time (mV-min)	Concentration Of rutin (Mg/Ml)
T78 (D)	123700.11	11700.00	0.05
T78 (A)	1095.00	9.90	0.000044
CP1 (D)	95611.00	10000.90	0.04
CP1 (A)	832.75	8.0	0.000035

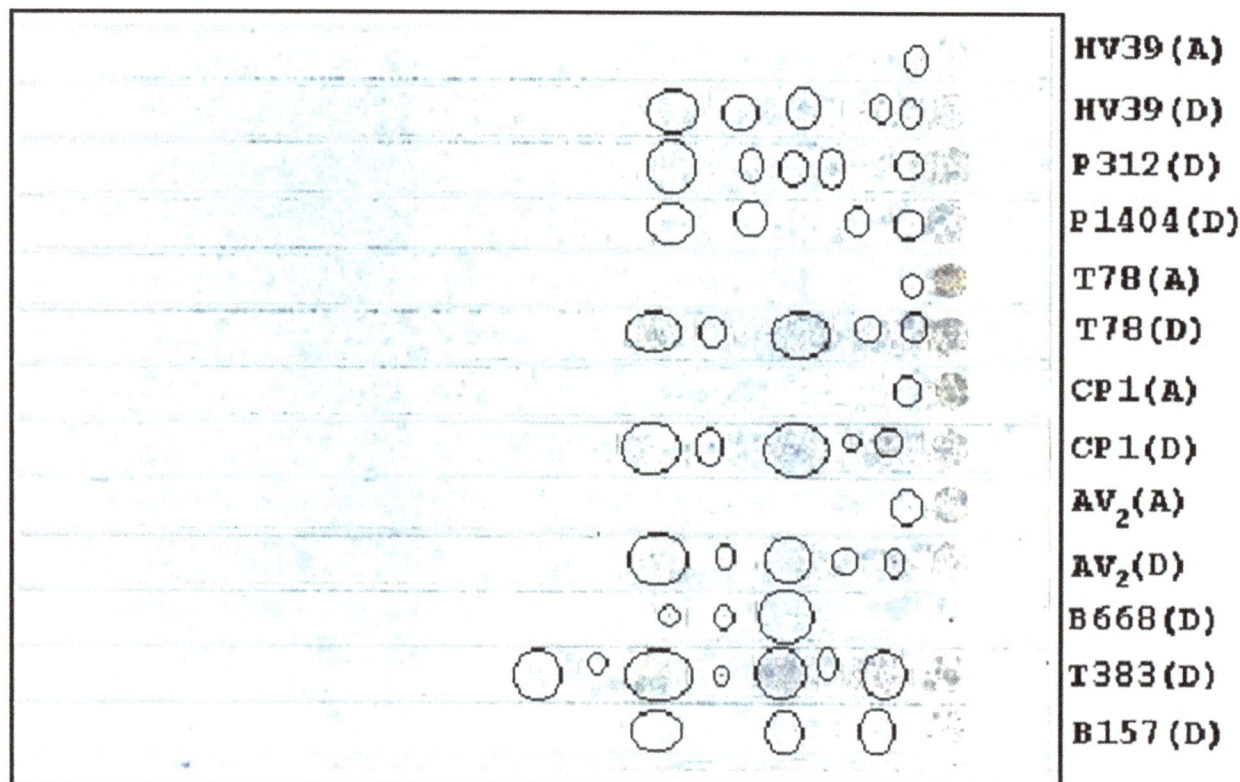

Figure 2. Thin layer chromatographic separation on plate of flavonoid glycoside in tea clones growing in high and low altitude. 1 = B157(D),2 = T383(D),3 = B668(D),4 = AV2(D),5 = AV2(A),6 = CP1(D),7=CP1(A), 8 = T78 (D),9 = T78(A),10 = P1404(D),11= P312(D),12 = HV39(D),13 = HV39(A).

Table 1b. Rutin content (%) in different tea clones.

Tea clones	Rutin content (%)
T78 (D)	0.65±0.001
T78 (A)	0.005±0.001
CP1 (D)	0.55±0.001
CP1 (A)	0.001±0.001

Estimation of total rutin (flavonoid glycoside) content (%) determined spectrophotometrically at 360 nm.

phenyl methane sulphonyl fluoride (PMSF), 1 M sucrose, 2% PVP, 5.6 mM β-mercaptoethanol, and centrifuged at 20,000 g for 20 min. Supernatant was taken for enzyme assay. One ml assay mixture contained 4 mM paranitrophenyl-β-D-glucopyranoside (PNPG), in sodium citrate buffer (pH 4.0) and 60 μl leaf extract. After incubating for 10 min at 40°C, the reaction was stopped by adding 3 ml of aqueous sodium carbonate (2% w/v) and the color, developed as a result of p-nitrophenol liberation, was measured

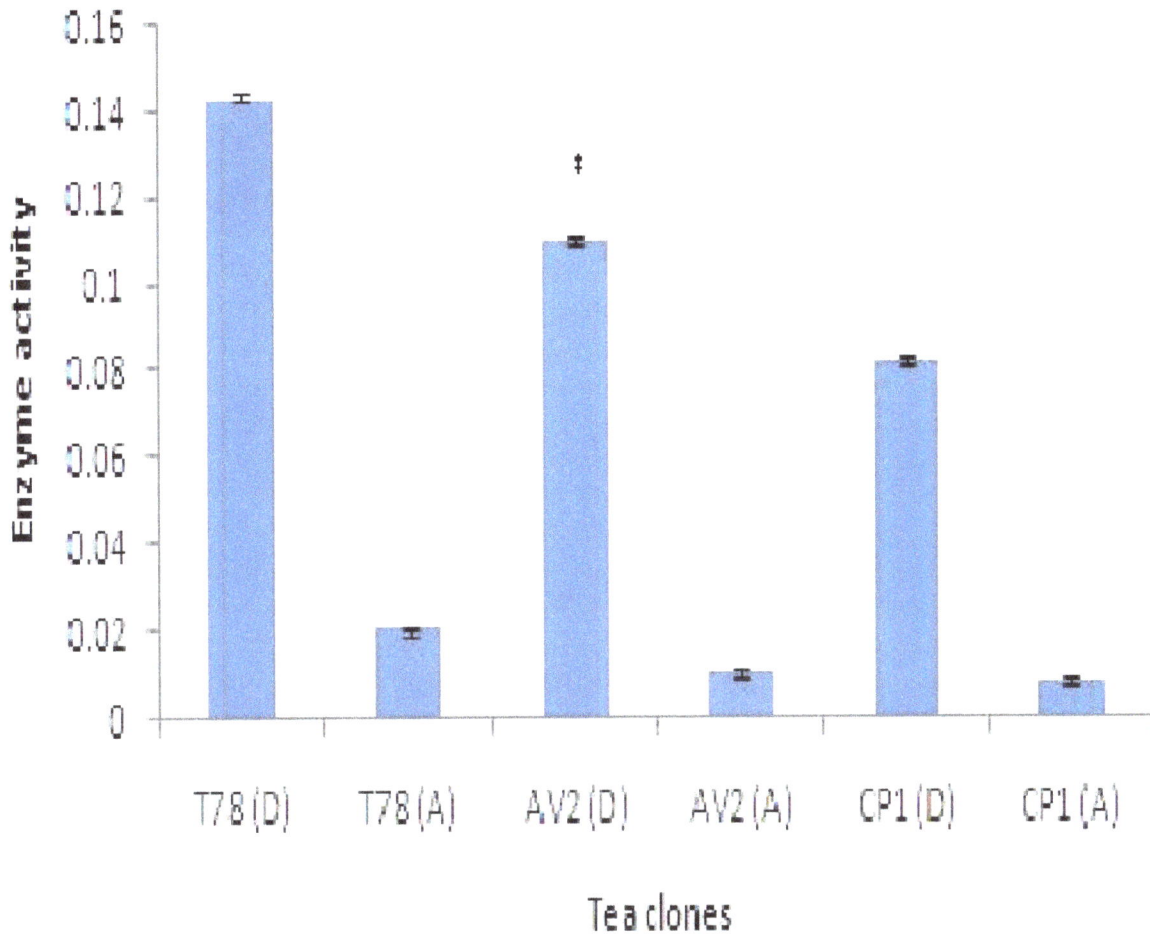

Figure 3. Spectrophotometric assay of enzyme phenylalanine ammonia lyase of tea clones viz. T78, AV2, CP1. D = Darjeeling, A = Assam. (P < 0.001, for S. D n = 6).

spectrophotometrically at 410 nm. The change in absorbance at 410 nm gives assessment of the enzyme activity. The data expressed as activity / mg protein is presented in Figure 6 (total protein in leaf extract was assessed according to the method of Bradford, 1976).

Assay for linalool

Percent content of linalool was measured according to reports in http://www.ffcr.or.jp/zaidan. Ten milliliters of leaf extract (200 mg leaf extracted in 10 ml of Tris-Cl buffer pH 7.5) was transferred into a flask and allowed to stand in ice water for 10 min; after this, 20 ml of dimethylaniline was added and shaken well. This was followed by addition of 10 ml acetyl chloride and 5 ml of anhydrous acetic acid and left to stand for 5 min in ice cold condition, allowed 30 min at room temperature, followed by heating in a water bath at 50°C for 4 h. After cooling, the contents were transferred to a separating funnel, and washed 3 times with 75 ml ice cold water. The oily layer was then washed with 25 ml of dilute sulfuric acid. Sodium hydroxide solution was added to alkalinize the washings until turbidity subsided. The extract was then washed with 10 ml of sodium carbonate solution until it become alkaline; then again, it was washed with 25 ml of sodium chloride solution until the solution become neutral. Oily phase was transferred into a dried flask. 2 g of anhydrous sodium sulfate was added, shaken and allowed to stand

for 30 min; the extract was then filtered. The filtrate was weighed and taken for assay. Using a blank and a standard linalool (Sigma, Aldrich), the percent content of linalool of the sample (Figure 7) was done.

Biostatistical analysis

In every assay, student's t-test was performed. P-values were tested in each case and in all experiments, standard deviation (S.D) values were varied according to the value of n (number of times experiments are done).

RESULTS AND DISCUSSION

Total flavonoid by high-performance liquid chromatography (HPLC) method

Spectrophotometric scans at 285 nm of the HPLC eluants reveal a varietal difference in total flavonoid (including flavonoid glycosides) content among the tea clones representing different varieties (Figure 1). The scans, covering a period of 0 to 55 min retention time in all the

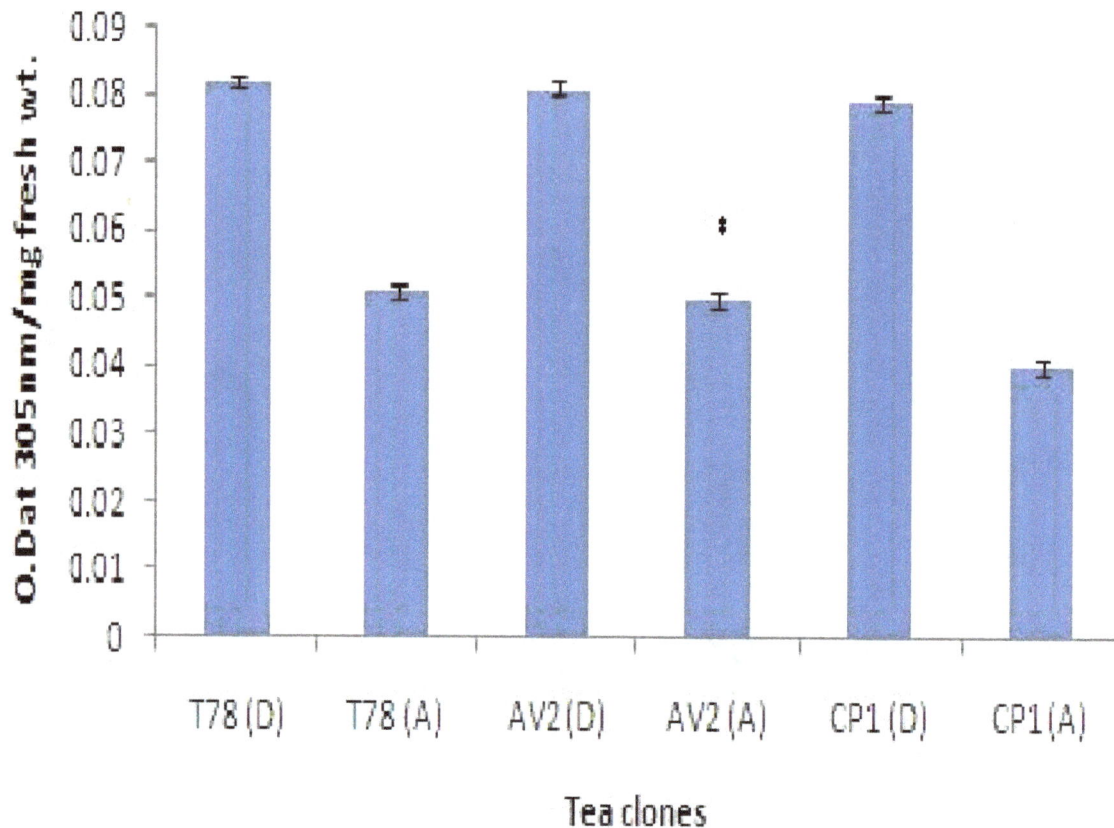

Figure 4. Spectrophotometric assay of total UV absorbing compounds of different tea clones viz. T78, AV2, CP1. D = Darjeeling, A = Assam. (P < 0.001, for S. D n = 6).

samples, show a near base-line separation, revealing clear varietal difference in flavonoids between the tea clones grown at each altitude viz. in Darjeeling (~4500 ft msl) and in clones of the same varieties in Assam (~350 ft msl). An enhancing effect of high altitude related high UV (that is the major environmental factor differing in these two cultivation sites) is further evident in the Darjeeling clones. Hofmann et al. (2000) have similarly reported that in *Trifolium repens*, where leaf quercetin glycoside, that is, rutin is a varietal expression, varying in amount in different cultivars, a pronounced UV-B induced increase in the flavonol glycosides is also evident. A quantitative estimate of peak area determined according to Schierle et al. (2004) within 0 to 55 min retention time is given in Table 1a. This data shows higher values in high altitude grown tea clones (A and B in Figure 1) superimposed on the varietal difference observed in each altitude. Studies on nine *T. repens* populations have also revealed UVB related variation in accumulation of flavonol glycoside; under enhanced UV radiation the content of quercetin glycoside (viz. rutin) was found to be about three-times more than in the controls (Hoffman et al., 2000) presumably due to UV light induced up-regulation of flavonoid glycoside synthesis (Logeman et al. 2000). For such synthesis, a UV photoreceptor mediated signal transduction pathway has also been

implicated (Pratt and Butler, 1970). HPLC scan of the standard rutin (Santa Cruz Biotechnology) sample in 25 min eluant (0.01 mg/ml, peak area 2227.5 mV-min at 25 min retention time), equivalent with concentration 0.01 mg/ml is given in Figure 1(marked as C). Comparison of these scans with that obtained for the authentic flavonoid glucoside viz. rutin sample shows clearly that amongst other types of flavonoids and flavonoid glycosides shown in the scans, rutin is a major component in the Darjeeling grown tea clones (Figure 1, marked A and B); in the Assam grown clones presence of rutin appears comparatively insignificant (Figure 1, marked A' and B').

Flavonoid glycosides visualized by TLC

For a specific study of flavonoid glycoside, a TLC method in methanolic leaf extracts with ferric salts for colour development is presented in Figure 2. Although qualitative, a clear difference could be observed with respect to flavonoid glycosides between the low altitude (Assam) and high altitude (Darjeeling) growing clones. Whereas the plants growing at high altitude showed about 5 to 6 spots, the same clones grown in low altitude showed only 1 spot. A comparison of the data on flavonoid glycosides obtained by different techniques viz.

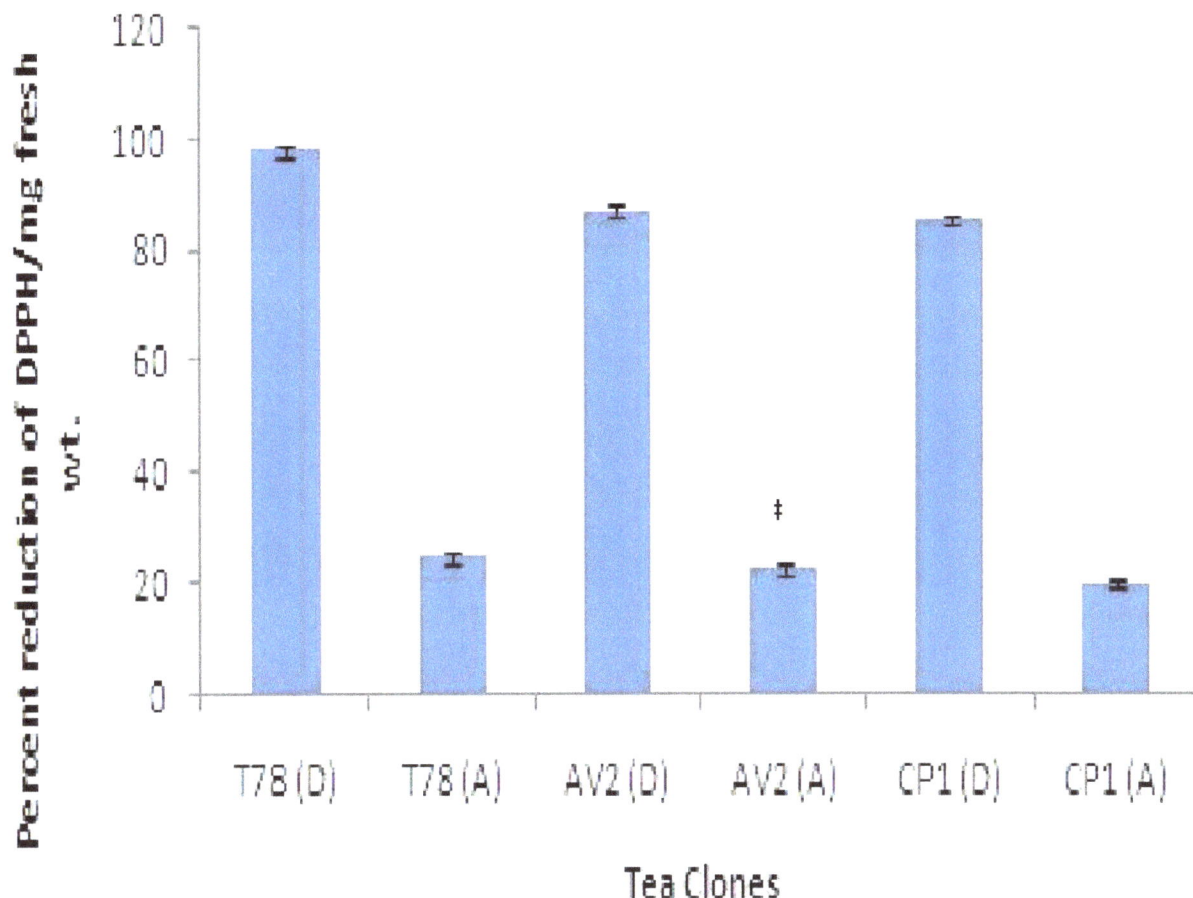

Figure 5. Spectrophotomatric assay of antioxidant potential in tea clones viz. T78, AV2, CP1 (D = Darjeeling, A = Assam) by percent reduction of DPPH recorded at 517   nm. (P < 0.001, for S. D, n = 6).

HPLC (Table 1a) and TLC (Figure 2) reveals that Darjeeling grown tea clones have greater accumulation of flavonoids and flavonoid glycosides that are known to serve as antioxidants and also as aroma precursors. It is pertinent to mention here that the market value of Darjeeling tea is internationally known to possess high antioxidant and aroma values (Lachman et al., 2003).

Spectrophtometric values (at 360 nm) for total rutin - a flavonoid glycoside, functioning as antioxidants show varietal difference in the clones growing at each altitude. For all the varieties, a superimposed enhancement due to UV over the genetic attribute in each variety was evident between clones at high and low altitude (Table 1b). The proportionately high value in clones of each variety at high altitude is presumably due to high altitude related high UV fluence. Studies on maize (Stapleton and Walbot, 1994) and on parsley (Logemann et al., 2000) have also shown higher flavonoid glycoside accumulation in plants growing under high (artificial) UV radiation than in the untreated control plants. Carrao-Panizzi and Bordingnon (2000) have also reported varietal difference in (iso) flavone glycosides is further altered by environment (in soybean cultivars).

Phenylalanine ammonia lyase activity (PAL) (EC number 4.3.1.24) activity

Phenylalanine ammonia lyase (PAL) activity exhibited a varietal difference in values at both altitudes - the values being higher (with respect to the value for the different varieties at low altitude) in the high altitude grown tea clones (Figure 3). The data suggest that phenylalanine ammonia lyase activity (PAL) (Figure 3), a key enzyme in the biosynthetic pathway for flavonoid production, although basically under genetic control, is further enhanced/up regulated at high altitude locations presumably due to altitude related high UV radiation. From studies on pea, Pluskota et al. (2005) have demonstrated UV stress induced enhancement in flavonoid biosynthesis through signal-transduced transcription (up-regulation) of genes for phenylalanine ammonia lyase, in the phenylpropanoid pathway/anthocyanin pathway. It may be noted this pattern of difference is also reflected in the value of accumulation of the flavonoids and its derivatives viz. flavonoid glycosides (such as, products of the anthocyanin pathway preceded by the phenylpropanoid

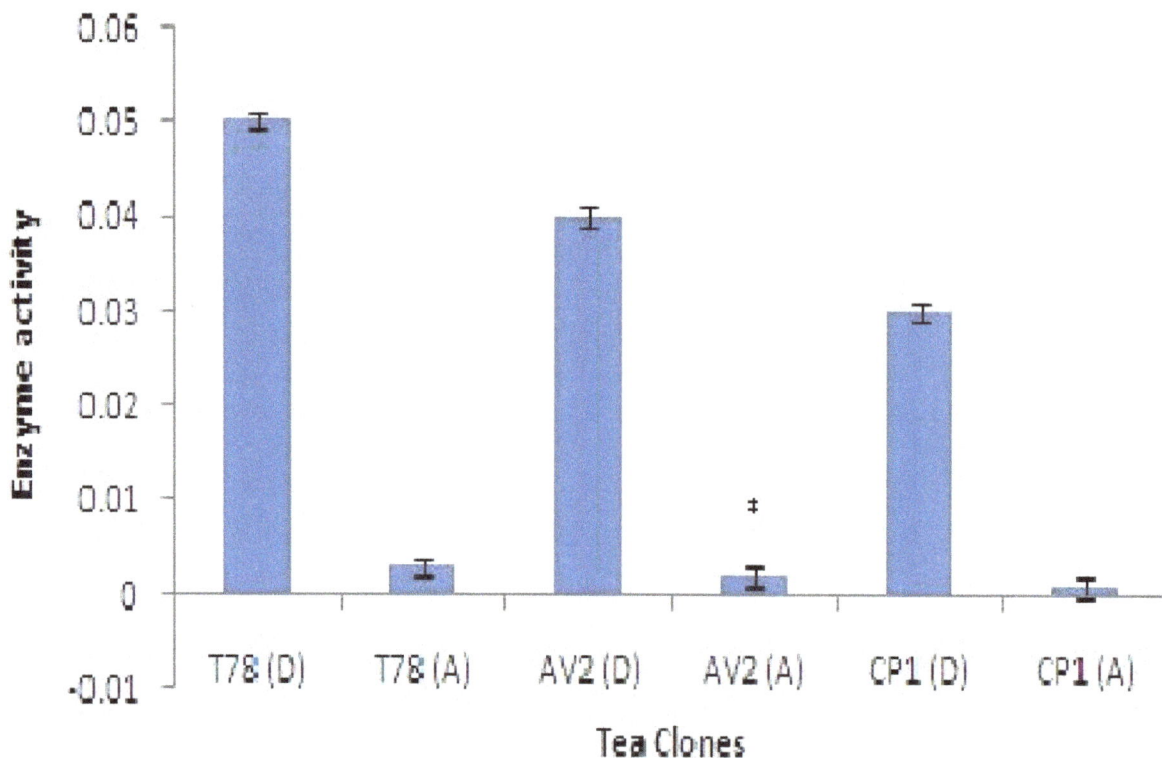

Figure 6. Spectrophotometric assay of β -D Glucosidase enzyme activity of tea clones viz. T78, AV2, CP1. D = Darjeeling, A = Assam. (P < 0.001, for S. D n = 6).

pathways involving PAL) as is recorded in Figures 1, 2 and 3 and Table 1.

Assay of UV absorbing compounds

Spectrophotometric assay (Mazza et al., 2000) at 305 nm of UV absorbing compounds (Figure 4) that represent an important role of the flavonoid group of compounds shows higher values in tea leaf of plants at high altitude (D) compared to plants of the same genotypes growing in low altitude (A) - a varietal difference between the clones still remain clearly evident at each altitude, appearing enhanced at high altitude. The higher values of UV absorbing was found to correlate with the higher content of flavonoids (Figure 1 and Table 1) that are known to function as UV absorbing compounds. Variation between genotypes with respect to UV absorbing compounds has also been reported in other field grown plants (Quaite et al., 1994). Caldwell (1968) has reviewed the possible roles of flavonoids in absorbing solar UV radiation, especially at high elevation.

Assay of total antioxidant potential

A varietal (genetic) difference in antioxidant potential between the varieties was evident at both the altitudes

- the values for each variety was found to be further enhanced at high altitude, showing higher values in the Darjeeling grown clones compared to that of the low altitude (Assam) grown clones of the same varieties (Figure 5). Antioxidant potential data (Figure 5) shows clearly that in addition to a varietal difference, the altitudinal difference apparently (due to UV fluence) plays a major role in determining antioxidant potential in tea leaf. This explains why Darjeeling tea exhibits higher (than Assam clones) antioxidant potential as is conventionally known (Lachman et al., 2003). This data may be compared with Figure 1 that shows high value for flavonoids (that are polyphenolic compounds) that, in addition to serving as UV screens, may also serve as antioxidants. It is pertinent to mention here that flavonoids, flavonoid glycosides and several intermediates in the phenylpropanoid pathway that serve as antioxidants are reported to exhibit anticancer/antiapoptitic functions; such functions have been reported to be higher in Darjeeling (high altitude at ~27ºN latitude) grown tea plants.

Assay of aroma releasing enzyme β-D glucosidase (EC number 3.2.1.21) activity

Spectrophotometric assay of β-D-glucosidase shows (Figure 6) higher specific activity (U = activity/μg protein)

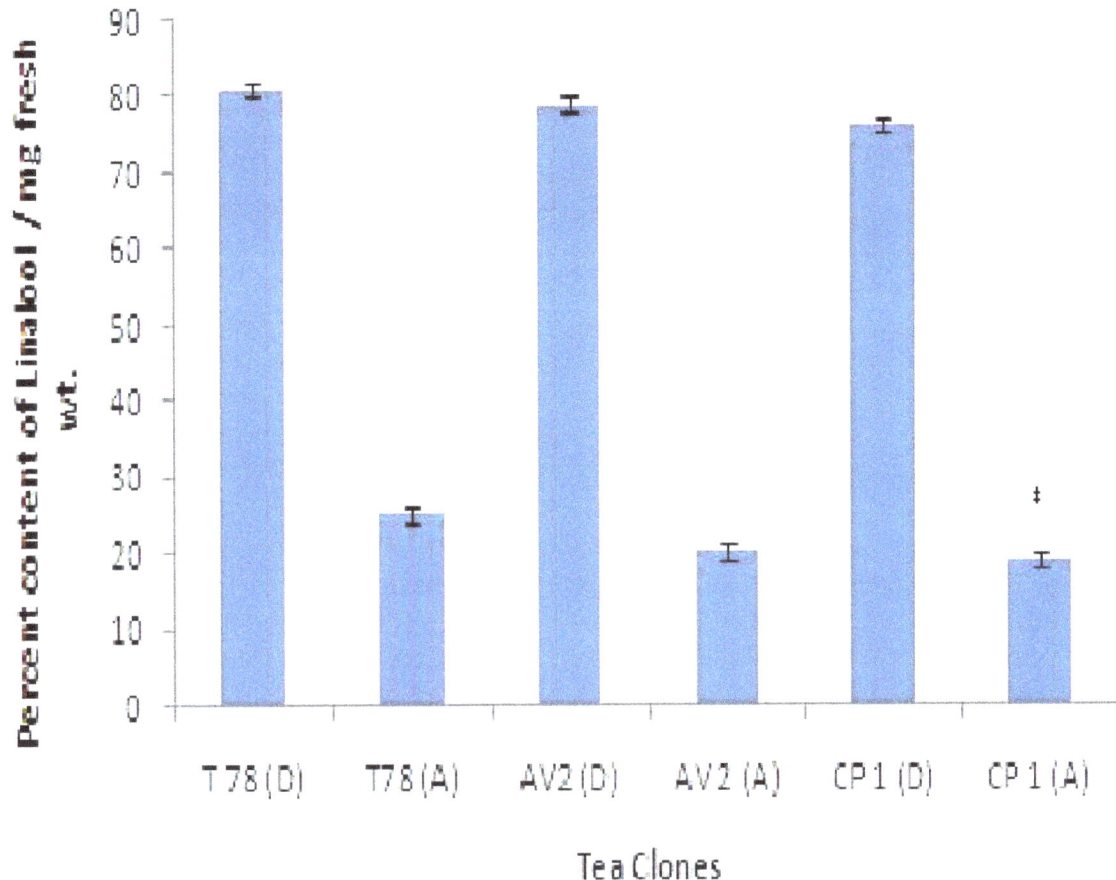

Figure 7. Percent content of linalool in different tea clones viz. T78, AV2, CP1. D = Darjeeling, A = Assam. (P < 0.001, for S. D n = 6).

in high altitude (Darjeeling) grown clones than in the same clones grown in low altitude (Assam) - the values appearing as superimposed enhancement over varietal attribute in each variety. The data reveals varietal difference at each altitude with T78 showing higher activity than CP 1 and AV2 at both the altitudes. The enhancement in values of the varieties at high altitude is presumably due to altitude related UV enhancement.

Assay of total linalool content

Spectrophotometric assay of aroma causing aglycon moiety (assayed in comparison to a standard linalool--Sigma Aldrich) known to be produced by activity of β-D glucosidase on a substrate linked β-D glucoside (Moon et al., 1996) provide the data in Figure 7. It is clear from the data that high accumulation of linalool in tea leaf is a function of high altitude environment over and above the varietal difference in values at each altitude. In comparison with data in Figure 6, it is evident that high altitude related UV fluence caused enhancement in activity of the enzyme β-D glucosidase, results in higher production of this aglycon moiety viz. linalool. Linalool

has been reported to be high in black tea, oolong tea and green tea (Ogawa et al., 1995). It appears that the high aroma known for Darjeeling orthodox tea (Lachman et al., 2003) is due to the high level of aglycon moiety, viz. linalool, occurring in fresh leaf of Darjeeling grown tea clones.

Conclusion

High accumulation of flavonoids (Figure 1) and flavonoid glycosides (Figure 1, Table1a,Table 1b, Figure 2), and higher activity of PAL *(EC 4.3.1.24)* (Figure 3) for production of flavonoids that function as UV absorbing compounds (Figure 4) and antioxidant (Figure 5) as well as higher activity of β-D glucosidase *(EC 3.2.1.21)* (Figure 6) that splits flavonoid glycosides to cause the production of aroma causing compounds viz. linalool (Figure 7), was found to be higher in high altitudes grown tea plants; the values are found to be comparable to a basic value that reflects a varietal difference, such observation was true for both altitudes. The data presented relate to tea plants growing at high altitudes (Darjeeling) and low altitude (Assam) - both places falling

PRIMARY   **SECONDARY METABOLISM**

METABOLISM

Acetyl co A   **UV RADIATION**

                                                                                          glycon

                                                                                          moieties

ACCase

Palmitate ◄—— **Malonyl**   Naringenin   ➤ Flavonols   ➤ Flavonoid
          COA CoA   **1** Chalcone   **2**   **3**   **4**

                                                            Glycosides

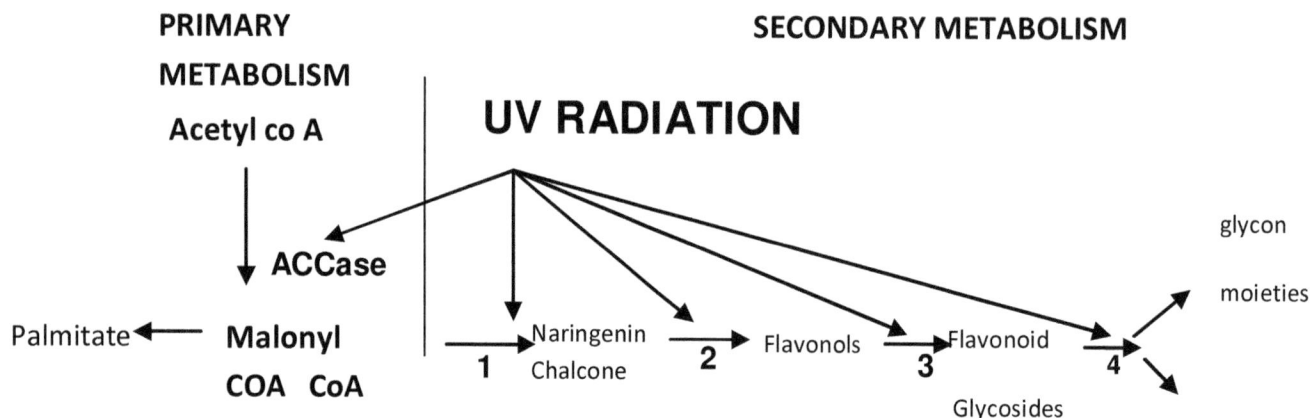

Scheme 1. Schematic presentation of UV involvement in secondary metabolism. 1: chalcone synthase; 2: 3′–O- Methyl transferees; 3: UDP-glucose flavone : flavonol 7- 0- glucosyltransferase; 4. β-D-glucosidase.

within the subtropical region of the Northern hemisphere viz. on ~27ºN. It is pertinent to mention here that experimental tea leaf were collected during April to June for several consecutive years and hence, the data presented here relate to tea leaf produced during the 1st flush of tea leaf in Darjeeling and Assam. This suggests that high aroma and high antioxidant potential known for Darjeeling tea is a location specific attribute presumably caused by UV mediated epigenetic effect viz. up-regulation of relevant genes under high altitude related high UV fluence.

This study establishes that although UV radiation is generally known to cause cell destruction, (representing a negative effect of UV on plant growth and development), UV stress may in turn up-regulate the production of cell protective and aroma causing compounds that may also serve as photoreceptors for signaling further production of the protective and quality compounds (as represented in Scheme 1). This report presents our comparative study on the flavonoid group of compounds and associated enzymes with respect to antioxidant and aroma (value addition) in leaf of tea plants growing in conventional tea cultivation sites at high altitude (Darjeeling) and low altitude (Assam), between which UV fluence presents the single major variation in environmental factors. The experimental data presented here establishes the biochemical status of Darjeeling tea leaf with reference to the "Darjeeling Tea" of repute. Such a study should also be useful in planning strategies for tea cultivation in non-conventional sites particularly in the face of a global climate change.

ACKNOWLEDGEMENTS

The authors gratefully acknowledge receiving experimental plant material from Mr. A. Lohia, Ging Tea Estate, Darjeeling, India, and from Tea Research Association (TRA), Jorhat, Assam India.

REFERENCES

Atanassova M, Bagdassarian V (2009). Rutin content in plant products. J. Univ. Chem. Technol. Metal., 44 (2): 201-203.

Balakrishnan V, Ravindran KC, Venkatesan K, Karuppusamy S (2005). Effect of UV-B supplemental radiation on growth and biochemical characteristics in Crotalaria Juncea L. seedling. EJEAF Che., 4 (6): 1125-1131

Bradford MM (1976). A rapid and sensitive for the quantification of microgram quantities of protein utilizing the principle of protein-dye binding. Anal. Biochem., 72: 284-254.

Cabrera S, Bozzo S, Fuenzalida HV (1995). Variations in UV radiation in Chile. J. Photochem. Photobiol. B: Biol. 28 (2): 137-142.

Caldwell MM (1968) Solar ultraviolet radiation as an ecological factor for alpine plants. Ecol. Monogr., 38: 243-268.

Carrao-Panizzi MC, Bordingnon JR (2000). Activity of beta-glucosidase and levels of isoflavone glucosides in soybean cultivars affected by the environment. Pesq Agropec Bras., 35: 873-878.

Cho MJ, Howard LR, Prior RL, Clark JR (2004). Flavonoid glycosides and antioxidant capacity of various blackberry, blueberry and red grape genotypes determined by high performance liquid chromatography / mass spectrometry. J. Sci. Food Agric., 84: 1771-1782.

Cockell CS, Knowland J (1999) Ultraviolet radiation screening compounds. Biol. Rev., 74: 311-345.

Conesa A, Punt PJ, Van den Hondel CAMJJ (2002) Fungal peroxidases: molecular aspects and applications. J. Biotechnol., 93: 143-158.

Das AK, Gogai MN, Gogoi R, Goswami MR (1994). Modification of CTC processing for quality improvement. Proceeding of the 32nd Tocklai Conference. pp. 294-299.

Franski R, Matlawska I, Bylka W, Sikorska M, Fiedorow P, Stobiecki M (2002). Differentiation of interglycosidic linkages in permethylated flavonoid glycosides from linked-scan mass spectra (B/E). J. Agric. Food Chem., 50: 976-982.

Goswami MR, Barbora BC (1994). Chemical factors influencing seasonal quality of clonal teas. Proceedings of the 32nd Tocklai Conference. pp. 281-293.

He J, Huang LK, Whitecross MI (1994). Chloroplast ultrastructure changes in Pisum sativum associated with supplementary ultraviolet (UV-B) radiation. Plant Cell Environ., 17: 771-775.

Hofmann RW, Swinny EE, Bloor SJ, Markham KR, Ryan KG, Campbell BD, Jordan BR, Fountain DW (2000). Responses of nine Trifolium repens L. populations to ultraviolet –B radiation: differential flavonol glycoside accumulation and biomass production. Ann. Bot., 86: 527-537.

Jiang CJ, Li YY (1999). Studies on testing conditions of β-D-glucosidase activity in tea. J. Anhui. Agric. Univ., 22: 212-215.

Kirsch JD (2001). Flavonoids: the good, the bad and the ugly. Free

Radicals Biol. Med., 77: 222.

Kliebenstein DJ, Lim JE, Landry LG, Last RL (2002). Arabidopsis UVR8 regulates ultraviolet- B signal transduction and tolerance and contains sequence similarity to human regulator of chromatin condensation. Plant Physiol., 130: 234-243.

Kreft S, Trukelj BA, Gaber IK, Kreft I (2002). Rutin in buckwheat herbs grown at different UV-B radiation levels: comparison of two UV spectrophotometric and an HPLC method. J. Exp. Bot., 53 (375): 1801-1804.

Kubasek WL, Shirley BW, Mckillop A, Goodman HM, Briggs W, Ausubel FM (1992). Regulation of flavonoid biosynthetic genes in germinating Arabidopsis seedlings. Plant Cell., 4: 1229-1236.

Lachman J, Orsak M, Pivec V, Dudjak J, Krym O (2003). Polyphenol content in green black and oolong tea (Camellia sinensis (L.)Kuntze) infusions in different times of tea maceration. Scientia Agric. Bohem., (Czech Republic). 34: 22-28.

Landry LG, Chapple CCS, Last RL (1995). Arabidopsis mutants lacking phenolic sunscreens exhibit enhanced Ultraviolet – B injury and oxidative damage. Plant Physiol., 109: 1159 – 1166.

Lesser MP (1996). Elevated temperatures and ultraviolet radiation cause oxidative stress and inhibit photosynthesis in symbiotic dinoflagellates. Limnol. Oceanogr., 41(2): 271-283.

Li J, Ou-Lee TM, Raba R, Amundson RG, Last RL (1993). Arabidopsis flavonoid mutants are hypersensitive to UV – B irradiation. Plant Cell., 5: 171-179.

Li YY, Jiang CJ, Wan XC, Zhang ZZ, Li DX (2005). Purification and partial characterization of β-glucosidase from fresh leaves of tea plants (Camellia sinensis (L.) O. Kuntze). Acta Biochem. Biophys. Sinica, 37: 363-370.

Logemann E, Tavernaro A, Schulz W, Somssich IE, Hahlbrock K (2000). UV light selectively induces supply pathways from primary metabolism and flavonoid secondary product formation in parsley. Proc. Nat. Acad. Sci., 97: 1903-1907.

Lois R, Buchanan BB (1994). Severe sensitivity to ultraviolet radiation in an Arabidopsis mutant deficient in flavonoid accumulation II. Mechanism of UV- resistance in Arabidopsis. Planta, 194: 504-509.

Matsuura M, Obata A, Fukushima D (1989). Objectionable flavor of soymilk developed during the soaking of soybeans and its control. J. Food Sci., 54: 602-605.

Mazza CA, Boccalandro HE, Giordano CV, Battista D, Scopel AL, Ballare CL (2000). Functional significance and induction by solar radiation of ultraviolet-absorbing sunscreens in field-grown soyabean crops. Plant Physiol., 122: 117-126.

Moon JH, Watanabe N, Ijima Y, Yagi A, Ina K, Sakata K (1996). Cis- and trans-Linalool 3,7-oxides and methyl salicylate glycosides and (Z)-3-hexenyl β-D-glucopyranoside as aroma precursors from tea leaves for oolong tea. Biosci. Biotech. Biochem., 60: 1815–1819.

Moriguchi T, Kita M, Tomono Y, Endo-Inagaki T, Omura M (2001). Gene Expression in flavonoid biosynthesis: Correlation with flavonoid accumulation is developing citrus fruit. Physiologia Plantarum., 111: 66-74

Murali NS, Teramura AH (1986). Effectiveness of UV-B radiation on the growth and physiology of field grown soybean modified by H_2O stress. Photochem. Photobiol., 44: 215-220.

Ogawa K, Moon JH, Guo WF, Yagi A, Watanabe N, Sakata K (1995). A study on tea aroma formation mechanism: Alcoholic aroma precursor amounts and glycosidase activity in part of the tea plant. Z Naturfor., 50:493-498.

Poole CF, Poole SK (1994). Instrumental thin layer chromatography. Anal. Chem., 66: 27-37.

Pluskota WE, Michalczyk DJ, Gorecki RJ (2005). Control of phenylalanine ammonia-lyase gene promoters from pea by UV radiation. ACTA Physiol. Plant., 27: 229-236.

Pratt LH, Butler WL (1970). Phytochrome conversion by ultraviolet light. Photochem. Photobiol., 11: 503-509.

Quaite FE, Takayanagi S, Ruffini J, Sutherland JC, Sutherland BM (1994). DNA damage levels determine cyclobutyl pyrimidine dimer repair mechanisms in alfalfa seedlings. Plant Cell., 6:1635-1641.

Robberecht R, Caldwell MM (1978). Leaf epidermal transmittance of ultraviolet radiation and its implication for plant sensitivity to ultraviolet-radiation induced injury. Oecologia, 32: 277-287.

Ribeiro AB, Silva DHS, Bolzani VS da Silva (2002). Antioxidant flavonol glycosides from Nectandra grandiflora (Lauraceae). Eclet Quim. (ISSN 0100-4670 versao impressa): 27 pecial Sao Paulo. 2002.

Ryan KG, Swinny EE, Winefield C, Markham KR (2002). Flavonoids and UV photo- protection in Arabidopsis mutants. Z. Naturfor., 56: 745-754.

Sakata K, Guo WF, Moon JH (1995). Molecular basis of alcoholic aroma formation in Oolong tea. In Proceedings of 95 International Tea-quality -- Human Health Symposium in Shanghai. Hangzhou Tea Society of China 1995. 175-187.

Saunders JA, McClure JW (1974). The suitability of a quanitative spectrophotometric assay for phynylalanine ammonia lyase activity in Braley, Buckwheat and Pea seedlings. Plant Physiol., 54: 412-413.

Schierle J, Pietch B, Fizet C (2004). Method for the Determination of Beta Carotene in Supplements and Raw Materials by Reversed-Phase Liquid Chromatography: Single Laboratory Validation. J. AOAC. Int., 87(5): 207-213.

Shahat AA, Cos P, Hermans N, Apers, S, De Bruyne T, Pieters L , Berghe DV, Vlietinck AJ (2003). Anticomplement and antioxidant activities of new accetylated flavonoid glycosides from Centaurium spicatum . Planta Med., 69: 1153-1156.

Stapleton AE, Walbot V (1994). Flavonoids can protect maize DNA from the induction of ultraviolet radiation damage. Plant Physiol., 105: 881-889.

Spano G, Rinaldi A, Ugliano M, Moio L, Beneduce L, Massa S (2005). A β-glucosidase gene isolated from wine Lactobacillus plantarum is regulated by abiotic stresses. J. Appl. Microbiol., 98: 855–861.

Strid A, Porra RJ (1992). Alterations in pigment content in leaves of Pisum sativum after exposure to supplementary UV-B. Plant and Cell Physiol., 33: 1015-1023.

Turunen M, Latola K (2005). UV-B radiation and acclimatization in timberline plants. Environ. Pollut., 137: 1205-1216.

22

Antidermatophytic activities of *Ixora brachiata Roxb*

B. Sadeghi-Nejad[1]* and S.S Deokule[2]

[1]Department of Mycoparasitology, Medical School, Joundi-Shapour University of Medical Sciences, Ahwaz, Iran.
[2]Department of Botany, University of Pune Ganeshkhind, Pune- 411007, India.

The *in vitro* antifungal activity of *Ixora brachiata Roxb.* leaf and root extracts were evaluated against three different genera of dermatophytes viz. *Microsporum, Trichophyton* and *Epidermophyton* by Dilution Agar Method. The crude extracts of *Ixora brachiata* root and leaf showed *in-vitro* antifungal properties and completely prevented the growth of tested dermatophytic species with minimum inhibitory concentration (MIC) values of *I. brachiata* leaf (IBL) and *I. brachiata* root (IBR) between 5.0 - 10 and 2.5 - 10 mg ml^{-1} medium, respectively. Minimum fungicidal concentration (MFC) values of *I. brachiata* leaf (IBL) and *I. brachiata* root (IBR) was also similar to 5.0 and 2.5 mg ml^{-1} of the medium, respectively. Results of phytochemical screening indicated that the leaf and root of *I. brachiata* gave positive test for starch, saponins, reducing sugars, anthraquinones, glycosides, phenols and proteins while they gave negative test for alkaloids. IBL gave positive test for tannins while IBR gave positive test for flavonoids. Detection of coumarins and triterpenes in IBL suggested that these compounds might be responsible for the anti-dermatophytic activity in this study.

Key words: Antidermatophytic activity, *Ixora brachiata Roxb.*

INTRODUCTION

Mycotic infections are probably the most common cause of skin disease in developing countries of tropical regions. Dermatophytosis is the most frequent superficial fungal infection in tropical and subtropical countries. The drugs used against dermatophytosis exhibit several side effects and have limited efficacy. Therefore, there is a distinct need for the discovery of new safer and more effective antifungal agents. The use of medicinal herbs in the treatment of skin diseases including mycotic infections is an age-old practice in many parts of the world (Irobi et al., 1993), because herbal remedies used in traditional folk medicine may help to overcome the growing problem of resistance to antifungal drugs and their relative toxicity. *Ixora brachaita* Roxb. belongs to the family *Rubiaceae*. It is a small tree 15 - 30 ft. high, found to be growing in high rainfall locality (Cooke, 1958).

Human infections particularly those involving the skin are increasing at an alarming rate, especially in tropical and subtropical developing countries, with dermatophytes as the most common pathogens (Fenner et al., 2005; Portillo, 2001; Mahesh et al., 2009). This increase is directly related to the growing population of immunocompromised individuals. Human mycoses are not always successfully treated, since the available many advance effect show recurrence or lead to the development of resistance. It is therefore, essential to research for more effective and less toxic new antifungal agents (Zacchino et al., 1999). According to Siddha literature, *I. brachaita* Roxb. have anti-inflamatory, aromatic and antipyretic properties. But the literature on antioxidant and antimicrobial properties are scanty. Since no review of literature are available on the antifungal effect of *I. brachiata*, thus, the present study was undertaken to evaluate the antifungal activity of ethanolic extracts of leaf and root against tested dermatophytic species.

MATERIALS AND METHODS

The leaves of *I. brachiata* were extracted in ethanol. To 10 g of each powdered material air dried was added 100 ml of 80% ethanol

*Corresponding author. E-mail: batsad4@yahoo.com.

(drug/solvent ratio=1:10 w/v) for maceration, and then kept on a rotary shaker for 72 h at room temperature (Fenner et al., 2005). Following filtration of the suspension through a Buckner funnel and Whatman filter paper #1, the crude ethanol extracts were evaporated in oven at 45°C.

Dermatophyte isolates

Five dermatophytic species vis. *Trichophyton mentagrophytes, Trichophyton rubrum, Microsporum canis, Microsporum gypseum* and *Epidermophyton floccosum* were used in the present study. They were collected from medical diagnosis laboratory, Ahwaz, Iran.

Preparation of fungal inoculum

For this, the suspension of conidia was prepared by using 0.85% sterile physiological saline which containing 0.05% Tween 80 (Sigma). The final suspension of conidia was counted with a hemocytometer cell counting chamber. The inoculum of conidia suspensions were obtained according to Shin and Lim (2004) and Wright et al. (1983) and adjusted to 10^5 conidia with colony-forming units ($CFUml^{-1}$).

Antifungal susceptibility testing

The antifungal activities of ethanol extracts were evaluated by the Agar Dilution Method (Fenner et al., 2005; Mitscher et al., 1972; Lucia et al. 2003). 1000 mg of the crude extract was dissolved in 1 ml of sterile DMSO served as stock solution (Fenner et al., 2005). For the assay, stock solutions of extracts were two-fold diluted with 0.85% sterile physiological saline to produce serial decreasing dilutions ranging from 0.078 - 20 mg ml^{-1}. 100 μl of the solution extracts and 50 μl of dermatophyte suspension of 10^5 $CFUml^{-1}$ were added to 5 ml Mycosel agar medium with 45°C and evenly fine mixed. The plates were incubated at 28 - 30°C up to 15 days for dermatophytic species. The antifungal agents, keteconazole (Janssen pharmaceutical) and griseofulvin (Sigma) were used as positive controls. Drug free solution (only with appropriate amount of DMSO) was also used as a blank control for verification of fungal growth. The leaf and root of the above extracts were further extracted with various polarities solvents like Diethyl ether, acetone, methanol and water. The antifungal activities of these extracts against *T. mentagrophytes* were tested by Disk Diffusion Method as described above.

Phytochemical study

In the present investigation the leaf and root of *I. brachiata* were evaluated qualitatively for the presence of saponins, reducing sugars, tannins, alkaloids, proteins, glycosides, anthraquinones and flavonoids. The ethyl acetate extracts of *I. brachiata* leaf and root were subjected to TLC by using precoated silica gel F_{254} plate. The mobile phase of Acetone/Ethyl acetate/Petroleum ether (0.5: 0.5:2.0) [AEP] was used for giving the best resolution of spots. High performance thin layer chromatography (HPTLC) fingerprint for same extract was obtained at UV- 254 nm and UV- 366 nm.

Statistical treatment of results

The analysis of data was performed with the SPSS program version 10. Analysis of variance tests were conducted using the general one-way ANOVA with post hoc comparison of mean values by LSD.

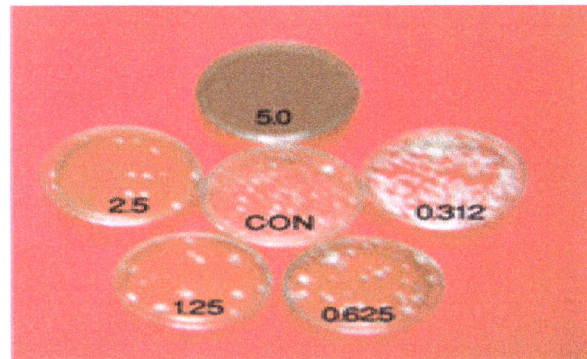

Figure 1a. Inhibitory effects of ethanolic extract of *I. brachiata* leaf on growth of *T. menta.* by Agar Dilution Method on Mycosel medium. Decreasing dilution ranging from 0.078 - 5.0 mg/ml medium. MIC = 5.0 mg/ml medium.

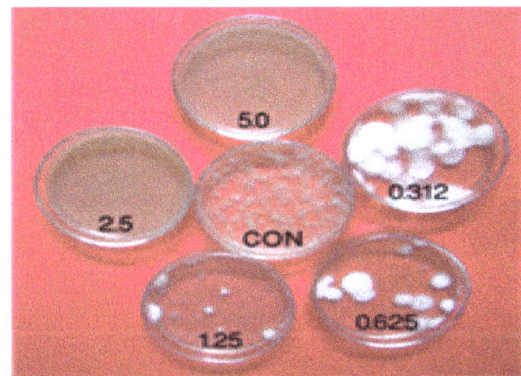

Figure 1b. Inhibitory effects of ethanolic extract of *I. brachiata* root on growth of *T. menta.* by Agar Dilution Method on Mycosel medium. Decreasing dilution ranging from 0.078 - 5.0 mg/ml medium. MIC = 2.50 mg/ml medium.

RESULTS

The ethanolic extracts of *I. brachiata* leaf and root completely prevented the growth of tested dermatophytic species with MIC values for IBL and IBR ranged between 5.0 - 10 and 2.5 - 10 mg ml^{-1} medium, respectively. MIC90 and MIC50 values equal 2.50 and 0.625 mg ml^{-1} medium for IBL and 1.250 and 0.312 for IBR (Figure 1a and 1b). MIC90s and MIC50s were similar in all tested clinical and standardized dermatophytic species of *T. mentagrophytes, M. canis, M. gypseum, T. rubrum* and *E. floccosum*. MFC values for IBL and IBR were also similar in all tested clinical and standardized dermatophytic species (5.0 and 2.5 mg ml^{-1} medium) respectively. The results are shown in Tables 1 and 2.

Results on phytochemical screening indicated that the leaf and root of *I. brachiata* gave positive test for starch,

Table 1. MICs (mg ml $^{-1}$) of the extracts.

Name of plant	Plant part used	MIC value (mg ml $^{-1}$)[a]				
Ixora brachiata Roxb		M.C.[b]	M.g.[c]	E.f.[d]	T.r.[e]	T.m.[f]
	Leaf	5.00	5.00	5.00	5.00	5.00
	Root	2.50	2.50	2.50	2.50	2.50
[g]Griseofulvin		12.5	100	25	50	100
[h]Keteconazole		25	6.25	0.78	25	6.25

Abbreviations: [a]*Microsporum canis* PTCC5069. [b]*Microsporum gypseum* PTCC5070. [c]*Epidermophyton floccosunm* EF-3. [d]*Trichophyton rubrum* TR-1. [e]*Trichophyton mentagrophytes* PTCC5054. IBL (*Ixora brachiata* leaf), IBR (*Ixora brachiata* root). MIC values are given as mean values (mg ml^{-1}) from the triplicate experiments. MIC values griseofulvin and keteconazole (μg ml $^{-1}$) as positive control.

Table 2. Minimum inhibitory concentration (MIC) and minimum fungicidal concentration (MFC) of IBL, IBR, Griseofulvin (GRS) and Keteconazole (KTZ) against dermatophytes by Agar Dilution Method

Dermatophytes No. of strains	Antifungal Compounds	MIC and MFC				
		Range	50%	90%	MFC	Geometric mean MIC
T. mentagrophytes (3) *T. menta.* PTCC5054	KTZ	0.78 - 6.25	1.56	6.25	12.5	3.52
	GRS	12.5 - 100	25	100	200	56.25
	IBL	0.312 - 2.500	0.625	2.500	5.000	1.46
	IBR	0.156 - 1.250	0.312	1.250	2.500	0.703
M. gypseum (3) *M. gypseum* PTCC5070	KTZ	0. 78 - 6.25	1.56	6.25	12.5	3.52
	GRS	12.5 - 100	25	100	200	56.25
	IBL	0.312 - 2.500	0.625	2.500	5.000	1.46
	IBR	0.156 - 1.250	0.312	1.250	2.500	0.703
M. canis (3) *M. canis* PTCC5069	KTZ	1.56 - 12.50	3.12	12.5	25	7.03
	GRS	3.12 - 25.00	6.25	25	50	14.06
	IBL	00.312 - 2.500	0.625	2.500	5.000	1.46
	IBR	0.156 - 1.250	0.312	1.250	2.500	0.703
T. rubrum (2)	KTZ	3.12 - 25.00	6.25	25	50	14.06
	GRS	6.25 - 50.00	12.5	50	100	28.13
	IBL	0.312 - 2.500	0.625	2.500	5.000	1.46
	IBR	0.156 - 1.250	0.312	1.250	2.500	0.703
E. floccosum (3)	KTZ	0.39 - 0.78	0.39	0.78	1.56	0.585
	GRS	3.12 - 25.00	6.25	25	50	14.06
	IBL	0.312 - 2.500	0.625	2.500	5.000	1.46
	IBR	0.156 - 1.250	0.312	1.250	2.500	0.703

Abbreviations: MIC values are reported as μgml^{-1}for KTZ (Keteconazole), GRS (Greseofulvin) and mg ml^{-1} for IBL (*Ixora brachiata* leaf), IBR (*Ixora brachiata* root) extracts. *T. Trichophyton, M. Microsporum, E. Epidermophyton.* 50 and 90%, MICs at which 50 and 90% of the isolates in the test panel respectively are inhibited. Values are given as mean from the triplicate experiments.

saponins, reducing sugars, anthraquinones, glycosides, phenols and proteins while they gave negative test for alkaloids. IBL gave positive test for tannins while IBR gave positive test for flavonoids (Table 3). In the present investigation, the organic solvents of acetone, methanol and water with different polarity did not show any efficacy for extraction from *I. brachiata* leaf and root but only Diethyl ether with semi-polarity had high affection with inhi-

bittion zone of 15 and 25 mm diameter against *T. mentagrophytes* for IBL and IBR, respectively. Results on High Performance Thin Layer chromatography (HPTLC) indicated that the ethyl acetate extract of *I. brachiata* leaf (Wagner, 1984) contains coumarin that it was observed in UV-254 nm with 8 peaks and in UV-366 nm with 9 peaks (Figure 2 a and 2b). The ethyl acetate extract of *I. brachiata* root contains triterpene and it was observed a

Table 3. Phytochemical screening of *Ixora brachiata* leaf and root extracts.

Name of the test carried out	Reagents used	*Ixora brachiata*	
		Leaf	Root
(A.) Water Extract			
Starch	I2-KI	+ve	+ve
Tannins	Acidic FeCl$_3$	+ve	-ve
Saponins	H$_2$SO$_4$ + Acetic unhydride	+ve	+ve
Proteins	Million's test	+ve	+ve
Anthraquinones	Benzene + 10%NH$_4$OH	+ve	+ve
Reducing sugars	Benedict's	+ve	+ve
(B.) Alcoholic Extracts			
Alkaloids	Mayer's	-ve	-ve
	Wagner's	-ve	-ve
	Dragendorff's	-ve	-ve
Flavonoids	HCl + Mg turnings	-ve	+ve
Glycosides	Benzene + hot ethanol	+ve	+ve

+ve: Present; -ve: Absent.

I. brachiata Leaf

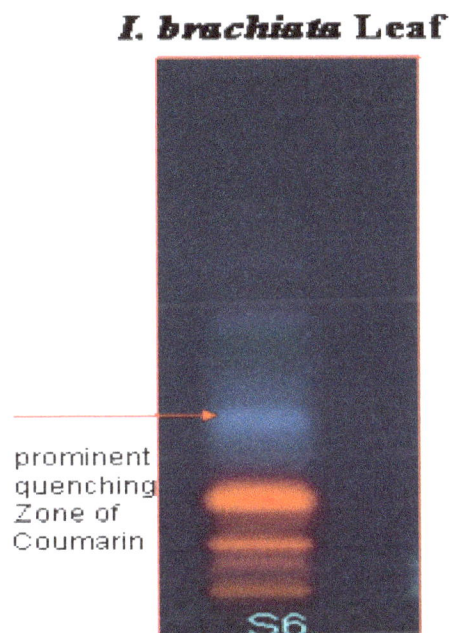

Figure 2a. Image in 366 nm after derivation with vanillin sulphuric acid.

I. brachiata Root

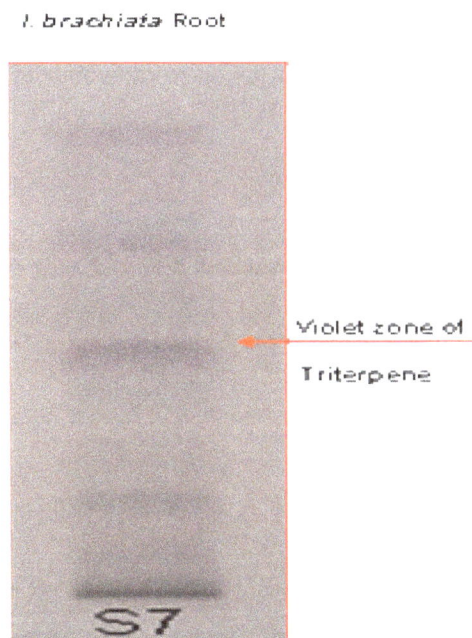

Figure 2b. Image in visible after derivation with vanillin sulphuric acid.

a violet zone in the visible region after derivation from Anisaldehyde – Sulphuric Acid (Figure 2a and 2b) with 10 peaks at UV-254 nm and 12 peaks at UV-366 nm.

DISCUSSION AND CONCLUSION

These results indicated that the ethanolic extract of *I. brachiata* possesses antifungal properties not only against standardized strains of clinically important dermatophytes but also against their clinical phytochemical studies on other species of *Ixora* such as *Ixora coccinea* which consists of anthocyanins in flowers, oleic and linoleic acids in root oil and octadecadienoic acid from root bark (Chopra et al., 1956) and saponins and tannins (Grainge et al., 1988). In previous reports it is seen that screening of ether extract of *I. coccinea* gave positive test for alkaloids, flavonoids, sapogenins, sterols, terpenes and that of methanol extract for alkaloids, phenols and sterols (Annapurna and Raghavan, 2003). These results are similar to those results obtained in the present investtigation from phytochemical screening of *I. brachiata* whereas it gave negative test for alkaloids.

Finally after detection and confirmation of triterpenes and coumarin by HPTLC in *I. brachiata*, it was suggested that these compounds might be responsible for the anti-dermatophytic activity in this plant which gave a positive test results by *in-vitro* isolates as suggested by Cowan (1999).

Based on the results of this study, we can consider ethanolic extract of I. brachiata as a new source for developing local antifungal agents. However, further studies are needed to determine the efficacy of active chemical constituent of this plant extract. Toxicological studies on the extract must also be performed to ensure the safety of the extract.

ACKNOWLEDGEMENT

The authors would like to thank Prof. B.B. Ghaugule Head of the Botany Department for providing necessary laboratory facilities and for encouragement to carry out this work.

REFERENCES

Annapurna J, Amarnath PVS, Amar Kumar D, Ramakrishna SV, Raghavan KV (2003). Antimicrobial activity of *Ixora coccinea* leaf. Fitoterapia. 74: 291–293.

Chopra RN, Nayar SL, Chopra IC (1956). Glossary of Indian medicinal plants. Council of Scientific and Industrial Research India (CSIR).

Publication and information directorate New Delhi-110012.: 57, 102, 139, 198 and 256.

Cooke T (1958). Flora of the Presidency of Bombay, Botanical Survey of India.Vol. I, II & III.

Dymock D, Warden CJH, Hooper D (1810). Pharmacographia Indica.(III): 74-75.

Fenner M, Sortinob SM, Ratesa R, Agnola S, Zacchino B (2005). Antifungal activity of some Brazilian *Hypericum* species. Phytomedicine 12: 236-240.

Lucia KHS, Cecilia MAO, Pedro HF, Juldasio GOJ, Ary Henrique SJ, Orinalda de Fatima LF, Maria do Rosario RS (2003). Antimicrobial Activity of *Hyptis ovalifolia* Towards Dermatophytes. Mem Inst Oswaldo Cruz, Rio de Janeiro. 98 (7): 963-965.

Grainge M, Ahmed S (1988). Handbook of plants with pest control properties. New York: Wiley.

Irobi ON, Darambola SO (1993). Antifungal activities of crude extract of *Mitracarpus villosus* (Rubiaceae). J. Ethnopharmacol. 40: 137-140.

Marco F, Pfaller MA, Messer S, Jones RN (1998). In vitro activities of voriconazole (UK-109,496) and four other antifungal agents against 394 clinical isolates of Candida spp. Antimicrob. Agent Chemother. 42:161–163.

Mitscher L, Leu R, Bathala M, Beal J (1972). Antimicrobial agents from higher plants. Introduction, Rationale Methodology. 35: 157–166.

Portillo A, Vila R, Freixa B, Adzet T, Canigueral S (2001). Antifungal activity Paraguayan plant usrd in traditional medicine. J. Ethnopharmacol. 76: 93-98.

Rebell G, Taplin D (1970). Dermatophytes, Their Recognition and Identification, University of Miami Press, Coral Gables, Florida.

Shin S, Lim S (2004). Antifungal effects of herbal essential oils alone and in combination with ketoconazole against Trichophyton spp. J. Appl. Microbiol. 97: 1289–1296.

Wagner H, Bladt S, Zgainski EM (1984). Plant Drug Analysis: A Thin Layer Chromatography Atlas. 2nd Edition, Springer- Verlag, New York: 305-327.

Wrigh L, Scott E, Gorman S (1983). The sensitive of mycelium, arthrospores and microconidia of *Trichophyton mentagrophytes* to imidazoles determined by *in-vitro* tests. J. Antimicrob. Chemother. 12: 317-323.

Zacchino S, Lo Pez S (1999). *In-vitro* evaluation of antifungal properties of phenylpropanoids and related compounds acting against dermatophytes. J. Nat. Prod. 62: 1353-1357.

α_1–Antitrypsin: Anti-inflammatory roles in exercise and atherosclerosis

Stuart .J. Semple[1]* and Andrew .J. McKune[2]

[1]Department of Biokinetics and Sport Science, University of Zululand, KwaDlangezwa, South Africa.
[2]School of Physiotherapy, Optometry and Sports Science, University of KwaZulu-Natal, South Africa.

α_1-Antitrypsin, also known as serum trypsin inhibitor, is an acute phase protein that is upregulated in response to tissue damage and infection. More specifically this glycoprotein affords the host protection against enzymes that are released by immune inflammatory cells. The most notable of these enzymes is neutrophil elastase. Neutrophil elastase has the ability to damage vasculature and in doing so may contribute to atherosclerosis and other chronic diseases in which inflammation is an integral component of the pathology. Exercise has recently been defined as anti-inflammatory in nature, however, the complex mechanism underlying this beneficial effect is not fully understood. This paper provides an overview of the roles that α_1-antitrypsin may play in atherogenesis, summarises the findings from exercise studies in which α_1-antitrypsin was measured, and proposes that transient exercise induced elevations in α_1-antitrypsin may potentially contribute to the anti-inflammatory effect of exercise.

Key words: Protease inhibitor, exercise, cardiovascular disease, inflammation.

INTRODUCTION

α_1-Antitrypsin (AAT) is categorized as an acute-phase protein that is up-regulated in response to tissue necrosis and inflammation (Baumann and Gauldie, 1994; Gabay and Kushner, 1999; Lisowska-Myjak, 2004). It rarely increases more than 4-fold, and exhibits a 4.5 day half life (Lisowska-Myjak, 2004). The primary function of this protein is to protect the lower respiratory tract of lungs from proteolytic attack by neutrophil elastase and other neutrophil-derived proteinases (Brantly et al., 1988; Carrell et al., 1982). The majority of research conducted on AAT has focused on the deficiencies thereof, however, as will be discussed, AAT may be linked to a broader range of physiological functions many of which may be implicated in chronic disease that is inflammatory in nature.

CELLS SYNTHESISING α_1-ANTITRYPSIN

In keeping with its role as an acute-phase protein, AAT synthesis has been shown to occur within hepatocytes (Brantly, 2002; Bhan, 1976). However, Coakley et al. (2001)

reported, it can also be actively secreted by neutrophils, mononuclear phagocytes and enterocytes. In addition to the aforementioned secretory cells, it has also been shown that epithelial cells can synthesise leukocyte protease inhibitors (Marchand et al., 1997; Cichy et al., 1997). A study by Cichy et al. (1997) demonstrated that cells originating from the respiratory tract epithelium produced AAT, and those inflammatory mediators, such as interleukin-1, contributed towards this expression. Lu et al. (2006) have also implicated skeletal muscle in the expression of AAT. In this study, recombinant adeno-associated virus serotype 1 was injected intramuscularly into mice. Immuno-localisation demonstrated that the AAT transgene was expressed in the skeletal muscles, and that it formed a complex with neutrophil elastase in a dose dependant manner. Although not fully understood, this finding highlights the potentially important role that AAT may play in regulating skeletal muscle homeostasis.

Deficiencies of α_1-Antitrypsin

The major function of AAT is to inhibit proteinase activity (Talamo, 1975). This involves 'neutralising' the tissue damaging effects, particularly of human neutrophil elastase

*Corresponding author. E-mail: ssemple@pan.uzulu.ac.za.

(HNE) (Luisetti and Seersholm, 2004; Sanford et al., 1999). HNE is packaged in neutrophil granules and is released by activated neutrophils as part of an inflammatory response (Coakley et al., 2001). In the lungs, the controlled release of HNE facilitates the movement of inflammatory cells through the extracellular stroma. However, excessive, uncontrolled production of HNE results in lung damage and destruction. The key regulatory protein of HNE in the lungs is AAT (Coakley et al., 2001). Therefore, a deficiency of AAT retards the effectiveness of the host to remove excessive HNE, leading to gradual destruction of connective tissue and loss of alveolar units. This damage manifests clinically as chronic obstructive pulmonary disease (COPD).

α_1-Antitrypsin and exercise

For some time now it has been accepted that exercise may retard the atherogenic process. Evidence supporting this includes findings that physical activity is associated with reductions in low-density lipoproteins and blood pressure, improved endothelial function, and increases in high-density lipoproteins (Stefanick et al., 1998; Schlager et al., 2011; Fagard, 2001, Leon and Sanchez, 2001). Strenuous, prolonged or unaccustomed physical activity has the capacity to elicit skeletal muscle damage (Clarkson and Trembley, 1988; Evans, 1987). It is well documented that an acute phase inflammatory response accompanies this damage and is characterised by the increased concentration of a number of plasma proteins and immune cells (Weight et al., 1991; Semple et al., 2004). Neutrophil elevations have been observed following moderate intensity physical activity (Avloniti et al., 2007). It has been proposed that the neutrophil elevations following acute exercise are linked to both muscle damage and oxidative stress (Tidball, 2005; Quindry et al., 2003). Although the precise role of neutrophils in muscle injury and repair processes requires clarification, it is generally agreed upon that AAT would play an important role in regulating neutrophil activity. Relatively few studies have investigated AAT responses to exercise. These are summarised in Table 1.

ANTI-INFLAMMATORY EFFECTS OF α_1-ANTITRYPSIN – POTENTIAL ROLES IN ATHEROSCLEROSIS

Atherosclerosis is a disease in which 'plaque' accumulates in between the layers that make up the walls of arteries. This process is referred to as atherogenesis, involves the progressive retention and oxidation of lipids within arteries such that the plaque mass or atheroma increases to a point where it can significantly occlude blood flow and/or result in thrombosis (Insull, 2009). The atherogenic process is now well defined as one in which immune system mediated chronic

inflammation plays a central role in its pathophysiology (Perrins et al., 2010). Exercise plays an important role in dampening this process through its anti-inflammatory actions (Mathur and Pederson, 2008), some of which may be mediated by AAT.

Histamine is a major pro-inflammatory vasoactive amine that is released from mast cells when they bind to IgE (Janeway et al., 2001; Roitt, 2001). There is recent evidence showing that histamine can exacerbate atherosclerotic lesions (Rozenberg et al., 2010). He and Xie (2004) showed that AAT inhibited IgE dependant histamine release from mast cells by 36.8%. Thus, at inflammatory sites, the presence of AAT may serve to blunt the inflammatory response by inhibiting histamine release. In doing so it may reduce the amount of low-density lipoprotein that accumulates within the atheroma.

AAT has also been shown to regulate aspects of complement-mediated inflammation. The membrane proteinase, p57, cleaves C3, enhancing inflammation (Ollert et al., 1990). AAT inhibits the activity of p57, suppressing C3 activity limiting inflammation (Rodriguez-Lima et al., 1998).

Similarly, Nita et al. (2005) have highlighted the anti-inflammatory role of Prolastin (a preparation of purified human AAT used for augmentation therapy) in regulating cytokine release from human neutrophils and monocytes. The neutrophils and monocytes were stimulated with lipopolysaccharide (either alone or in conjunction with Prolastin) and the release of pro-inflammatory cytokines tumour necrosis factor- α (TNF-α), interleukin 1β (IL-1β) and interleukin-8 (IL-8) were determined. The Prolastin 'treated' monocytes showed a significant decrease in TNF-α and IL-1β production compared to controls. Prolastin significantly decreased IL-8 production by neutrophils. The authors concluded that Prolastin inhibits the effects of endotoxin (LPS) and thus reduces the inflammatory response. Endotoxins from bacteria found within atheroma's have been implicated in triggering inflammatory responses (Triantafilou et al., 2007).

Exercise induced AAT elevations – Heart/vascular health benefits

From the studies included in Table 1, it is apparent that in 50% of the studies, plasma AAT increased significantly following exercise. An additional study showed a substantial (32%), yet non-significant elevation. Two studies (20%) showed no changes, one showed a decrease, and in one it is unclear if the absolute plasma/serum concentration changed. From these results it seems as if the trend is for exercise to induce elevations in AAT. Its primary role may be to limit the potential damage associated with exercise induced leukocytosis and the accompanying damage inflicted by these activated neutrophils which release harmful enzymes (Correale et al., 2008). However, it is plausible

Table 1. Effects of exercise on α_1–antitrypsin.

	Participants	Intervention	Observation
Haralambie (1970)	Ten physically active, medical students (22 to 26 y)	2 h seated ergometer exercise performed between 140 to 150 W.	AAT increased significantly ($p < 0.001$) from 284 ± 33.4 mg / 100 ml before the exercise to 313 ± 40.2 mg / 100 ml after the exercise.
Liesen et al. (1977)	Eight well trained males (24 ± 2 y)	Prolonged (3 and 2 h) runs spaced 2 weeks apart. A smaller group partook in a 9 week endurance training program.	Moderate elevations in AAT were observed following the runs. The athletes exhibited 'elevated' resting levels of AAT following the endurance training.
Gleeson et al. (1995)	Eight healthy, untrained adults (28 ± 8 y)	40 min bench stepping exercise at 15 steps per minute on a 47cm bench.	AAT exhibited no significant changes compared to pre exercise concentrations.
Fallon et al. (2001a)	Elite female netball (n = 14) and soccer (n = 18) players	Routine moderate and heavy training weeks.	Compared to resting concentrations AAT showed significant ($p < 0.05$) elevations following routine moderate intensity training in soccer and netball players.
Fallon (2001b)	Seven males and one female (47 ± 7 y)	6-day ultra-marathon track race.	No significant changes observed for AAT at any of the time points. However increases up to 32% during the race from resting (pre-race) concentrations.
Dufaux and Order (1989)	Healthy, moderately trained males (n = 8; 20-28 y)	2.5 h treadmill running. The subjects covered a distance between 25 to 33 km. The mean running speed was $80.1 \pm 6.5\%$ of the speed at which blood lactate reached 4 mmol.l^{-1}	AAT was significantly ($p < 0.01$) elevated 1h into the run, as well as immediately after and at 1 h and 3 h after the run.
Petibois et al. (2001)	Elite rowers (n = 13; 24 ± 4 y)	AAT was measured at rest and during exercise (18 km of rowing, 80% of VO_2max) weekly from the 1st –8th week, and then after 10, 13, 15, 18, 20, 23, 28, 33, 37, 41 and 47 weeks.	No significant ($p > 0.10$) changes in AAT were observed at rest and during exercise for the entire study period.
Mila-Kierzenkowska et al. (2010)	Elite / Olympic female kayakers (n = 9; 23 ± 3 y)	Ten day intense combination training (strength, endurance and water sessions)	AAT was significantly lower after day six ($p < 0.01$) and day 10 ($p < 0.01$) compared with pre training levels.
Zhang et al. (1993)	Rheumatoid arthritis patients (n = 5; 35-77 y)	Participants walked as "briskly as possible" for 10 min.	Synovial fluid AAT activity significantly ($p < 0.05$) decreased following the exercise. Plasma AAT concentration was significantly higher than that found within the synovial fluid.
Semple et al. (2006)	Professional cyclists (n = 17; 28 ± 1 y)	Two prolonged stages (194 and 164 km) of a cycling tour.	AAT was significantly ($p < 0.02$) elevated after the 194 km stage.

that a secondary, 'spill over effect' is to indirectly improve vascular or heart health by limiting endothelial damage. Ikari et al. (2001) have shown that AAT is a critical factor in protecting the extracellular matrix of vascular smooth cell from being degraded by proteinases and also inhibits the caspase activation and thereby functions as an antiapoptotic factor. These antiprotease and antiapoptotic functions are two anti-inflammatory mechanisms whereby AAT may impart heart health benefits by protecting the vasculature.

Additional mechanisms are those linked to regulating cytokine responses. AAT inhibits gene expression of the potent inflammatory cytokine tumor necrosis factor-α (Subramaniyam et al., 2008) and induces the release of interleukin-1 receptor antagonist from macrophages (Tilg et al., 1993). The majority of evidence in the literature supports the anti-inflammatory actions associated with AAT despite the fact that there is evidence that oxidised AAT may contribute to or exacerbate inflammation (Scott et al., 1999). It is unclear whether or not acute or chronic exercise may affect the levels of oxidised/modified AAT and thereby impact on the inflammatory processes. Similarly the opposing mechanism whereby AAT may impart or modulate atherogenic processes requires elucidation as authors have proposed conflicting theories (Correale et al., 2008).

In summary, AAT is the most abundant proteinase inhibitor. It exhibits pronounced anti-inflammatory actions and is integrally involved as an acute-phase protein in modulating aspects of the inflammatory response. As with many immune/biochemical proteins it is arguable that the exercise induced changes may be mode, duration, intensity and population dependant. Together these factors make it difficult to precisely describe and quantify the AAT response to exercise. Despite this, it does seem as if exercise elevates AAT. It is unclear however if transient exercise induced elevations in plasma translate into increases in intravascular AAT where inflammatory pathologies manifest in the form of atherosclerosis. If so this protein may be a crucial role player in combating cardiovascular disease. Lack of evidence also makes it difficult to determine if persistent up or down regulation of ATT accompanies chronic training or if the response is purely transient following each session. The latter, which seems more plausible based on the available evidence, would suggest that AAT benefits are only imparted if individuals exercise regularly (that is, on a daily basis), a concept upon which current exercise guidelines and recommendations are based in order for individuals to derive optimal health benefits. Recently, exercise has received considerable attention as an anti-inflammatory 'modality'. The aim of this paper was to highlight the potential roles that AAT may play in this complex phenomenon which to date has only focussed on selected immune cells and proteins. Strong evidence implicates the fact that AAT modulates inflammation; however, the mechanism whereby exercise induced elevations in AAT may create an impact on inflammatory

disease remains speculative.

REFERENCES

Avloniti AA, Douda HT, Tokmakidis SP, Kortsaris AH, Papadopoulou EG, Spanoudakis EG (2007). Acute effects of soccer training on white blood cell count in elite female players. Int. J. Sports Physiol. Perform., 2(3): 239-49.

Baumann H, Gauldie J (1994). The acute phase response. Immunol. Today. 15: 74-80.

Bhan AK, Grand, RJ, Colten HR, Alper CA (1976). Liver in alpha1-antitrypsin deficiency: Morphologic observations and in vitro synthesis of alpha1-antitrypsin. Paediatr. Res., 10: 35-40.

Brantly M (2002). alpha1-Antitrypsin: Not just an antiprotease. Am. J Res. Cell Mol. Biol., 27: 652-654.

Brantly M, Nukiwa T, Crystal RG (1988). Molecular basis of α_1-antitrypsin deficiency. Am. J. Med., 84:13-31.

Carrell RW, Jeppsson JO, Laurell CB, Brennan SO, Owen MC, Vaugham I, Boswell DR (1982). Structure and variation of human α_1-antitrypsin. Nature, 298: 329-334.

Cichy J, Potempa J, Travis J (1997). Biosynthesis of alpha1-proteinase inhibitor by human lung-derived epithelial cells. J. Biol. Chem., 272: 8250-8255.

Clarkson PM, Trembley I (1988). Exercise-induced muscle damage, repair, and adaptation in humans. J. Appl. Physiol. 65: 1-6.

Coakley RJ, Taggart C, O'Neil S, McIvaney NG (2001). Alpha1-antitrypsin deficiency: Biological answers to clinical questions. Am. J. Med. Sci. 321: 33-41.

Correale M, Brunetti ND, De Gennaro L, Di Biase M (2008). Acute phase proteins in atherosclerosis (acute coronary syndrome). Cardiovasc. Hematol. Agents Med. Chem., 6(4): 272-7.

Dufaux B, Order U (1989). Plasma elastase alpha-1-antitrypsin, neopetrin, tumour necrosis factor, and soluble interleukin-2 receptor after prolonged exercise. Int. J. Sports Med., 10: 434-438.

Evans WJ (1987). Exercise-induced skeletal muscle damage. Physician Sports Med., 15: 89-100.

Fagard RH (2001). Exercise characteristics and the blood pressure response to dynamic physical training. Med. Sci. Sports Exerc., 33 (6 suppl): S484–S492.

Fallon KE (2001b). The acute phase response and exercise: The ultramarathon as prototype exercise. Clin. J. Sports Med., 11: 38-43.

Fallon KE, Fallon SK, Boston T (2001). The acute phase response and exercise: court and field sports. Brit. J .Sport Med., 35: 170-173.

Gabay C, Kushner I (1999). Acute phase proteins and other systemic responses to inflammation. New Engl. J. Med., 340: 448-454.

Gleeson M, Almey J, Brooks S, Cave R, Lewis A, Griffiths H (1995). Haematological and acute-phase responses associated with delayed onset muscle soreness. Eur. J. Appl. Physiol., 71: 137-142.

Haralambie G (1970). Changes of serum glycoprotein levels after long-lasting physical exercise. Clin. Chim. Acta, 27: 475-479.

He SH, Xie H (2004). Modulation of histamine release from human colon mast cells by protease inhibitors. World. J. Gastroentero., 10: 337-341.

Ikari Y, Mulvihill E, Schwartz SM (2001).alpha 1-Proteinase inhibitor, alpha 1-antichymotrypsin, and alpha 2-macroglobulin are the antiapoptotic factors of vascular smooth muscle cells. J. Biol. Chem., 276(15): 11798-803.

Insull W Jr. (2009). The pathology of atherosclerosis: plaque development and plaque responses to medical treatment. Am. J. Med., 122 (1 Suppl): S3-S14.

Janeway CA, Travers P, Walport M, Shlomchik M (2001). Immunobiology. The Immune System in Health and Disease. Garland Publishing, New York.

Leon AS, Sanchez OA (2001). Response of blood lipids to exercise training alone or combined with dietary intervention. Med. Sci. Sports Exerc., 33(6 suppl): S502–S515.

Liesen H, Dufaux B, Hollman W (1977). Modifications of serum glycoprotein's following prolonged physical exercise and the influence of physical training. Eur. J. Appl. Physiol. O., 37(4): 243-254.

Lisowska-Myjak B (2004). AAT as a diagnostic tool. Clin. Chim. Acta

352(1-2):1-13.

Lu Y, Choi YK, Campbell-Thompson M, Li C, Tang Q, Crawford JM, Flotte TR, Song S (2006). Therapeutic level functional human alpha1-antitrypsin (hAAT) secreted from murine muscle transduced by adeno-associated virus (rAVV1) vector. J. Gene Med., 8(6): 730-735.

Luisetti M, Seersholm N (2004). Epidemiology of alpha-antitrypsin 1 deficiency. Thorax, 59: 164-169.

Marchand V, Tournier JM, Polette M, Nawrocki B, Fuchey C, Pierott D, Burlet H, Puchelle E (1997). The elastase-induced expression of secretory leukocyte protease inhibitor is decreased in remodelled airway epithelium. Eur. J. Pharmacol., 336: 187-196.

Mathur N, Pedersen BK (2008). Exercise as a mean to control low-grade systemic inflammation. Med. Inflam., 109502: 1-6.

Mila-Kierzenkowska C, Wozniak A, Boraczynski T, Jurecka A, Augustynska B, Wozniak B (2010). The effect of whole-body cryostimulation on the activity of lysosomal enzymes in kayaker women after intense exercise. J. Thermal. Biol., 36(1): 29-33.

Nita I, Hollander C, Westin U, Janciauskiene S (2005). Prolastin, a pharmaceutical preparation of purified human alpha1-antitrypsin, blocks endotoxin-mediated cytokine release. Respir. Res., 6: 12.

Ollert MW, Frade R, Fiandino A, Panneerselvam M, Petrella EC, Barel M, Pangburn MK, Bredehorst R, Vogel CW (1990). C3-cleaving membrane proteinase. A new complement regulatory protein of human melanoma cells. J. Immunol., 144: 3862-3867.

Perrins CJ, Bobryshev YV (2010). Current advances in understanding of immunopathology of atherosclerosis. Virchows Archiv epub ahead of print.

Petibois C, Cazorla G, Deleris G (2001). The biological and metabolic adaptations to 12 months training in elite rowers. Int. J. Sports Med., 24: 36-42.

Quindry JC, Stone WL, King J, Broerder CE (2003). The Effects of Acute Exercise on neutrophils and plasma oxidative stress. Med. Sci. Sports .Exerc. 35(7): 1139-1145.

Rodriguez-Lima F, Hermann J, Jean D, Frade R (1998). Alpha1-proteinase inhibitor is the serum regulator of the activity of p57, a C3-cleaving proteinase present in human erythrocyte membranes. Biochim. Biophys. Acta, 1402(2): 131-138.

Roitt I, Brostoff J, Male D (2001). Immunology. Elsevier Science Limited, Edinburgh.

Rozenberg I, Sluka SH, Rohrer L, Hofmann J, Becher B, Akhmedov A, Soliz J, Mocharla P, Borén J, Johansen P, Steffel J, Watanabe T, Lüscher TF, Tanner FC (2010). Histamine H1 receptor promotes atherosclerotic lesion formation by increasing vascular permeability for low-density lipoproteins. Arterio. Thromb. Vasc. Biol., 30(5):923-30.

Sanford AJ, Chagani T, Spinelli JJ, Pare PD (1999). Alpha1-Antitrypsin genotypes and the acute-phase response to open heart surgery. Am. J. Respir. Crit. Care. Med., 159: 1624-1628.

Schlager O, Giurgea A, Schuhfried O, Seidinger D, Hammer A, Gröger M, Fialka-Moser V, Gschwandtner M, Koppensteiner R, Steiner S (2011). Exercise training increases endothelial progenitor cells and decreases asymmetric dimethylarginine in peripheral arterial disease: A randomized controlled trial. Atherosclerosis. [Epub ahead of print].

Scott LJ, Russell GI, Nixon NB, Dawes PT, Mattey DL (1999). Oxidation of alpha1-proteinase inhibitor by the myeloperoxidase-hydrogen peroxidase system promotes binding to immunoglobulin A. Biochem. Biophys. Res. Comp., 255: 562-567.

Semple SJ, Smith LL, McKune A.J, Neveling N, Wadee AA (2004). Alterations in acute-phase reactants (CRP, rheumatoid factor, complement, Factor B, and immune complexes) following an ultramarathon. S Afr J Sports Med., 16: 17-21.

Semple SJ, Smith LL, McKune AJ, Hoyos AJ, Mokgethwa B, San Juan AF, Lucia A, Wadee AA (2006). Serum concentrations of C-reactive protein, alpha - 1antitrypsin, and complement (C3, C4, C1 esterase inhibitor) before and during the Vuelta a Espana. Br. J. Sports Med., 40: 124-127.

Stefanick ML, Mackey S, Sheehan M, Ellsworth N, Haskell WL, Wood PD (1998). Effects of diet and exercise in men and postmenopausal women with low levels of HDL cholesterol and high levels of LDL cholesterol. N. Engl. J. Med., 339: 12–20.

Subramaniyam D, Virtala R, Pawlowski K, Clausen IG, Warkentin S, Stevens T, Janciauskiene S (2008). TNF-α-induced self expression in human lung endothelial cells is inhibited by native and oxidised α1-antitrypsin. Int. J. Biochem. Cell. Biol. 40: 258-271.

Talamo RC (1975). Basic and clinical aspects of alpha1-antitrypsin. Paediatrics, 56: 91-99.

Tidball JG (2005). Inflammatory processes in muscle injury and repair. Am. J. Physiol. Regul. Integr. Comp. Physiol., 288(2):345-53.

Tilg H, Vannier E, Vachino G, Dinarello CA, Mier JW (1993). Anti-inflammatory properties of hepatic acute phase proteins: Preferential induction of interleukin 1 (IL-1) receptor antagonist over IL-1B synthesis by human peripheral blood mononuclear cells. J. Exp. Med., 178: 1629-1636.

Triantafilou M, Gamper FG, Lepper PM, Mouratis MA, Schumann C, Harokopakis E, Schifferle RE, Hajishengallis G, Triantafilou K (2007). Lipopolysaccharides from atherosclerosis-associated bacteria antagonize TLR4, induce formation of TLR2/1/CD36 complexes in lipid rafts and trigger TLR2-induced inflammatory responses in human vascular endothelial cells. Cell Microbiol., 9(8):2030-2039.

Weight LM, Alexander D, Jacobs P (1991). Strenuous exercise: analogous to the acute-phase response? Clin. Sci., 81: 677-683.

24

Antioxidant screening of ethanolic and aqueous extracts of *Organum vulgare* L. *in-vitro*

Rubina Majid[1*], Latief Ahmad[2] and M. A. Zargar[1]

[1]Department of Biochemistry University of Kashmir J&K India.
[2]Division of Agronomy SKUAST-Kashmir J&K India.

The present study was envisaged to assess the rationality for the use of traditionally invogue herb *Organum vulgare* as an anti-oxidant agent. Potential antioxidative activity of *O. vulgare* was evaluated using various *in vitro* methods including post mitochondrial supernatant (PMS) and microsomal lipid peroxidation, DNA sugar damage, 2,2-diphenyl-1-picrylhydrazyl (DPPH) radical scavenging and FTC/TBA methods. Both ethanolic and aqueous extracts exhibited good antioxidant and radical scavenging properties but the effects were pronounced in ethanolic extracts of *O. vulgare*. The extracts strongly inhibited DNA damage. The extracts showed significantly remarkable scavenging effects in DPPH free radical scavenging assay and the activity indicated a marked correlation with phenolic content. From the results the extracts (that is, aqueous and ethanolic extracts of *O. vulgare* might be valuable antioxidative sources.

Key words: Antioxidant, radical scavenging, *Organum vulgare*, 2,2-diphenyl-1-picrylhydrazyl (DPPH).

INTRODUCTION

Organum vulgare L. is a sub-species of a widespread wild oregano found in Greece, Turkey and in South and East Asia - appears in almost all of Europe and Asia, Northwest Africa, the Iberian Peninsula and Macaronesian region (Castroviejo et al., 2010). In India, it grows at high altitudes in the Himalaya usually in rocky areas and in the Kashmir valley where it is properly known as (*watpan*).

Origanum Linn. (Labiatae)

A small genus of perennial herbs or undershrubs, Origanum is distributed in the Mediterranean region and extra tropical Asia. One species *O. vulgare* Linn. common or wild Marjoram. Hindi-Sathra; Punjab-Mirzanjosh; Kashmiri-Baber occurs in India. An aromatic, branched perennial herb 30-90 cm high, found in the temperate Himalayas from Kashmir to Sikkim, at altitudes of 1500-3600 m. Leaves broadly ovate, entire or rarely toothed; flowers purple or pink, in corymbose cymes; nutlets smooth, brown.

O. vulgare is very common in Shimla hills and in Kashmir valley. It is hardy and can be grown in all warm garden soils. It is propagated by seeds, cuttings, layers and root division. It can be sown during October in the plains and during March and April in the hills. The plant possesses aromatic, thyme like flavor. The leaves and tops cut prior to blooming are used to flavor foods in the same way as sweet Marjoram (*Majorana hortensis*). The plant is used in Punjab as a pot herb; it is eaten also as vegetable in Lahul. It was formerly employed to flavor ale and beer, before hops were introduced in the brewing industry.

The herb contains a volatile oil (0.15-0.40%), tannin (0.8%) and a bitter principle. The oil of European origin (specific gr.[150], 0.868-0.910; [α] D,-20° to -70°] possesses an aromatic, spicy, somewhat basil like odour and contains thymol (upto 7%). Carvacrol, free alcohols (C, 13%), esters (as geranyl acetate), free alcohols (2-3%) and a bicyclic sesquiterpene (12.5%). Steam distillation of the whole plant from Kashmir gave pale yellow oil (yield 0.2%) with a pleasant smell and the following characteristics:

Sp.gr.$^{27°}$, 0.8812; n$^{27°}$,1.4795;[α]$^{27°D}$,-1.5°; acid value,

---

*Corresponding author. E-mail: rubina_ku@yahoo.co.in.

2.5; ester value, 10.4 (after acetylation, 102.7); Phenol content, nil; free sol in 90% alcohol. It contained dl-pinene, dipentene, linalool, bi and tricyclic sesquiterpenes and palmitic acid. The oil called oil of origanum in trade is really thyme oil (from *Thymus vulgaris* Linn.).Oil of *O. vulgare* is often confused with sweet marjoram oil (from *Marjorana hortensis*) which is, however dextrarotatory (upto +40°).

The oil possesses carminative, stomachic, diuretic, diaphoretic and emmenagogue properties. It is given as a stimulant and tonic in colic and diarrhea. It is applied in chronic rheumatism, toothache and earache (Wealth of India). Due to the spasmolytic action of the oil, it is used in whooping cough and bronchitis. In homeopathy it is used for hysteric condition. It is used as an external application in healing lotions for wounds, usually in conjunction with other herbs. The oil has been employed in veterinary ointments. It is used in gargle and bath. It stimulates growth of hair. It is also used in cosmetic and soap industry. Its usage in the treatment of Rheumatic pain has evolved considerable interests in the recent past (Mukeerjee et al., 1940).

The whole herb of *O. vulgare* have been used for centuries in Indian system of medicine (Alves-Pereira and Fernandes-Ferreira, 1998) and the effects of herb on arthritis, diabetes and cancer (Wealth of India, 1966) have been reported. Chemical investigations have shown the presence of carvacrol, ursolic acid, caffeic acid, terpinolene, alpha pinene, camphene, myrecene etc. In view of the ethano botanical uses of *O. vulgare* as described above, the antioxidant potential of the extracts of plant together with their radical scavenging activities were studied. Phenolic content of the extracts were also determined.

MATERIALS AND METHODS

Plant material that is, *O. vulgare* was collected from different places of Kashmir valley and authenticated by a taxonomist. All the chemicals used in this study were of analytical grade and were procured from the standard commercial sources in India. Bovine serum albumin, hydrogenperoxide, tertiary butyl hydroperoxide (E.Merk), thiobarbituric acid, folins ciocalteus phenol reagent (CDH India), calf thymus DNA (Sigma Aldrich), ethanol (Bengal chemicals), ascorbic acid, ferric nitrate, trichloroacetic acid, sodium carbonate, sodium dihydrogen monophosphate, sodium hydrogen diphosphate, EDTA (Hi-media). Perchloric acid, sodium potassium tartarate and sodium hydroxide, were obtained from Thomas Baker India. 2, 2 diphenyl picryl hydrazyl (DPPH) was procured from Sigma Aldrich. Ammonium thiocyanate (Qualigens), ferrous chloride (BDH-Analar), Linoleic acid was procured from Sigma Aldrich.

Collection and preparation of extract

During collection the whole herb (*O. vulgare*) was authenticated identified and collected from higher reaches of Kongdoori, Afarwath areas of Gulmarg and Thajwas glacier of Sonamarg in the month of May-June. The plants were identified by the courtesy of library and expert facilities of the KASH (Kashmir University Herbarium) in centre of plant taxonomy (COPT), University of Kashmir, Srinagar.

The voucher specimen was deposited under herbarium no. Kash-bot/KU/org-Rb-001 at the Centre.

The authentically identified plant material (leaves and stem of *O. vulgare*) was shade dried. It was powdered and then subjected to different extraction procedures. The absolute ethanolic extract was prepared using soxhlet extractor. The extract was dried under reduced pressure using a rotary flash evaporator. The percentage yield of absolute ethanolic extract was 18 and 22 g.

The aqueous extract was prepared by decoction method. The powdered material suspended in just boiled distilled wate r(10 g/50 ml) and kept overnight (18-20 h). The extract was separated from the residue using a muslin cloth, and kept in autoclaved screw capped glass bottle in refrigerator. The residue was re-extracted in further 50 ml distilled water and the decoction was prepared as above. The supernatant was mixed with the earlier one and stored. The total volume of water used to prepare the decoction was thus 100 ml. The percentage yield for aqueous extract was 8-10 g. All the extracts were re-dissolved in autoclaved DDW and stored at 4°C for experimental use.

Preparation of post mitochondrial supernatant and microsomes

The post mitochondrial supernatant (PMS) and microsomes were prepared from the liver of the Male wistar rats. Liver from the freshly killed animals were perfused and kept in an ice cold normal saline 0.9% NaCl and extraneous material was removed. All operations were performed out in an ice at temperature of about 4°C. Tissue was blotted between the folds of a filter paper and weighed 10% (w/v), minced homogenate was prepared in Tris HCl buffer (50 mM) containing 0.15 KCl, pH 7.4. The homogenate was filtered through a muslin cloth and centrifuged at 6000 rpm for 10 min at 4°C to separate nuclear debris. The supernatant so obtained was centrifuged at 15000 rpm for 20 min at 4°C to get the PMS. The PMS fraction was then used as a model for lipid per-oxidation.

Microsomes were obtained by centrifuging a portion of PMS as obtained in an ultracentrifuge (Sorvall) at 105000X g for 60 min at 4°C. The pellet obtained was considered microsomes. The pellet was washed and dissolved in a phosphate buffer (0.1 M pH 7.4) containing KCl (1.17%).These were stored at 4°C for experimental use.

Lipid peroxidation assay (PMS and microsomes)

The assay for lipid peroxidation was done by using the method of Wright et al. (1981) with little modifications. The reaction mixture in a total volume of 1.0 ml contains 0.5 ml of PMS or microsomes (3 mg protein/ml), 0.1 ml of ferric nitrate (20 mM), 0.1 ml of ascorbic acid (500 mM). Various concentrations of the plant extracts were added wherever needed. The reaction was stopped by the addition of 25% trichloroacetic acid (TCA). Tubes were centrifuged at 5000 rpm for 5 min.To the supernatant 1 ml of 1.67% thiobarbutaric acid (TBA) was added to each tube. All the tubes were then immediately cooled. Amount of TBARS formed in each sample was assessed by measuring the absorbance at 535 nm using spectrophotometer (Shimadzu 1601) against a reagent blank.

Lipid peroxidation was also performed using cumene hydroperoxides oxidants. Lipid peroxidation was induced by incubating PMS/microsomes for one hour at 37°C in presence of 5 mM tertiary butyl hydroperoxide. After the addition of TCA and TBA, the absorbance was measured at 535 nm.

DNA sugar damage thiobarbituric acid reactive species (TBARS) assay

The sugar damage was assayed by the method of Gutteridge and

Wilkinson (1983). The hydroxyl radical was generated by using ferric nitrate (Fe^3), ascorbic acid (reducing agent), and hydrogen peroxide.

The reaction mixture in a total volume of 2 ml contained 1 ml of calf thymus DNA (1 mg/ml), 0.57 ml of Tris HCl buffer (0.001 M, pH 7.5), 0.2 ml of Fe_2NO_3 (2 mM), 0.2 ml of Ascorbic acid (100 mM) and 0.03 ml of H_2O_2 (30 mM). Various concentrations of plant extract (1000, 500 and 250 µg/ml) were added, wherever needed. The reaction mixture was incubated at 37 °C in a shaking water bath for 24 h. After incubation was over, the deoxyribose degradation was assessed by theTBARS. To reaction mixture 1 ml of 1.67% of thiobarbituric acid (TBA) was added. Tubes were kept in a boiling water bath for 10 min. Tubes were cooled and centrifuged at 10,000 g for 5 min. The supernatant TBARS showing a characteristic absorption at 535 nm was read on spectrophotometer.

Radical scavenging activity using 1, 1-diphenyl-2-picrylhydrazyl (DPPH) assay

The DPPH assay was performed according to the method of Yamaguchi et al. (1998). An aliquot (200 µl) of the various concentrations of the extract (1000, 500 and 250 µg/ml) was mixed with 800 µl of Tris-HCl buffer (100 mM, pH 7.4). To this was added 1 ml of 500 µM DPPH in ethanol, and the mixture was vortexed vigorously. The tubes were then incubated at room temperature for 20 min in the dark, and the absorbance was taken at 517 nm %DPPH scavenging activity was calculated as:

$$\frac{\text{Control absorbance} - \text{Extract absorbance}}{\text{Control absorbance}} \times 100$$

Ferric thiocyanate (FTC) assay

This assay was carried out as described in the method of Kikuzaki and Nakattani (1993). A mixture of 4.0 mg of test sample (extract of O. vulgare) in 4 ml of absolute ethanol, 4.1 ml of 2.5% linoleic acid in absolute ethanol, 8.0 ml of 0.02 M phosphate buffer (pH 7.0) and 3.9 ml of water contained in a screw-cap vial was placed in an oven at 40 °C in the dark. The final concentration of sample was 0.02% w/v. To 0.1 ml of this mixture, 9.7 ml of 75% (v/v) ethanol and 0.1 ml of 30% ammonium thiocyanate was added. Three minutes after the addition of 0.1ml of 2.0×10^{-2}M ferrous chloride in 3.5% HCl to the reaction mixture, the absorbance was measured at 500 nm at every 24 h interval until one day after absorbance of the control reached its maximum value.

Thiobarbituric acid (TBA) assay

This test was conducted according to the method of Kikuzaki and Nakattani (1993). The same samples prepared for FTC method were used. To 2.0 ml of the sample solution, was added 1.0 ml of 20% aqueous TCA and 2.0 ml of aqueous thiobarbituric acid solution. The final sample concentration was 0.02% w/v. The mixture was placed in boiling water bath for 10 min. After cooling, it was centrifuged at 3000 rpm for 20 min. Absorbance of the supernatant was measured at 532 nm. Antioxidant activity was recorded based on absorbance on the final day. In both methods, antioxidant activity is described by percent inhibition.

$$\% \text{ Inhibition} = \frac{\text{Absorbance of control} - \text{Absorbance of sample}}{\text{Absorbance of control}} \times 100$$

Determination of total phenolics

The amount of total phenolics in extracts was determined according to Singletons procedure (Singleton and Rossi, 1965). To the sample solution in (0.5 ml duplicates) were added 2.5 ml of folinciocalteus reagent (0.124 g/ml) and 2 ml of sodium carbonate (7.5%). The reaction mixtures were allowed to stand for 120 min. Absorption at 675 nm was measured by UV-VS spectrophotometer. The total phenolic content was expressed as gallic acid equivalents (GAE) in mg/gm of dry material.

PMS oxidation in the presence of various extracts of O. vulgare

Figure 1 represents the effects of ethanolic and aqueous extracts of the O. vulgare on the PMS oxidation induced by Fe^{3+}/A.A in the presence of hydrogen peroxide.

In the presence of ethanolic extract

At a concentration of 250 µg/ml, the value of MDA decreased from 17 nmoles to 9.8 nmoles in Fe^{3+}/A.A/H_2O_2 oxidant system. At a higher concentration of 500 and 1000 µg/ml of the same extract, the value of peroxidation decreased to 7.0 and 4.3 nmoles respectively.

In the presence of aqueous extract

At a concentration of 250, 500 and 1000 µg/ml the extract decreased the value of MDA formation from 17 to 13.7 nmoles, 11.4 and 9.7 nmoles respectively (Figure 1).

Microsomal lipid peroxidation in the presence of various extracts of O. vulgare

Figure 2 represents the effect of alcoholic and aqueous extracts of O. vulgare on Fe^{3+}/A.A mediated oxidant damages in the presence of hydrogen peroxide.

In presence of ethanolic extract

The values observed are 4, 3.2 and 2.0 nmoles at extract concentration of 250, 500 and 1000 µg/ml respectively (Figure 2).

In the presence of aqueous extract

At a concentration of 250, 500 and 1000 µg/ml, the aqueous extract decreased the value from 9.7 to 6.4 nmoles, 5.3 and 4.2 nmoles respectively (Figure 2).

Effect of O. vulgare extracts on deoxyribose damages

Figure 3 represents the effects of the ethanolic and aqueous extracts of O. vulgare extracts on deoxyribose sugar damages calculated through estimation of TBARS.

Effect of absolute ethanolic extract

With the pretreatment of extracts at a concentration of 250, 500 and 1000 µg/ml the TBARS formation decreased from 15 to 6.8 nmoles, 4.7 and 3.0 nmoles respectively (Figure 3).

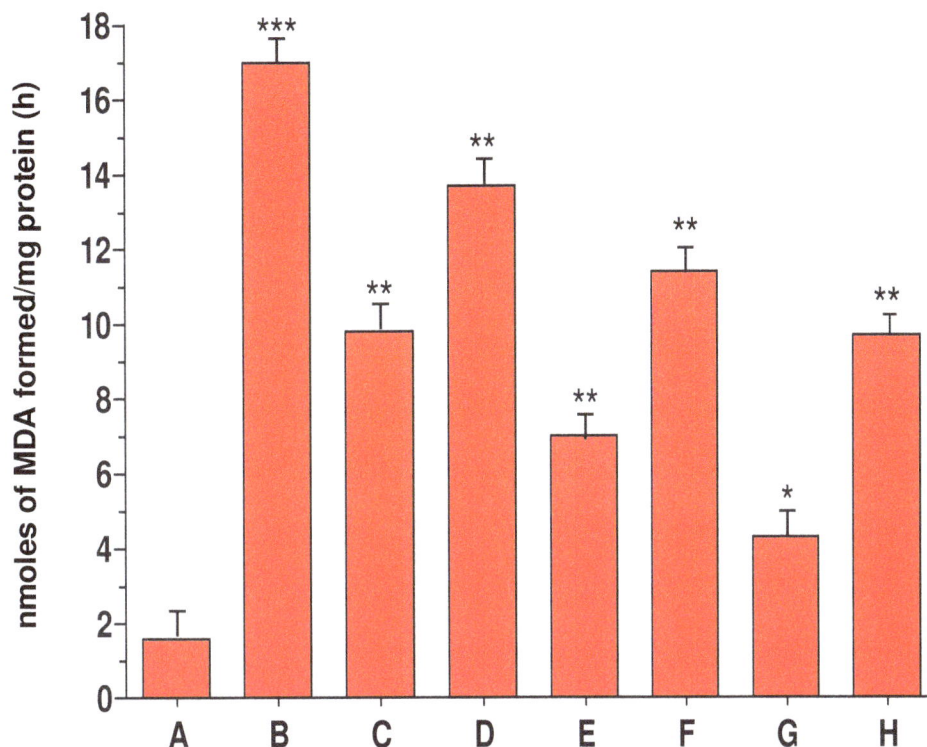

Figure 1. Effect of ethanolic and aqueous extracts of *O.vulgare* on ferric nitrate/ascorbic acid mediated induction of PMS membrane lipid peroxidation in the presence of hydrogen peroxide. A represents PMS (4 mg/ml) alone (control), B represents PMS, ferric nitrate (20 mM) and ascorbic acid (500mM) and hydrogen peroxide (30 mM), C represents B+250 µg/ml of *O.vulgare* (absolute ethanolic extract), D represents B+250 µg/ml of *O vulgare* (aqueous extract), E represents B+500 µg/ml of *O vulgare* (ethanolic extract), F represents B+500 µg/ml of *O vulgare* (aqueous extract), G represents B+1000 µg/ml of *O. vulgare* (ethanolic extract) and H represents 1000 µg/ml of *O. vulgare* (aqueous extract).Each value represents mean ± S.E of six experiments,*** P< 0.001 with respect to their control, ** P< 0.01 with respect to their control,*P<0.05 with respect to their control.

Effect of aqueous extract

The value of TBARS at 250, 500 and 1000 µg/ml decreased to 8.7, 6.0 and 4.9 nmoles respectively in the presence of aqueous extracts of *O. vulgare* (Figure 3).

DPPH radical scavenging activity

Another way of measuring antioxidant activity through free radical abrogating potential of our testing plants is by determining the free radical inhibitory ability of the extracts of *O. vulgare*. The results are depicted in Table 1. The 1, 1 Di phenyl 2, picryl hydrazyl radical scavenging activity shown by the extracts is concentration dependent. With the increase in concentration, the radical scavenging activity increases in both absolute ethanolic and aqueous extracts of *O. vulgare*. The maximum percentage inhibition is shown by absolute ethanolic extract of *O. vulgare* at a concentration of 1000 µg/ml. Vitamin C was taken as a reference compound which shows percent inhibition of 92% at a concentration of 1000 µg/ml.

Antioxidant activity assay (ferric thiocyanate assay)

The FTC method measures the amount of peroxide produced

during the initial stages of oxidation which are the primary products of oxidation. As shown in Figure 4 all tested extracts exhibited varying antioxidant activity when compared with Vitamin E (α-tocopherol) in the FTC method by using *O. vulgare* (absolute ethanolic) and aqueous extracts, the absorbance values ranged from 0.005-0.007 which shows a percent inhibition of 88.09-83.3 respectively (Table 2). The percent inhibition observed for Vit E was 92.3%.

The TBA assay measures the total peroxide content at a later stage of lipid oxidation, involving the quantitation of the secondary products formed from oxidation. The results of the TBA assay agreed well with that of the FTC assay. As shown in Table 2 absolute ethanolic extract of *O. vulgare* showed a high percentage inhibition of (84.6%) as in FTC assay while the aqueous extract showed percentage inhibition of 82.05%.

Antioxidant potential due to phenolics

The total concentration of phenolic compounds in the extracts was determined using a series of gallic acid standard solutions (1 mg/ml) as described by Singleton and Rossi (1965) but with some modifications. Results indicate the higher amounts of gallic acid equivalents in ethonolic extract of *O. vulgare*. Aqueous extracts also possess good phenolic content (Table 3).

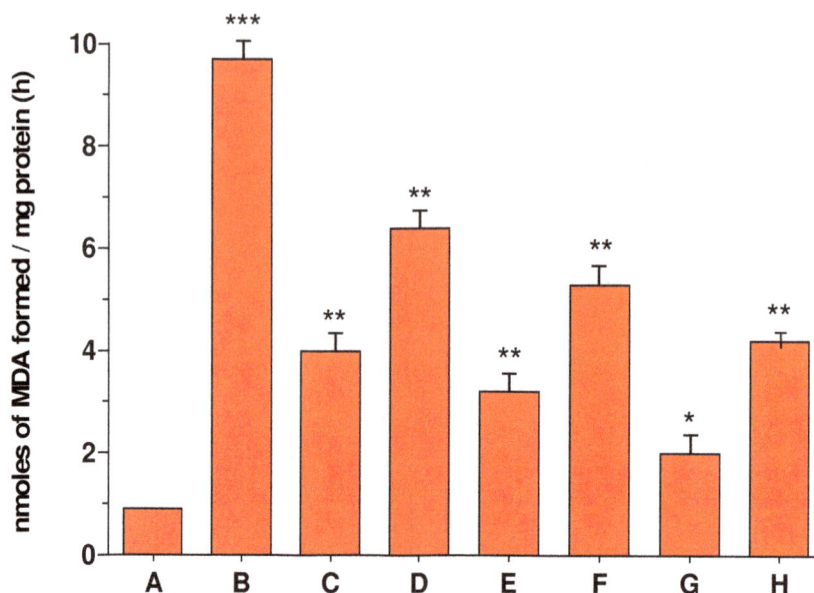

Figure 2. Effect of ethanolic and aqueous extracts of *O. vulgare* on microsomal lipid peroxidation induced by Ferric nitrate/Ascorbic acid in presence of various peroxides. A represents microsomes alone (control), B represents microsomes, ferric nitrate (20 mM) and ascorbic acid (500 mM) and hydrogen peroxide (30 mM), C represents B+250 µg/ml of *O. vulgare*(absolute ethanolic extract), D represents B+250 µg/ml of *O. vulgare* (aqueous extract), E represents B+500µg/ml of *O. vulgare* (ethanolic extract), F represents B+500µg/ml of *O. vulgare* (aqueous extract), G represents B + 1000µg/ml of *O. vulgare* (ethanolic extract) and H represents 1000µg/ml of *O. vulgare* (aqueous extract). Each value represents mean ± S.E of six experiments, *** P< 0.001 with respect to their control, ** P< 0.01 with respect to their control,*P<0.05 with respect to their control.

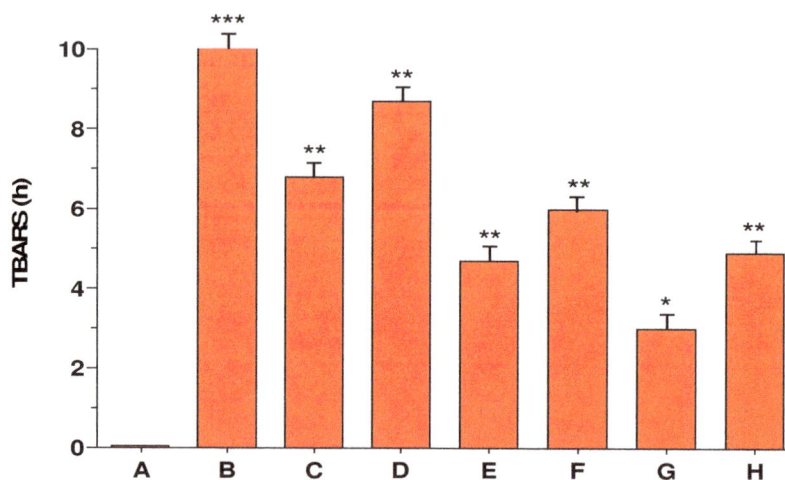

Figure 3. Effect of absolute ethanolic and aqueous extracts of *O. vulgare* on DNA damage induced by Ferric nitrate/Ascorbic acid alone and in presence of various peroxides. A represents DNA alone (control), B represents DNA +Ferric nitrate/Ascorbic acid and Hydrogen peroxide (30 mM), C represents B+25 0 µg/ml of *O. vulgare* (absolute ethanolic extract), D represents B + 250 µg/ml of *O. vulgare* (aqueous extract), E represents B + 500µg/ml of *O. vulgare* (ethanolic extract), F represents 500 µg/ml of *O. vulgare* (aqueous extract), G represents B+ 1000 µg/ml of *O. vulgare* (ethanolic extract) and H represents B + 1000 µg/ml of *O. vulgare* (aqueous extract). Each value represents mean ± S.E of six experiments, *** P< 0.001 with respect to their control,** P<0.01 with respect to their control, *P< 0.05 with respect to their control.

Table 1. DPPH radical scavenging activity of absolute ethanolic and aqueous extracts of *O. vulgare*.

Sample	Percent inhibition
DPPH alone	
DPPH+ ethanolic *O. vulgare*	
1000 µg/ml	79.6
500 µg/ml	69.5
250 µg/ml	54.0
DPPH+ aqueous *O. vulgare*	
1000 µg/ml	77.8
500 µg/ml	70.2
250 µg/ml	62.0
DPPH+Vit.C	
1000 µg/ml	92
500 µg/ml	89.8
250 µg/ml	85.6

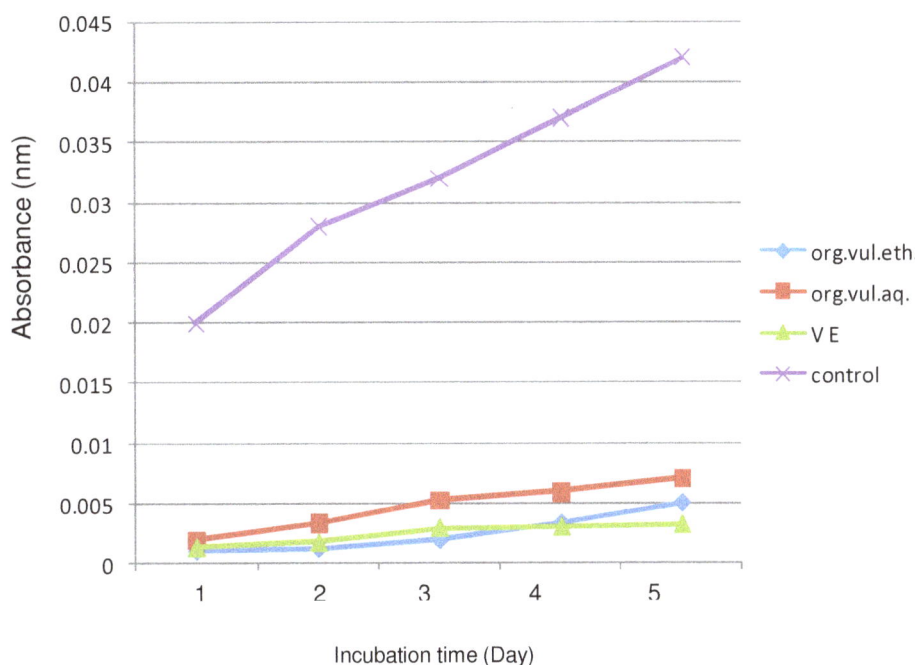

Figure 4. Antioxidant activity of ethanolic and aqueous extracts of *Origanum vulgare* as measured by FTC method.

DISCUSSION

Oxidative agents are highly reactive intermediates (ROS, RNS) which interact with several extracellular and intracellular molecules and with each other, thus generating a complex network of responses culminating in an outcome that may be detrimental or beneficial for the host (Virgillio, 2004).

Our data on experiments with PMS and microsomes clearly reflects that the extracts isolated from *O. vulgare* display effective free radical scavenging property as signified by the suppression of the lipid peroxidation initiated by Fe^{3+}/A.A and hydrogen peroxide. Concentration dependent percentage inhibition of lipid peroxidation was observed with both ethanolic and aqueous extracts. The herb of *O. vulgare* has been shown to possess volatile oil, tannins, thymol, carvacrol, free alcohols, esters, and bicyclic sesquiterpenes. The antioxidant property of

Table 2. Comparison of absorbance values and percent inhibition of linoleic acid peroxidation as measured by the FTC and TBA antioxidant assays.

Sample	Absorbance* (FTC)	Percent inhibition	Absorbance* (TBA)	Percent inhibition
O. vulgare (ethanolic)	0.005	88.09	0.006	84.6
O. vulgare (aqueous)	0.007	83.3	0.007	82.05
Vitamin E	0.0032	92.3	0.0037	90.5
Control	0.042	0	0.039	0

*Absorbance reading on the 5th day (one day after control reached maximum).

Table 3. Total phenolic content μg equivalents of gallic acid/mg of plant extract.

Plant	Total phenol (μg GAE/mg extract)
O. vulgare (ethanolic)	105.4±0.2
O. vulgare (aqueous)	51.5±0.10

the extract could be attributed to these compounds present in this plant. Tannins and carvacrol has been reported with antioxidant activity (Mukerjee et al., 1940). The antioxidant properties of substances possessing reactive phenolic groups can be explained by chain breaking activity of polyphenolic, which act as H-atom donors to peroxy radical, involving termination of radical chain formation (Flatmark and Romslo, 1975).

Various studies suggest that cyclic reduction and oxidation of iron with the perpetual production of free radicals are involved in mediating the DNA damage. The OH attacks the C4 sugar moiety of the DNA, abstracts H-atom from it and form C4 centered radical. The addition of an oxygen molecule generates the peroxyl radical. The successive rearrangement leads to sugar cleavage by the β-elimination. The extracts of the plants have the ability to inhibit free radical production or through scavenging properties can be helpful in diminishing Fe^{3+}/A.A hydroperoxide DNA damages.

The percentage DPPH scavenging activities of the extracts were concentration dependent. Significant DPPH radical scavenging activity was evident at all the tested concentrations of the plant extracts. The DPPH free radical scavenging by the plant extracts is due to their hydrogen donating ability due to their rich contents of polyphenols.

In the FTC and TBA antioxidant assays, the low absorbance values corresponding to a good percent of inhibition for alcoholic and aqueous extracts of *O. vulgare* indicate their good antioxidant potentials. The antioxidant activity of these plants could not be easily attributed to a single compound or a single class of compounds. However, flavonoids and its glycosoids are known to be good antioxidants and the presence of these compounds in our test extracts would be certainly contributing to this antioxidant activity.

Although average content of total phenolics has been determined in both test extracts and it cannot be excluded that the scavenging and antioxidant activity could be attributed to their presence but there is a possibility of a synergistic effect with other metabolites. Our data suggest enough evidence to support the enormous antioxidant potential of the extracts of our testing plants.

ACKNOWLEDGEMENT

Authors are immensely thankful to Indian Institute of Integrative Medicine Jammu, Department of Biochemistry Jamai Hamdard New Delhi, Department of Biotechnology, Department of Botany University of Kashmir and Department of Floriculture SKAUST- Kashmir for providing all the facilities and constant encouragement during this period of work.

REFERENCES

Castroviejo S (2010). *Flora Iberica. Plantas vasculares de la Península Ibérica e Islas Baleares.* Real Jardín Botánico, CSIC. 12: 410-414. Madrid.

Wright JR, Colby HD, Miles PR (1981). Cytosolic factors which affect microsomal lipid peroxidation in lung and liver. *Arch. Biochemistry Biophys.* 206: 294-304.

Flatmark T, Romslo I (1975). Energy dependent accumulation of iron by isolated rat liver mitochondria.Requirement of reducing equivalents and evidence for a unidirectional flux of Fe (II) across the inner membrane. J. Biol. Chem., 250: 6433-6438.

Gutteridge JMC, Wilkinson S (1983).Copper salt dependent hydroxyl radical formation damage to protein acting as antioxidant. *Biochem._Biophys.Acta.* 23(759): 38-41.

Mukerjee KB (1940). D.E.P., V, 494; Fl. Br. Ind., IV, 648; 14 (I), 94; Pl. 759A. *Rec. Bot.Surv.*India.

Kikuzaki H, Nakattani N (1993). Antioxidant effects of some ginger constituents. J. Food Sci., 58: 1407-1410.

Singleton VL, Rossi IA (1965). Colorimetry of total phenolics with phosphomolybdic- phosphotungstic acid reagents. *Am. J. Enolo. Vitic.,* 16: 144-215.

Virgillo DF (2004). New pathways for reactive oxygen species generation in inflammation and potential novel pharmacological targets. *Curr. Pharm. Des.* 10: 1647-1652.

Alves-Pereira MS, Fernandes-Ferreira M (1998). Essential oils and hydrocarbons from leaves and calli of *O.vulgare* ssp. virens. Phytochemistry. 48(5): 795-799.

Wealth of India (1966). Raw materials volume A-B, O-P.

Yamaguchi T, Takamura H, Matoba T, Terao J (1998). HPLC method for the evaluation of the free radical scavenging activity of foods by using 1, 1 dipheny l-2-picryl hydrazyl. *Biosci. Biotechnol. Biochem.* 62: 1201-1204.

25

An evaluation of antioxidants and oxidative stress in Iraqi patients with thyroid gland dysfunction

Salwa H. N. Al-Rubae'i* and Abass K. Al-Musawi

Chemistry Department, College of Science, Al-Mustansiriya University, Baghdad, Iraq.

The present study evaluates the effects of hypothyroidism and hyperthyroidism states on antioxidant vitamins (A, E, C, β-carotene) and uric acid in Iraqi patients before treatment. Lipid peroxidation, an index of oxidative stress was elevated in hyperthyroidism but reduced in hypothyroidism patients as compared to control. The results showed a highly significant decrease in the sera levels of Vitamins A, E and C in all patients with thyroid dysfunction as compared to control. A highly significant decrease in β-carotene levels in patients with hyperthyroidism and a highly significant increase in β-carotene levels in patients with hypothyroidism were compared to control. The level of uric acid was elevated in hyperthyroidism but reduced in hypothyroidism patients as compared to control. In hypothyroidism patients, there was a significant negative correlation between the levels of thyroid hormones, Vitamins A, E, β-carotene and uric acid with concomitant increase in MDA levels, whereas a significant positive correlation was observed between Vitamin C and MDA levels. In hyperthyroidism patients, there was a significant negative correlation between MDA levels and TT3, β-carotene, Vitamin A, and Vitamin E, while a significant positive correlation with TT4, Vitamin C, and uric acid was found. No changes in TSH were observed. The results of this study reveal the importance of monitoring the levels of those antioxidant vitamins in thyroid dysfunction patients before therapy, especially when the disease is more severe.

Key words: Thyroid gland dysfunction, antioxidant vitamins, lipid peroxidation, oxidative stress.

INTRODUCTION

Free radicals and disorders of the antioxidant defense system have a pathogenic impact on human tissues and hence are seen as important factors in the development of various diseases (Mahadik et al., 2001; McCord, 2000). Free radicals are atoms, ions or molecules with one or more unpaired electrons in their outer orbits and therefore have an extremely high reactivity. The main free radicals in human tissues are superoxide, hydroxyl, hydrogen peroxide, singlet oxygen, and nitric oxide (Gutteridge, 1995). Free radicals are produced in the normal cell metabolism, in biochemical reactions involving oxygen, for the purpose of destroying bacteria and other living organisms taken into the cell by phagocytosis. However, they may also be overproduced by exposure to radiation, tobacco, and other pollutants or following hyperoxia, excessive exercise, and ischemia.

Excessive concentration of free radicals in the cell environment may lead to cell damage and death. This damage may be prevented or alleviated by the presence of antioxidant molecules (Patil et al., 2006). Malondialdehyde (MDA) is a natural product of peroxidation of unsaturated fatty acids with three or more double bonds. The interaction between the thyroid hormones and Vitamin A metabolism has long been established (Morley et al., 1978). Vitamin A in plasma binds to a specific protein known as retinol binding protein- RBP, and it has been showed that plasma RBP is complex with the thyroxine binding pre-albumin (Garein and Higueret, 1983). Furthermore, the role of the thyroid hormone in absorption and conversion of carotenoides into Vitamin A is one of the earlier studies pursued (Umesh et al., 1999). In this study, the changes in serum levels of Vitamin A, E, C, β-carotene, and uric acid were determined in hypo- and hyperthyroidism before treatment. The results were correlated with those of MDA in the sera of the corresponding patients. Vitamin E, as the major chain-broking antioxidant, inhibits lipid peroxidation, thus preventing membrane damage and modification of low density lipoproteins. It is generated by the water soluble Vitamin C. Carotenoids efficiently scavenge singlet molecular oxygen and peroxyl radicals. There is increasing evidence from epidemiological studies, animal experiments, and *in vitro* investigations that an increased intake of antioxidants is associated with a diminished risk for several diseases (Stahl and Sies, 1997). The aim of this study was to investigate the dynamics of oxidative stress and antioxidant status markers in both patients with hypothyroidism and hyperthyroidism before treatment by measuring the level of vitamins (A, E, C, β-carotene) and uric acid in Iraqi patients and then finding the correlation between all these parameters with lipid peroxidation, given by MDA level's determination.

MATERIALS AND METHODS

Subjects

Ethical approval (Appendix) was sought and approved by the Ethical Committee of the Chemistry Department, College of Science, Al-Mustansiriya University. We studied patients with newly diagnosed and untreated hypothyroidism (8 males and 27 females), mean aged 44 ± 10 years. A total of 40 patients, 14 males and 26 females (mean aged 41 ± 9 years) with hyperthyroidism were enrolled in this study. A total of 40 healthy volunteers 15 males and 25 females (mean aged 44 ± 11 years) served as controls with normal serum TSH. To eliminate the factors which might affect free radical antioxidant activity, we excluded all smoking and alcohol-drinking subjects, as well as individuals suffering from chronic or acute diseases, such as hypertension, diabetes mellitus, diseases of the liver, kidney, and endocrine and immunological disorders from both patient groups and healthy controls.

Analysis of samples

Fasting blood samples were collected and placed into containing tubes. After centrifugation at 1500 × g for 5 min the serum were removed and retained for assay of the level of Vitamin C and all the parameters, respectively. Serum samples were stored at 20 °C until analysis. Serum concentration of total triiodothronine (TT3), total thyroxin (TT4) and TSH were measured. Levels of TSH, TT3, and TT4 were measured by mini-VIDIS assay using kit supplied by Biomerieux Marcy-l′Etoile/ France.

Vitamins A, E, C and β- carotene determination

The method for Vitamin A and β- carotene determination is based on the Neeld-Pearson procedure in which trifluoroacetic acid is reacted with conjugated double bond system of organic solvent extracted compounds to produce a blue color (A620). The results determined from the calibration curve are expressed in mg/dl (McComic, 1986).

Vitamin C determination is based on the oxidation of ascorbic acid in serum by Cu^{2+} to form dehydroascorbic acid that react with the acidic 2,4-dinitrophenylhydrazine to form a red bis-hydrazone which is measured as A520. The level determined from the calibration curve is expressed in mg/dl (McComic, 1986).

The principle of Vitamin E determination is the extraction of tocopherols into hexane after precipitation of proteins with ethanol. Tocopherol is oxidized to tocopherol quinone by the addition of ferric chloride reagent, and the Fe^{2+} in the resultant $FeCl_2$ is complex with α, α - dipyridyl to produce a red color which measured as A510. The results are determined from the calibration curve is expressed in mg/dl (Pesce and Kaplan, 1987).

Measuring of serum uric acid levels

Uric acid was measured with an enzymatic colorimetric assay using a kit supplied by Giesse Diagnostics, Italy.

Measuring of serum MDA levels

Malondialdehyde formed from the breakdown of poly unsaturated fatty acids serves as a convenient index of peroxidation reaction. The thiobarbituric acid method of Buege and Aust (1978) was used to measure MDA, which reacts with thiobarbituric acid to yield a pink color. Absorbances were determined at 532 nm.

Statistical analysis

All data were expressed as mean ± standard deviation (mean ± SD). Statistical analysis was performed using LSD, considering p < 0.05 as the lowest limit of significance. Statistical analysis was performed using a software program (SPSS 10 for Windows, USA). One-way analysis of variance (ANOVA) was used to compare means with least significant difference (LSD).

RESULTS

TT3 displayed highly significant depletion in hypothyroidism patients compared with control group, as shown in Table 1, the results also show a highly significant increase in the levels of TT3 in hyperthyroidism patients compared to control. A similar trend of significance was noticed in the serum level of TT4 in hypothyroidism and hyperthyroidism patients respectively. On the other hand there was a highly significant increase in TSH value of hypothyroidism patients and a significant decrease in hyperthyroidism patients when compared to control group. Table 1 shows that there is no significant difference in the age of both hypothyroidism and hyperthyroidism patients when compared to control group.

Vitamin A shows a highly significant decrease in both hyperthyroidism and hypothyroidism compared with that of control group as shown in Table 2. A similar trend of significance was noticed in the serum level of Vitamins E and C in different groups. A highly significant decrease in serum β-carotene occurs in hyperthyroidism, while a highly significant increase in serum β-carotene in hypothyroidism group as compared with control group, respectively. Also, Table 2 shows a highly significant increase in the levels of serum uric acid and MDA occurs in hyperthyroidism, while a highly significant decrease in hypothyroidism group as compared with control group,

Table 1. Thyroid function in patients with hypothyroidism, hyperthyroidism, and controls.

Group description	Control	Hypothyroidism	P	Hyperthyroidism	P
No	40	35	-	40	-
Mean age (years±SD)	44±11	44±10	NS	41±9	NS
Sex ratio (men:women)	15:25	8:27	-	14:26	-
TT_3 (µmol/L)	1.635±0.0446	0.702±0.274	<0.0001	3.037±0.691	<0.0001
TT_4 (µmol/L)	90.339±14.147	40.128±14.264	<0.0001	166.316±44.430	<0.0001
TSH (µIU/ml)	2.084±1.058	8.416±2.794	<0.0001	0.191±0.324	<0.002

*NS : Non significant, **the mean difference is significant at the p < 0.05 level.

respectively.

Table 3 shows ANOVA analysis and the results of correlation between oxidative stress index (represented by MDA level) and concentration of antioxidant vitamins, and uric acid in hyperthyroidism and hypothyroidism patients.

In hyperthyroidism patients, a highly significant correlations was noticed between MDA and Vitamin E (P < 0.0001). Also, a highly significant correlation was observed between MDA and β- carotene (P < 0.004), MDA and Vitamin C (P < 0.007), MDA and Vitamin A (P < 0.009) and MDA and uric acid (P < 0.019) while there is a non significant correlation between MDA and thyroid hormones.

In hypothyroidism patients a highly significant correlation was observed between MDA and Vitamin E (P < 0.006). Also, a highly significant correlation was observed between MDA and β- carotene (P < 0.002), MDA and Vitamin C (P < 0.014), MDA and Vitamin A (P < 0.025) and MDA and uric acid (P < 0.012) while there is only significance between MDA and TSH (P < 0.05) but not with other thyroid hormones.

DISCUSSION

The present study reveal some correlation between thyroid hormones and oxidative stress. Oxidative stress results from an imbalance between formation and neutralization of reactive oxygen species (ROS) / reactive nitrogen species (RNS). Lipid peroxidation reaction leads to formation of MDA (Del Rio et al., 2005). The body has several mechanisms to counteract these attacks by using DNA repair enzymes and /or antioxidants (Pacher et al., 2007; Genestra, 2007; Halliwell, 2007; Willcox et al., 2004). If not regulated properly, oxidative stress can induce a variety of chronic and degenerative disease as well as the aging process and some acute pathologies (Huy et al., 2008). In hyperthyroidism, patients have an increase in TT3 and TT4 and simultaneously decrease of TSH. While the condition was a reverse in hypothyroidism patients, which showed a constant decrease of TT3 and TT4 and simultaneously increase in TSH. Elevated TT_3 and TT_4 concentrations are indicative

of hyperthyroidism and low levels are indicative of hypothyroidism, a low TSH in the presence of elevated thyroid hormones is logical because secretion of TSH from the anterior pituitary is regulated by negative feedback from the serum free thyroid hormone concentration (Stockigt, 2003). Many vitamins, enzymes, organic molecules and trace elements play a major role in scavenging those free radicals generated from food oxidation and many pollutants. Beta-carotene serves as an important antioxidant in keeping cells healthy and also serving as pool that is converted to Vitamin A when needed (Russell, 2004). The results obtained an increase level of β- carotene in patients with hypothyroidism as compared to control group, because individuals with hypothyroidism may lack the carotenoids that is needed to be converted into Vitamin A. Also, the alteration in serum carotene levels found in hypothyroid patients is not the direct consequence of a lack of thyroid hormone in the metabolism of vitamin A, but an indirect effect of thyroid disease. Our results are in good agreement with Umesh et al. (1999). The decreased level of β-carotene in hyperthyroidism as compared to the control group is in agreement with Solati et al. (2007) because of a change in the basal metabolism of this group. Results in Table 2 also showed a highly significant decrease (p < 0.0001) in Vitamins A, E and C concentration in both hypothyroidism and hyperthyroidism patients, when a comparison was done with the control group. Vitamin A is a potent antioxidant and acts as a scavenger of free radicals either independently or as a part of large enzyme system. Vitamin A deficiency (VAD) has multiple effects on thyroid function in animals (Arthur et al., 1999):

(1) In the thyroid, VAD decreases thyroidal iodine uptake and iodine incorporation into thyroglobulin and increases thyroid size (Nockles et al., 1984),
(2) In the periphery, VAD increases circulating thyroid hormone concentrations (Morly et al., 1978),
(3) In the pituitary, VA status modulates thyrotropin (thyroid- stimulating hormone) TSH production by Retinoid X receptor (RXR)-mediated expression of pituitary TSHβmRNA (Wolf, 2002).

Clinical and experimental studies showed an elevated

Table 2. Serum levels of antioxidant vitamin A, E and C, β- carotene, uric acid, and (MDA) in different cases of thyroid dysfunction.

Group type (No. of studies)	Component	Mean	SD	SE	P
(Hyper) (N=40)		20.4	6.182	0.977	<0.0001
(Hypo) (N=35)	Vit.A (mg/dl) ×10-2	21.9	4.279	0.723	<0.0001
(C) (N=40)		33.4	7.534	1.19	-
(Hyper)		34.7	18.5	2.92	<0.0001
(Hypo)	Vit.E (mg/dl) ×10-2	66.6	18.2	3.07	<0.0001
C		109	31.5	4.99	-
(Hyper)		124.4	30.1	4.77	<0.0001
(Hypo)	Vit.C (mg/lL) ×10-2	134.1	44.9	7.59	<0.0001
C		146.7	49.6	7.85	-
(Hyper)		11.7	1.774	0.281	<0.0001
(Hypo)	β- carotene (mg/dl) ×10-2	20.2	5.766	0.975	<0.0001
C		15.7	2.037	0.322	-
(Hyper)		37.6	1.91	30.2	<0.0001
(Hypo)	Uric acid (mmol/L) ×10-2	20.2	2.747	46.4	<0.0001
C		25.0	1.997	31.6	-
(Hyper)		163.1	18.8	2.98	<0.0001
(Hypo)	MDA (μmol/L) ×10-2	81.6	20.6	3.48	<0.0001
C		108.7	13.3	2.11	-

Hyper: hyperthyroidism, Hypo: hypothyroidism, C: healthy control group

free radical level in hyperthyroidism. Hyperthyroidism is a hyper metabolic state accompanied by an increase in the total consumption of oxygen, fostering formation of reactive oxygen species and other free radicals, or the occurrence of oxidative stress (Abalovich et al., 2003). For these reasons, the antioxidant Vitamin A had been consumed as a result of excessive production of free radicals (Bourdel-Marchasson et al., 2001). Furthermore, it has also been reported recently that hyperthyroidism enhances tumor growth *in vivo* (Ferreira et al., 2007). In light of the present knowledge, this may be attributed not only to the aforementioned oxidative stress, as it is an important factor in cancer etiology (Hussain et al., 2003), but also to the stimulation of glucose turnover observed in patients with hyperthyroidism (Laville and Riou, 1984), as exacerbated glucose consumption is a cancer hallmark (Ferreira, 2010).

Interestingly, Vitamin A decreases tissue responsiveness to thyroxine hormones, as evidenced by downregulation of Na-K-ATPase activity in the liver along with the decrease in size of the thyroid gland (Garcin et al., 1983). Similarly, it has been shown that Vitamin A enhances the conversion of T4 to T3 (Garcin et al., 1983). Our results were in agreement with Solati et al. (2007).

Vitamin E was reported to be an important factor in quenching free radicals and increasing of the capability of the immune system (Ersan et al., 2006). We can extrapolate from the lower Vitamin E level in thyroid dysfunction that a higher rate of free radical metabolism is occurring. Lowered Vitamin E level is presumably due to its use in preventing free radical damage that seems more extensive in thyroid dysfunction patients (Garcin et al., 1983). Mano et al. (1998) found in their study patients with various thyroid disorders that they presented elevated Vitamin E levels in their thyroid tissue. Researchers concluded that Vitamin E acts as a scavenger in thyroid follicular cell dysfunction. Additional studies have demonstrated that active oxygen radicals inhibit the activity of an enzyme responsible for the conversion of T4 to the active hormone T3 and that sufficient Vitamin E levels may mitigate that effect (Brzezinska-Slebodzinska and Pietras, 1997). Vitamin E, as an antioxidant, might have indirectly caused the destruction of H_2O_2, the required oxidizing agent for iodide oxidation, thus leading to a decrease in thyroid hormone biosynthesis (Zamora et al., 1991). Our findings are consistent with the past researches that highlighted the importance of the effects of Vitamin E in oxidative stress and as component of the antioxidant defense system (Kumar et al., 1992).

Vitamin C is considered the most powerful natural

Table 3. Correlation coefficients and the significant levels of different serum chemical components in patients with hyperthyroidism or hypothyroidism.

Component vs. MDA	Hyperthyroidism					Hypothyroidism				
	Slope	Intercept	R^2	R	P	Slope	Intercept	R^2	r	P
TT_3 (µmol/L)	-1.6327	6.0904	0.1205	-0.347*	0.28	-0.5635	1.1393	0.118	-0.334*	0.43
TT_4 (µmol/L)	106.91	5.5299	0.1346	0.367*	0.020	-18.828	57.934	0.1212	-0.348*	0.04
TSH (µIU/ml)	-0.0105	0.9594	3E-05	-0.006	0.972	-5.5817	13.581	0.1125	-0.335*	0.05
B-Carotene (mg/dl)	-4.9575	2.2193	0.1960	-0.443**	0.004	1.3658	0.5232	0.2533	-0.503**	0.002
Vitamin A (mg/dl)	-1.2308	1.8598	0.1655	-0.407**	0.009	-1.4921	1.1118	0.1438	-0.379*	0.025
Vitamin E (mg/dl)	-0.5275	1.7806	0.2899	-0.538**	0.0001	-0.4350	1.0666	0.2067	-0.455*	0.006
Vitamin C (mg/dl)	0.3051	1.2495	0.1783	0.422**	0.007	0.0915	0.6665	0.1685	0.411*	0.014
Uric acid (mmol/L)	1.5356	1.1049	0.1355	0.368*	0.019	-1.9988	1.1766	0.1770	-0.421*	0.012

*Correlation is significant at the 0.05 level, **correlation is significant at the 0.01 level.

antioxidant (Weber et al., 1996), which is capable of "scavenging" reactive oxygen species by reducing free radicals to more stable species (Gumuslu et al., 2000).

Our results were in good agreement with those obtained by Mohan et al. (2004) and Aliciğüzel et al. (2001) as these studies described low levels of Vitamin C in hyperthyroidism and increase oxidative stress at the same time, it also indicate that antioxidant vitamin become oxidized and it is eventually consumed in exerting its antioxidant action. The decrease in serum levels of antioxidant vitamins was greater in Iraqi individuals of thyroid dysfunction in comparison with western population. This can be attributed to nutritional differences among different societies and to the difference in concentration of air, water and food pollutants among those populations.

Uric acid is the major end-product of metabolism of all nitrogen containing compounds. The results show in Table 2, a highly significant increase (p < 0.0001) in uric acid concentration in hyperthyroidism patients and a highly significant decrease (p < 0.0001) in hypothyroidism patients were detected in comparison with the control group. Uric acid is considered as one of the

antioxidants that are directly scavenging oxygen radicals, singlet oxygen, oxo-haem oxidants and hydroxyl radicals. Another important property of uric acid is its ability to inhibit ascorbate oxidation, as well as lipid peroxidation. In contrast to other antioxidant scavenger reactions, the inhibition of ascorbate oxidation and lipid peroxidation provided by uric acid does not involve uric acid oxidation (Davies et al., 1986). The raised concentration of uric acid may be due to increase purine synthesis or increased degradation of puric nucleotides or decreased secretion on the other (Sato et al., 1995). Our results were in agreement with Vrca et al. (2004) which found an increased level of uric acid in the serum of patients with hyperthyroidism disease and correlated well with the concentration of thyroid hormones. Also, they found that the concentration of uric acid in the serum of patients with hypothyroidism was lower compared to the control group. The increase concentration of uric acid in hyperthyroidism is a consequence of the response of the organism to oxidative stress and mobilization of protective antioxidative mechanism (Vrca et al., 2004).

A highly significant change in MDA levels in patients with thyroid dysfunction compared with

control group was observed in Table 2. It was stated in the several studies that not only hyperthyroidism, but also hypothyroidism led to changes in oxidant and antioxidant systems (Brzezińska-Słebodzińska, 2001). Pathological disorders in thyroid gland bring about functional changes in different organs of the body. Findings obtained in both *in vivo* and *in vitro* studies point out that thyroid hormones have a strong impact on oxidative stress (Rasim et al., 2005).

Table 3 shows a good negative correlation of this component with TT3, TT4, and TSH in hypothyroidism patients, while there was a negative relationship between TT3 and MDA, a positive relationship between TT4 and MDA and no change was observed between TSH and MDA in hyperthyroidism patients. In hypothyroidism, a decrease in free radical production is expected because of the metabolic suppression brought about by the decrement in thyroid hormones levels (Pereira et al., 1994). On the other hand, hyperthyroidism is characterized by an increasing cellular metabolic rate, and thus an increased amount of free radicals (Castitho et al., 1998), and an increase in peroxides levels (Morini et al., 1991). Previous clinical and experimental studies showed a changed in free radical level (with different results) in hypothyroidism and hyperthyroidism. Some of the studies show a significant increase (Chattopadhyay et al., 2003; Sawant et al., 2003). While some other showed a significant decrease (Yilmaz et al., 2003; Brzezińska-Slebodzińska, 2001), or no significant differences (Dariyerli et al., 2004; Gredilla et al., 2003).

Table 3 reveal the correlation between MDA and Vitamins A, E, C, β- carotene and uric acid in patients with hypothyroidism and hyperthyroidism patients. These correlations represent the direct effect of MDA on antioxidant components level. The results show a positive correlation between MDA and β-carotene in hypothyroidism patients. Our findings indicate that the increased levels of MDA and β- carotene are associated with a reduced thyroid function patients. Many individual with hypothyroidism cannot convert β-carotene to Vitamin A, because β-carotene can quench the singlet oxygen without damage to itself and this can be used over and over gain (Passwater, 1984). This is related with β-carotene structure which consists of a long string of double bound with single bound in between. Thus, β-carotene can absorb the singlet oxygen's energy and speared it throughout this long chain of bonds. β-carotene then releases the energy as heat and returns to its usual state (Gaby and Singh, 1991). Table 3 also shows a negative correlation between MDA and β-carotene in hyperthyroidism patients. This result revealed that increasing the oxidative stress will be increasing the breakdown of the measured carotenoids contributing to the lower circulating concentration found in this study. Indeed, if the major mechanism by which inflammation is reduced breakdown, β-carotene concentration in the present study might then be expected, in that the concentration of β-carotene would be very low (Quasim et al., 2003; Galloway et al., 2000). A significant inverse correlation between MDA and Vitamin A was apparent in Table 3 in both cases, suggesting a deficiency in Vitamin A or its consumption as an antioxidant secondary to the excessive production of free radicals (Marchasson et al., 2001). In the present study, a highly significant inversed linear correlation between MDA and Vitamin E levels, and a significant positive correlation between MDA and Vitamin C levels was recorded in hypothyroidism and hyperthyroidism patients. Vitamins C and E are diet-derived antioxidants of major physiological importance (Krajcovicova-Kudlackova et al., 2004). Vitamin C reacts directly with superoxide, hydroxyl radical and singlet oxygen, and it reduces the tocopherol radical back to α-tocopherol (Hamilton et al., 2000). Vitamin E converts the peroxyl radical to the much less reactive hydroperoxides, thus inhibiting the propagation step in lipid peroxidation (Esterbauer and Ramos, 1995). Newer vitamin research has suggested that antioxidant vitamins, such as Vitamins C and E, can reduce the oxidative stress caused by hypothyroidism (Sarandol and Tas, 2005; Oner and Kukner, 2003). Results in Table 3 show a

negative significant correlation between MDA and uric acid levels in hypothyroidism patients, and a positive significant correlation between MDA and uric acid levels in hyperthyroidism patients. The positive correlation may be attributed to the two opposing direction of uric acid production in hyperthyroidism and its consumption (an antioxidant) which lead to a net increase in this variable with increasing in lipid peroxidation status in hyperthyroidism patients. This happens because the enzyme xanthine oxidase shows an enhanced activity with increased lipid peroxidation process caused by enhanced free radical formation together with higher supply of substrates and an insufficient defense antioxidant (Krajcovicova-Kudlackova et al., 2004), which lead to a final increase in the level of the end- product of purine catabolism. It has been suggested that Vitamin E has the potential to inhibit xanthine oxidase, the enzyme involved in urate synthesis (Shaheen et al., 1996).

Finally, from all the aforementioned observations it can be concluded that increased generation of reactive oxygen species and concomitant impairment of the antioxidant system occurs in patients with hyperthyroidism, and particularly in patients with hypothyroidism. These findings indicate that thyroid hormones have a strong impact on oxidative stress and the antioxidant system.

REFERENCES

Abalovich M, Liesuy S, Gutierrez S, Repetto M (2003). Peripheral parameters of oxidative strees in Graves's disease: The effect of methimazole and 131 iodine treatment. Clin. Endocrinol., 59(3):321-327.

Alicigüzel Y, Özdem SN, Özdem SS, Karayalcin U, Siedlak SL, Perry G, Smith MA (2001). Erythrocyte, plasma, and serum antioxidant activities in untreated toxic multinodular goiter patients. Free Radic. Biol. Med., 30(6):665-70.

Arthur JR, Beckett M, Mitchell JH (1999). Interactions between selenium and iodine deficiencies in man and animals. Nutr. Res. Rev., 12:55-73.

Brzezińska-Slebodzińska E (2001). Fever induced oxidative stress: the effect of thyroid status and the 5'-monodeiodinase activity, protective role of selenium and vitamin E. J. Physiol. Pharmacol., 52(2): 275-284.

Bourdel-Marchasson I, Delmas Beauvieux MC, Peuchant E, Richard-Harston S, Decamps A, Reignier B, Emeriau JP, Rainfray M (2001). Antioxidant defences and oxidative stress markers in erythrocytes and plasma from normally nourished elderly Alzheimer patients. Age Ageing, 30(3): 235-241.

Brzezinska-Slebodzinska E, Pietras B (1997). The protective role of some antioxidants and scavengers on the free radicals-induced inhibition of the liver iodothyronine 5'-monodeiodinase activity and thiols content. J. Physiol. Pharmacol. 48(3): 451-59.

Buege JA, Aust SD (1978). Microsomal lipid peroxidation. Methods Enzymol., 52: 302-310.

Castitho RF, Kowaltowski AJ, Vercesi AE (1998). 3, 5, 3'-triiodothyronine induces mitochondrial permeability transition mediated by reactive oxygen species and membrane protein thiol oxidation. Arch. Biochem. Biophys. 345(1): 151-57.

Chattopadhyay S, Zaidi G, Das K, Chainy GBN (2003). Effects of hypothyroidism induced by 6-n-propylthiouracil and its reversal by T3 on rat heart superoxide dismutase, catalase and lipid peroxidation. Indian J. Exp. Biol., 41: 846-849.

Dariyerli N, Toplan S, Akyolcu MC, Hatemi H, Yigit G (2004).

Erythrocyte osmotic fragility and oxidative stress in experimental hypothyroidism. Endocrine, 25: 1-5.

Davies KJ, Seranian A, Muakkassah KFS, Hoshhstein P (1986). Uric acid- iron complex. A new aspect of the antioxidant Function of uric acid. Biochem. J., 235: 747-754.

Del Rio D, Stewart AJ, Pellegrini N (2005). A review of recent studies on malondialdehyde as toxic molecule and biological marker of oxidative stress". Nutr. Metab. Cardiovasc. Dis., 15 (4): 316–28.

Ersan S, Bakir S, Ersan EE, Dogan O (2006). Examination of free radical metabolism and antioxidant defense system elements in patients with obsessive-compulsive disorder. Prog. Neuropsychopharmacol. Biol. Psychiatry, 30: 1039-42.

Esterbauer H, Ramos P (1995). Chemistry and pathophysiology of oxidation of LDL. Rev. Physrol. Biochem. Pharmacol., 127: 31-64.

Ferreira E, Estrela da Silva A, Serakides R, Gomes MG , Cassali GD (2007). Ehrlich tumor as model to study artificial hyperthyroidism influence on breast cancer. Pathol. Res. Pract., 203: 39-44.

Ferreira LMR (2010). Cancer metabolism: The Warburg effect today. Exp. Mol. Pathol., 89: 372-80.

Gaby SK, Singh VN (1991). β-carotene, Vitamin Intake and Health: A Scientific Review, Marcel Dekker.; N.Y., p30.

Galloway P, McMillan DC, Sattar N (2000). Effect of the inflammatory response on trace elements and vitamin status. Ann. Clin. Biochem., 37: 289-97.

Garein H, Higueret P (1983). The thyroid hormones in vitamin A-deficient rats: Effect of retinoic acid supplementation. Ann. Nutr. Metab., 27: 495-500.

Genestra M (2007). Oxyl radicals, redox-sensitive signalling cascades and antioxidants. Cell Signal., 19: 1807-19.

Gredilla R, Lopez Tones M, Portero-Otin M, Pamplona R, Barja G (2003). Influence of hyper and hypothyroidism on lipid peroxidation, unsaturation of phospholipids, glutathione system and oxidative damage to nuclear and mitochondrial DNA in mice skeletal muscle. Acta Vet. Hung., 51: 343-51.

Gumuslu S, Korgun DK, Bilmen S, Yargilcoglu p, Agar A (2000). Effect of sulfur dioxide inhibition on plasma vitamin C and ceruloplasmin in ageing rats. Ind. Health, 38; 319-22.

Gutteridge JMC (1995). Lipid peroxidation and antioxidants as biomarkers of tissue damage. Clin. Chem., 41: 1819–28.

Halliwell B (2007). Biochemistry of oxidative stress. Biochem. Soc. Trans., 35: 1147-50.

Hamilton JMJ, Gilmore WS, Benzie IFF, Mulholland CW, Strain JJ (2000). Interactions between vitamin C and vitamin E in human subjects. Br. J. Nutr., 84: 261-67.

Hussain SP, Hofseth LH, Harris CC (2003). Radical causes of cancer. Nat. Rev. Cancer, 3: 276-85.

Huy LAP, He H, Pham-Huy C (2008). Free Radicals, Antioxidants in Disease and Health. Int. J. Biomed. Sci., 4(2): 89-96.

Krajcovicova-Kudlackova M, Paukova M, Dusinska M (2004). Lipid peroxidation in relation to vitamin C and vitamin E levels. Cent. Eur. J. Publ. Health, 12(1): 46-48.

Kumar CT, Reddy VK, Prosad M, Thyagaraju K, Reddanna P (1992). Dietary supplementation of vitamin E protects heart tissue from exercise-induced oxidant stress. Mol. Cell Biochem. 111: 109-15.

Laville M, Riou J (1984). Glucose metabolism in experimental hyperthyroidism: intact in vivo sensitivity to insulin with abnormal binding and increased glucose turnover. J. Clin. Endocrinol. Metab., 58: 960-65.

Mahadik SP, Evans D, Lal H (2001). Oxidative stress and role of antioxidant and omega-3 essential fatty acid supplementation in schizophrenia. Prog Neuropsychopharmacol. Biol. Psychiatry, 25: 463–93.

Marchasson IB, Delmas-Beauvieux MC, Penchan E, Rrchard-Harston S, Decamps A, Reignier B, Emeriau JP, Rainfray M (2001). Antioxidant defences and oxidative stress markers in erythrocytes and plasma from normally nourished elderly Alzheimer patients. Age Ageing, 30: 235-41.

McCord JM (2000). The evolution of free radicals and oxidative stress. Am. J. Med., 108(8): 652–9.

McComic DB (1986). Vitamins. In: Tietz NW, editor.Textbook of clinical chemistry. Philadelphia, PA : WB Saunders Company, pp 932-33, 960-62 .

Mohan KKM, Bobby Z, Selvaraj N, Kumar DA, Chandra KB, Sen SK, Ramesh R, Ranganathan P (2004). Possible link between glycated hemoglobin and lipid peroxidation in hyperthyroidism. Clin. Chim. Acta., 342: 187-92.

Morini P, Casalino E, Sblanco C, Landriscina C (1991). The response of rat liver lipid peroxidation, antioxidant enzyme activities and glutathione concentration of the thyroid hormone. Int. J. Biochem., 23: 1025-30.

Morley JE, Damassa DA, Bordan J, Pekrary AE, Hersham JM (1978). Thyroid function and vitamin A deficiency .Life Sci., 22: 1901-6.

Nockles CF, Ewing DL, Phetteplace H (1984). Hypothyroidisms: an early signs of vitamin A deficiency in chickenes. J. Nutr., 114: 1733-36.

Oner J, Kukner A (2003). Effect of vitamin E on follicular cell proliferation and expression of apoptosis-associated factors in rats with 6-N-propyl-2-thiouracil-induced goitrogenesis. Folia Histochem. Cytobiol., 41(4): 213-217.

Pacher P, Beckman JS, Liaudet L (2007). Nitric oxide and peroxynitrite in health and disease. Physiol. Rev., 87: 315-24.

Passwater RA (1984). Beta Carotene, the Backstage Natnent Now Universally Recognized for cancer prevention. Keats Publishing Inc., New Canaan Conn., p18.

Patil SB, Kodliwadmath MV, Kodliwadmath MV (2006). Lipid peroxidation and nonenzymatic antioxidants in normal pregnancy. J. Obstes. Gynecol. Indian, 56(5): 399-401.

Pereira B, Rosa LF, Safi DA, Bechara EJ, Curi R (1994). Control of superoxide dismutase, catalase and glutathione peroxidase activities in rat lymphoid organs by thyroid hormones. J. Endocrinol., 140: 73-77.

Pesce AJ, Kaplan LA (1987). Methods in clinical chemistry. St Louis, MO: Mosby Company, p 586-587.

Quasim T, McMillan DC, Talwar D, Sattar N, O'reilly DST, Kinsella J (2003). Lower concentration of carotenoids in the critically-ill patient are related to a systemic inflammatory response and increased lipid peroxidation. Clin. Nutr., 22(5): 459-62.

Rasim M, Abdulkerim KB, Esma O, Leyla A, Isik T (2005). Hyperthyroidism causes lipid peroxidation in kidney and testis tissues of rats: Protective role of melatonin. Neuroendocrinol. Lett., 26(6): 806-10.

Russell RM (2004). The enigma of beta-carotene in carcinogenesis: What can be learned from animal studies. J. Nutr., 134 (1): 262 S- 68 S.

Sarandol E, Tas S (2005). Oxidative stress and serum paraoxonase activity in experimental hypothyroidism: Effect of vitamin E supplementation. Cell Biochem. Funct., 23(1): 1–8.

Sato A, Shirota T, Shinoda T, Komiya I, Aizawa T, Takemura Y, Yamada T (1995). Hyperuricemia in patients with hyperthyroidism due to Graves disease. Metabolism, 44: 207-11.

Sawant BU, Nadkarni GD, Thakare UR, Joseph LJ, Rajan MG (2003). Changes in lipid peroxidation and free radical scavengers in kidney of hypothyroid and hyperthyroid rats. Indian J. Exp. Biol., 41: 1334-37.

Shaheen AA, Abdelfattah AA, Siefelvasr M (1996). Influence of verapramil on the efficacy of vitamin E in preventing the ischaemia-reperfusion induced biochemical derangement in cerebral cortex of rat. Drug Res., 47: 670-73.

Solati SM, Attaei L, Azizi F (2007). Lipid oxidation, antioxidants and paraoxonase enzyme activity in patients with subclinical thyrotoxicosis. Ghudad –I Darunriz Va Mitabulim –Iran, 8(4): 317-23.

Stahl W, Sies H (1997). Antioxidant Defense: Vitamins E and C and Carotenoids. Diabetes, 46(Suppl.2): S14-S18.

Stockigt J (2003). Assessement of thyroid function: towards an integrated laboratory-clinical approach. Clin. Biochem. Rev., 24(4): 109-22.

Umesh C, Shobhita C (1999). The Status of Retinoid in Women Suffering from Hyper- andnHypothyroidism: Interrelationship between vitamin A, β-carotene and Thyroid Hormones. Int. J. Vit. Nutr. Res., 69(2): 132-35.

Vrca VB, Skreb F, Cepelak I, Mayer L (2004). Supplementation with antioxidants in the treatment of Graves' disease: the effect on the extracellular antioxidative parameters. Acta Pharm., 54: 79-89.

Weber P, Bendich A, Schalch W (1996). Vitamin C and human health are view of recent data relevant to human requirements. Int. J. Nutr.

Res., 66: 19-30.

Willcox JK, Ash SL, Catignani GL (2004). Antioxidants and prevention of chronic disease. Crit. Rev. Food Sci. Nutr., 44: 275-295.

Wolf G (2002). The regulation of the thyroid-stimulating hormone of the anterior pituitary gland by thyroid hormone and by 9-cis-retinoic acid. Nutr. Rev., 60: 374-77.

Yilmaz, S, Ozan S, Benzer F, Canatan H (2003). Oxidative damage and antioxidant enzyme activities in experimental hypothyroidism. Cell Biochem. Funct., 21: 325- 30.

Zamora R, Hidalgo FJ, Tappel AL (1991). Comparative antioxidant effectiveness of dietary ft-carotene, vitamin E, selenium and coenzyme Ql0 in rat erythrocytes and plasma. J. Nutr., 121: 50-56.

APPENDIX

Ethical Committee approval

بسم الله الرحمن الرحيم

MINISTRY OF HIGHER EDUCATION
& SCIENTIFIC RESEARCH
AL-MUSTANSIRIYA UNIVERSITY
COLLEGE OF SCIENCE

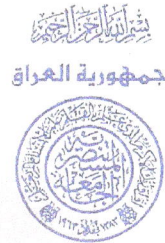

جمهورية العراق

وزارة التعليم العالي والبحث العلمي
الجامعة المستنصرية
كلية العلوم

No.: 136
Date: 24/5/2011

العدد:
التاريخ   /   /   /

Ethical committee approval

Dear Ese Asoro

We are the ethical committee of the chemistry department, college of science, Al-Mustansiriya University. We have studied the project of the M.Sc. student Abass K. Al-Musawi entitle " An Evaluation of Antioxidants and Oxidative Stress in Iraqi Patients with Thyroid Gland Dysfunction" under supervision of Dr. Salwa H.N. Al-Rubae'i and we approval the execution of the project on 20/5/2007 and the student Abass was finished his work and discussed his thesis on 25/6/2009 and have an excellent degree on the thesis. All above documents are in Arabic language if you want as to send them. We provided Dr. Salwa H.N. Al-Rubae'i by this ethical approval because she has desiring to published the paper in African Journal of Biochemistry Research.

Professor
Dr.Redha I. H. Al-Bayati
24/5/2011

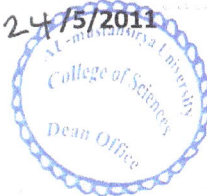

Assistant Professor
Dr. Ramzie R. Al-Ani
24/5/2011

Assistant Professor
Dr. Hussein I. Abdallah
24/5/2011

26

Correlation between moderate *Plasmodium falciparum* malarial parasitaemia and antioxidant vitamins in serum of infected children in South Eastern Nigeria

I. Onyesom[1]*, R. C. Ekeanyanwu[2] and N. Achuka[2]

[1]Department of Medical Biochemistry, Delta State University, Abraka, Nigeria.
[2]Department of Chemical Science, Novena University, Ogume, Delta State, Nigeria.

The levels of antioxidant vitamins were estimated in *Plasmodium falciparum* malarial infected children aged 0 to 12 years. 113 children with *P. falciparum* infection were selected based on laboratory evidence and clinical symptoms. 87 apparently healthy children with no malarial parasitaemia were included as the control subjects. *P. falciparum* parasitaemia and serum levels of antioxidant vitamins (A, C and E) were determined using standard procedures. The results obtained showed that the mean malarial parasitaemia was $6203.01 \pm 1216.79/\mu l$ and the mean serum antioxidant vitamin concentrations were 23.23 ± 8.40 µl/dl for vitamin A, 0.49 ± 0.18 mg/dL for vitamin C and 0.78 ± 0.32mg/dL for vitamin E for the *P. falciparum* malarial infected children. The control children had higher concentrations of vitamins A (51.80 ± 12.41 mg/dL, $X^2 = 60.713$, $P<0.05$), C (1.01 ± 0.16 mg/dl, $X^2 =0.031$, $P>0.05$) and E (0.96 ± 0.21 mg/dl, $X^2 =0.039$, $P>0.05$). The degree of malarial parasitaemia and serum concentration of vitamin E were positively correlated ($r=0.42$) but vitamins A ($r= -0.05$) and C (-0.06) were negatively correlated. Children within 0-5 years of age had higher malarial parasitaemia ($7379.82\pm 918.99/\mu l$), and these children had lower concentrations of vitamins A (21.27 ± 8.68 µg/dL) and C (0.45 ± 0.19 mg/dL) when compared with children between 6 to 12 years (vitamin A= 25.19 ± 8.12 µg/dl and vitamin C = 0.53 ± 0.16 mg/dL). Results suggest that the degree of malarial parasitaemia in especially children between 0 to 5 years could compromise immunity (as judged by the correlation with and reduction in vitamin E). Malarial infection among children (0 to 12 years) decreased the serum antioxidant vitamin levels, and this could lower free radical defense and contribute to the morbidity and mortality of malaria among children in this region. Health care providers should recognize these effects in planning malarial treatment and control programmes. Changes in serum antioxidant levels during post-treatment period should be investigated and documented.

Key words: *Plasmodium falciparum,* malaria, antioxidant vitamins, Owerri, fever.

INTRODUCTION

Malaria is a vector-borne infectious disease caused by protozoan parasites. It is widespread in tropical and sub-tropical regions, including parts of America, Asia and Africa. Each year, there are approximately 350-500 million cases of malaria (WHO, 2008) killing between one and three million people, the majority of whom are young children in Sub-Saharan Africa (Snow et al., 2005). 90% of malaria-related deaths occur in Sub-Saharan Africa (Greenwood et al., 2005). Usually, people get malaria by being bitten by infective female *Anopheles* mosquito. *Anopheles* mosquito can transmit malaria and they must have been infected through a previous blood meal taken on an infected person. When a mosquito bites an infected person, a small amount of blood is taken which contains microscopic malarial parasites. The disease, malaria is caused by protozoan parasites of the genus *Plasmodium* (Yoshida et al., 2007). Antioxidant vitamins (A, C and E)

*Corresponding author. E-mail: onyesominno@yahoo.co.uk.

have various identified roles in cells. Vitamin A is essential for normal immune function and has been shown to influence both anti-body response and cell mediated immunity (Semba, 1998). The changes in vitamin A concentration were accomplished by almost identical changes in serum retinal binding protein (RBP) concentration (Lapidaries et al., 1987). In malaria infected persons, low vitamin A concentration has been reported (Galloway et al., 2000; Adelekan et al., 1997; Metzger et al., 2001). The low concentration of vitamin A seen in malaria sufferers were attributed to inflammatory response (Thurnham, 1996) and redistribution of vitamin A into extra vascular spaces to allow increased bioavailability to tissues.

Strong antioxidants such as dietary carotenoids, vitamins E and C have been shown to modulate immune function in humans (Hughes, 1999; Meydam and Berharka, 1998). Vitamin C is a negative inflammatory reactant. Plasma vitamin C concentrations correlated inversely with white cell count, alpha-1-acid glycoproteins and IL-6, all of which are markers of inflammation (Winkerloofer- Roob et al., 1996). The synergistic combination of vitamins C and E may be further enhanced by the addition of vitamin A.

It has been reported that antioxidants such as vitamins A, C and E would provide protection against the oxidative stress induced by malaria infection (Adelekan et al., 1996). To gain insight into this, the antioxidant profile among children in Owerri, Imo State, Nigeria, diagnosed with *P. falciparum* malaria was investigated, and the correlation between antioxidant concentrations and moderate malarial parasitaemia was studied.

MATERIALS AND METHODS

Study location

The study was conducted in Owerri, Imo State, Nigeria, between April and September 2009. Owerri town lies on latitude 5.485°N and longitude 7.035°E and is located in the rainforest belt of Imo State; endemic for *P. falciparum* malaria parasite which is transmitted by the female *Anopheles* mosquito. It has a rainy period of April to November which is when the mosquito bites are more rampant. The rainforest belt where the state is located is also a very good habitat for mosquito.

Subjects

The study subjects consisted of 113 children who attended the Paediatric Clinic of the Federal Medical Centre (FMC), Owerri, Nigeria. These subjects were children between 0 to 12 years, infected with *P. falciparum* malaria parasite who were reported ill with fever (temperature >37.5°C), headache, vomiting, diarrhea, respiratory distress and other clinical signs and symptoms of malaria as previously documented (WHO, 2000). The children who did not meet these criteria were excluded from the study. Apparently healthy children (87) who were symptomatic and negative for *P. falciparum* in their peripheral blood were used as control individuals. The scope, nature and objectives of the investigation were thoroughly explained to the parents or guardians

of the children for their consent which was sought and obtained.

Collection of blood specimen

Venous blood samples were obtained from the subjects using a syringe. 5 ml of blood was obtained from patients and control subjects by venepuncture and placed into a clean blood container. Serum was obtained by centrifuging the whole blood sample at 3000 rpm for 10 min at room temperature (29 to 31°C). The serum was decanted into Bijou bottle and stored frozen until required for analyses.

Determination of serum antioxidant vitamins

The concentrations of serum vitamin A were determined using Carr-Price reagent (Kaser and Sketol, 1943). Serum vitamin C level was estimated using 2,4-dinitrophenylhydrazine method (Roe and Kuether, 1943). Serum levels of vitamin E was analysed using a micro-method (Quaife et al., 1949.)

Malaria parasite count

P. falciparum parasitaemia level was determined in blood films by Giemsa stain. The level of parasitaemia was graded as low (1 to 999/ μl), moderate (1000 to 9999/ μl) and severe (>10,000/ μl).

RESULTS

The results obtained are shown in Table 1 which shows a summary of the changes in serum antioxidant vitamins (A, C and E) levels induced by moderate *P. falciparum* malarial infection. The mean malarial parasitaemia was 6203.01 ± 1216.79/ μl. The mean serum antioxidant concentration of vitamin A for the malarial infected children was 23.23 ± 8 to 40 μg/dL but the control children had higher mean levels of vitamin A (51.80 ± 12.41 μg/dL). This difference was statistically significant (P<0.05). The mean concentration of vitamins C (1.01 ± 0.16 mg/dl) and E (0.96 ± 0.2 mg/dL) for the non-malarial infected (control) children were not statistically significant when compared with values (0.49 ± 0.18 mg/dL and 0.78 ± 0.32 mg/dL) for the infected children. Malarial parasitaemia and vitamin A or C were negatively correlated (r= -0.05 and -0.06, respectively). The level of vitamin E was positively correlated with malarial parasitaemia (r= 0.42).

Table 1 also shows that children between 0 to 5 years had a higher *P. falciparum* load (7379.82 ± 918.99/ μl) in their peripheral blood smear. These children also had lower vitamins A (21.27 ± 8.68 μg/dL, P<0.05), C (0.45 ± 0.19 mg/dL) and E (0.69 ± 0.22 mg/dL) when compared with the patients between 6 to 12 years.

DISCUSSION

The antioxidant vitamin levels in malarial patients were lower than the levels for the control children. The lower values observed in antioxidant vitamin levels in

Table 1. Serum antioxidant vitamin profile and malarial parasitaemia for children in different age groups.

Age group (yr)	0-5	6-12	Average	0-5	6-12	Average
Degree of P. falciparum malarial parasitaemia (/µL)	Moderate (7379.82 ± 918.99)	Moderate (5026.19 ± 1514.58)		Nil (Control)	Nil (Control)	
Number of subject (n)	51	62		44	43	
Antioxidant vitamin						
Vitamin A (µg/dL)	21.27 ± 8.68*	25.19 ± 8.12*	23.23 ± 8.40*	51.60 ± 12.51	52.00 ± 12.30	51.80 ± 12.41
Vitamin C (mg/dL)	0.45 ± 0.19	0.53 ± 0.16	0.49 ± 0.18	0.93 ± 0.16	1.08 ± 0.16	1.01 ± 0.16
Vitamin E (mg/dL)	0.69 ± 0.22	0.86 ± 0.41	0.78 ± 0.32	0.91 ± 0.30	1.01 ± 0.11	0.96 ± 0.21

Values are expressed as mean ± SD for 'n' subjects. *Significantly different from comparable control value ($p<0.05$).

malaria may be attributed to increased utilization of the host's serum antioxidants by the malaria parasites to counteract oxidative damages (Akpotuzor et al., 2007). It was observed that vitamin A concentration in P. falciparum infected children was significantly lower (P<0.05) than that of the control subjects (Table 1). This observation confirms earlier reports by Nmorsi et al. (2007) and Thurnham and Singkamani (1991). This study further implicates P. falciparum infection as an important component of vitamin A deficiency. This observation is regarded valid considering the role of vitamin A in immune function which influences antibody responses and cell mediated immunity (Nmorsi et al., 2007; Semba, 1998). The lower concentrations of vitamins A and C observed among the younger (0 to 5 years) infected children correlated with higher malarial parasitaemia.

From the present study, the level of serum vitamin E for P. falciparum malarial infected children was observed to be lower when compared with the non-infected children. This agrees with the investigation of Nmorsi et al. (2007) conducted in Ekpoma, Edo State, Nigeria. The low concentration of antioxidant vitamins E and C in infected children may be in part due to increased utilization of serum antioxidant or increased destruction during the malarial infection. Their transfer to the red blood cell membrane to counteract the increased oxidative stress during the acute phase of the disease by inhibiting membrane lipid peroxidation may be a contributing factor (Nmorsi et al., 2007).

Also, it was observed that the children within the first five years of age had lower concentrations of vitamin E than those older than 5 years who had lower parasitaemia (Table 1). However, previous studies by Nmorsi et al. (2007) showed that children within the first five years of age had lower parasitaemia. Therefore, they concluded that these micronutrients which increase with higher malarial parasitaemia may have protective effects against malaria in the Ekpoma region. This lends support to an earlier hypothesis that antioxidants (such as vitamin E) could offer protection against the oxidative stress induced by malarial infection (Clerc, 1992). However, Metzger et al. (2001) observed that low concentrations of vitamin E in serum were not associated with parasite clearance, which is not consistent with the hypothesis that low vitamin E status is protective against malaria (Levander, 1992). Overall, the depressed antioxidant concentrations in the children who had malaria indicated the impact of P. falciparum infection in the antioxidant vitamin status of children in Owerri, Imo State, Nigeria. This observation adds to accumulating reports (Nmorsi et al., 2007; Cooper et al., 2002; Metzger et al., 2001; Galloway et al., 2000). This observation can be further proven valid by the deduction of Akpotuzer et al. (2007) who indicated that antioxidants are used to counteract the effects of free radicals generated in the presence of malaria. This may also explain the negative correlation reported between moderate parasitaemia and antioxidant vitamins (A and C) concentrations among the uninfected children.

This pattern of antioxidant status is a reflection of the malarial pathogenesis, which involves the invasion of human erythrocytes by the malarial parasite. This brings about metabolic changes in the host cells which may then become vulnerable to damage due to toxic metabolites derived from both host and parasites. Reactive oxygen species generated in the host-parasite interaction causes the lysis of erythrocytes and alteration of antioxidants (Nmorsi et al., 2007; Erel et al., 1997; Allison and Enguii, 1983) leading to the development of malarial anaemia (Nmorsi et al., 2007; Kremsner, et al., 2000; Clark and Hunt, 1983).

From the observations in this study, the serum concentrations of antioxidant vitamins were reduced in malarial infection and this may contribute to overall reduction in total antioxidant levels and capacity of malaria infected children. The reduction of these vitamin antioxidants in (the stages of) malaria infection may expose children to free radical attack. To reverse this condition and reduce morbidity due to *P. falciparum*, it is necessary to recommend antioxidant agents (particularly vitamins) as a component drug for the treatment of malarial infection. Dietary modifications, including foods rich in antioxidants (such as vegetables, fruits etc) should be encouraged. The outcome of such recommended supplementation and diet manipulation should be investigated, so that health care providers can be better advised.

REFERENCES

Adelakan DA, Adeodu OO, Thurnham DI (1997). Comparative effect of malaria and malnutrition on plasma antioxidant vitamin in children Ann. F. Trop. Paed., 17: 223-227.

Akpotuzor JO, Udoh AE, Etukudo MH (2007). Total antioxidant status, vitamin A, C and ß-carotene levels of children with *Plasmodium falciparum* in University of Calabar Teaching Hospital (UCTH) Calabar. Pak. J. Nutr., 6(5): 485-489

Allison AC, Engui K (1983). The role of cell mediated immune response in resistance to malaria with special reference to oxidant stress. Ann. Rev. Immunol., 1361-392

Clark IA, Hunt NH (1983). Evidence for reactive oxygen intermediate causing hemolysis and parasite death in malaria. Infect. Immun., 39(1): 1-6.

Clerc M (1992). Observations surles vitamins anti-oxydantes etou anti redicalaries en medicine tropicate. Bull. Acad. Nat. Med., 176: 1393-1406.

Cooper R, Labacavias D, Louw ME (2002). Serum vitamin A and E concentrations in acute *P. falciparum* malaria modulators or markers of severity. Am. J. Clin. Nutr., 53: 84-96

Das BS, Thurnham DI, Das DB (1996). Plasma alpha tocopherol, retinol and carotenoids in children with *falciparum* malaria. Am. J. Clin. Nutri. 64: 94-100.

Erel KA, Avie S, Aktepe N, Buhit V (1997). Oxidative stress and antioxidant status of plasma and erythrocytes in patients with vivax malaria. Clin. Biochem., 30: 631-639

Galloway P, Mcmillian C, Scvattar N (2000). Effect of the inflammatory response on trace elements and vitamin status. Ann. Clin. Biochem., 37: 289-297.

Greenwood BM, Bojang K, Whitty CJ, Targett GA (2005). Malaria. Lancet, 365: 1487-1498.

Huges DA (1999). Effects of carotenoid on human immune function. Proc. Nutri. Soc., 58: 713-718.

Kaser E, Sketol I (1943). Determination of vitamin A using Carr-Price reagent. In : Practical Clinical Biochemistry. H. Varley and A.H Gowenlock (Eds), Elsevier, Amsterdam, pp. 216-223.

Kremsner PG, Gieve B, Leu B, Luckner D, Schmiol D (2000). Malarial anaemia in African children associated with high oxygen radical production. Lancet, 355: 40-41.

Labadaroies D, Brink PA, Weich HF, Visser L, Louw ME, Shepherd GS (1987). Plasma vitamin A, E, C and B6 levels in myocardial infaction. Afr. Med. J., 71: 561-563.

Levander AO (1992). Selenium and sulfur in antioxidant protective system: relationships with vitamin E and malaria. Proc. Soc. Exp. Biol. Med., 20: 255-259.

Metzger AM, Gelasuis A, Schankar G, Ndeezi G, Melikiang P, Semba R (2001). Antioxidant status and acute malaria in children in Kampala, Uganda. Am. J. Trop. Med. Hyg., 63: 15-19.

Meydani SN, Beharka AA (1998). Recent development in vitamin E and immune response. Nutr. Rev., 58: 49-58.

Nmorsi OPG, Ukwandu NCD, Egwunyenga AO (2007). Antioxidant status of Nigerian children with *Plasmodium falciparum* malaria. Afr. J. Microbiol. Res. Oct., 61-64.

Quaife ML, Scrimshaw NS, Lowry OH (1949). A micromethod for assay of total tocopherols in blood serum. J. Biol. Chem., 180: 1229-1235.

Roe E, Kuether N (1943). Serum vitamin C estimation. In :Practical Clinical Biochemistry. H. Varley and A.H Gowenlock (Eds), Elsevier, Amsterdam, pp. 254-263.

Semba RD (1998). The role of vitamin A and related retinoids in immune function. Nutr. Rev., 56: 38-48.

Snow RW, Guerra CA, Noor AM, Myint HY, Hayi SI (2005). The global distribution of clinical episodes of *Plasmodium falciparum* malaria. Nature, 434(7030): 214-217.

Thurnham DI (1996). Antioxidants and prooxidants in malnourished populations. Proc. Nutr. Soc., 49: 173-185.

Thurnham DI, Singkamani R (1991). The acute phase response and vitamin A status in malaria. Trans. R. Soc. Trop. Med. Hyg., 85(2): 194-199.

Winkerloofer-Roob BM, Elleemuter H, Fruhwith M, Schledge-Haueter SE, Kloschsorui G, Van't MA (1997). Plasma vitamin C concentrations in paitents with cystic fibrosis: evidence of associations with long inflammation. Am. J. Clin. Nutr., 65: 1858-1866

World Health Organisation, WHO (2000). Severe *P. falciparum* malaria. Tran. R. Soc. Trop. Med. Hyg., 94: 51-59.

Yoshida S, Shimada Y, Kondoh D (2007). Hemolytic C type lectin, CEL-III from sea cucumber expressed in transgenic mosquitoes impairs malaria parasite development. Plos. Pathog., 3(12): e192.

27

Prevention of cadmium-induced alteration in rat testes and prostate lipid patterns by α-tocopherol

M. A. Adaikpoh* and F. O. Obi

Department of Biochemistry, Faculty of Life Sciences, University of Benin, P. M. B 1154, Benin City, Nigeria.

Cadmium induced testicular damage has been investigated in α-tocopherol (Vitamin E) pretreated and non-pretreated male rats exposed to a single sub-lethal dose of cadmium in form of CdCl$_2$. Graded doses of vitamin E (75, 150, and 750 mg kg^{-1} body wt.) were administered daily to rats in separate groups by gavage for 4 weeks while 3 mg Cd kg^{-1} body wt was administered subcutaneously, 24 hr to the termination of the study. Relative to the Cd - free control rats, cadmium significantly ($P < 0.05$) increased total cholesterol (CHL) levels in the testes and prostate but did not change its level in plasma. It also decreased TPL/CHL and phosphatidylcholine (PC) / phosphatidylethanolamine (PE) ratios in testes and increased sphingomyeline (SPM) / phosphatidylethanolamine (PE) ratios in the testes. However, cadmium administration increased the PC/PE and SPM/PE ratio but reduced the TPL/CHL ratio in the prostate. It appears that increased cholesterol levels within the testes and prostate and attendant membrane rigidity may be one mechanism by which cadmium causes damage to the testes and prostate. It also appears that low - medium doses of α-tocopherol can effectively protect the testes and prostate against Cd - induced damage.

Key words: Cadmium, α-tocopherol, cholesterol, phospholipids, rat.

INTRODUCTION

Most animals with scrotal testes are susceptible to cadmium – induced testicular toxicity (King et al., 1999). Although only about 1 - 2% of an acute cadmium dose is usually taken up by the testes, testicular toxicity is almost invariably evident. It has been reported that as low as 1 - 2 mg Cd kg^{-1} body wt. can cause testicular damage without pathological changes to other organs (Prozialeck et al., 2006). Exposure to cadmium has been reported to reduce male fertility in both humans and rodents (Benoff et al., 2000).

Several reports refer to the role of cholesterol in sperm capacitation and the acrosome reaction process (Khorasani et al., 2000). Hypercholesterolemia results in quantitative and qualitative alterations in sperm membrane lipids leading to an impaired sperm capacity for capacitation and acrosome reactions (Shimamoto and Sofikitis, 1998). In addition, these reports further revealed secretory dysfunction of stimulated leydig cells in a hypercholesterolemic environment.

Although cadmium is a well known testicular toxicant,

its mechanism of toxicity on this organ has not been completely elucidated. Among the proposed mechanisms for its toxicity on the testes are; circulatory failure due to vascular damage and decreased utilization of Zn by spermatogenic cells due to competitive action of cadmium (Amara et al., 2008; Lee, Dixon, 1973). There is paucity of information on the effect of cadmium on the lipids of the testes. Consequently, there is a lack of information also on the role of cadmium - induced lipid changes in testicular function. The aim of the present study was therefore, to extend our investigation on the mechanism of cadmium-induced testicular toxicity by studying the lipid pattern in cadmium exposed and cadmium free rats and the effect of vitamin E, if any, on the lipid pattern.

MATERIALS AND METHODS

Thirty adult male albino rats (Wistar strain; 150 ± 20 g) purchased from the Laboratory Animal Unit of Lagos University Teaching Hospital (LUTH) were used in this study. The rats were allowed a 2 week acclimatization period. Thereafter, they were randomly divided into six groups of 5 rats each. They received water and chow (BFFM Ltd, Ewu, Nigeria) *ad libitum* throughout the period of the ex-

---

*Corresponding author. E-mail: tinadaikpoh@yahoo.com.

periment. They were housed in cages with wire mesh floor (33 x 20 x 13) to prevent coprophagia. Rats in group 1 (control) were cadmium and vitamin E free (- Cd -Vit). Rats in group 2 received only cadmium (+Cd -Vit). Those in group 3 received only 750 mg vitamin E kg^{-1} body wt (-Cd+V750) while those in groups 4, 5 and 6 received 75, 150 and 750 mg vitamin E kg^{-1} body wt respectively before cadmium. Vitamin E was administered daily for 4 weeks by gavage but the cadmium in form of CdCl$_2$ dissolved in normal saline was administered to the rats at a dose of 3 mg kg^{-1} body wt (sc), 24 h to the termination of the experiment. These treatments were carried out in accordance with the principles of laboratory animal care (NIH publication no. 85 - 93, revised 1985). At the end of the 4 weeks experimental study period, animals were necropsized under chloroform (BDH, Poole, England) anesthesia. The thoracic and abdominal regions were opened and blood was obtained by cardiac puncture and put into heparinized tubes, for plasma preparation. The testes and prostate were excised, freed of connective tissue and weighed.

Extraction of lipids from testes

Total lipid was extracted from known weight of testes by the method of Bligh and Dyer (1959), as modified by Jensen (1976). After the removal of the tunica albuginea, the testes were homogenized in a mechanical homogenizer using 20 volumes of chloroform methanol mixture (2:1, v/v). The extract was filtered on a Buchner funnel through solvent-washed filter paper. Filter paper and residue were re-homogenized and extracted with the same chloroform methanol mixture, using half of the volume applied in the initial extraction. The filtration and re-extraction procedures were repeated once more, this time using chloroform methanol (1:2 v/v). The solvent composition of the combined extracts was adjusted by addition of chloroform and distilled water in order to attain a chloroform-methanol-water ratio of 16:8:1. The extract was then washed with 0.9% aqueous sodium chloride. The organic and aqueous layers were finally separated after centrifuging at low temperature (2000 rpm, 5°C). The washed extracts were concentrated in a rotary evaporator and the residue was dissolved in 2.0 ml chloroform: methanol mixture (2:1). At all stages during the extractions, the vessels containing lipid material were flushed with nitrogen.

Biochemical analysis

The amount of total lipid was determined by the method of Zollner and Kirsh (1962). In this method, lipids were allowed to react with sulphuric acid and phosphovanilin reagent to form a pink coloured complex which is measured spectophotometrically at 530 nm.

Total cholesterol was estimated in both the lipid extract and plasma by the enzymatic end-point method using commercially available kits (Randox , UK) while total phospholipids was determined by the method of Fiske and Subarrow (1925).

Individual phospholipid types were separated by thin layer chromatography (Curzner and Davidson, 1967). Spots corresponding to specific phospholipids were recovered by scraping and quantified by the method of Fiske and Subarrow (1925). Recovered phospholipid fractions and reference standards (1 - 5 µg P/ tube) were digested with perchloric acid. Digests were then incubated with molybdate and ascorbic acid solutions and the absorbance of the coloured complex formed was read at 800 nm.

Statistical analysis

Results were expressed as means ± (STD). Analysis of variance (ANOVA) was used to test for differences between treatment effects while Turkey multiple comparison tests was used to test for significant differences between the treatment means. Values were considered significant at $P < 0.05$.

RESULTS

Twenty four hours after dosing with Cd, testicular total cholesterol levels, were significantly ($p < 0.05$) increased in the groups that were treated with only Cd and both Cd and 750 mg vitamin E Kg^{-1} body wt (Table 1) when compared with the control group (-Cd –Vit). Also When testicular total cholesterol of the rats that were treated with only Cd were compared with those that were treated with both Cd and vitamin E, a significant ($p < 0.05$) reduction was observed only in the group that was treated with both Cd and 150 mg vitamin E Kg^{-1} body wt. Treatment with only 750 mg vitamin E kg^{-1} body wt (-Cd +V750) had a similar effect as cadmium on total cholesterol. In the prostate, total cholesterol of the rats that were treated with only Cd (+Cd-Vit), was also significantly ($p < 0.05$) higher than the control. However, pre-treatment of rats with vitamin E before Cd treatment reduced prostate total cholesterol to levels that were not significantly different from control. Treatment with the highest dose of vitamin E without cadmium (-Cd +V750) significantly increased total cholesterol levels in all the tissues investigated in this study when compared with the control. Table 1 also shows that cadmium did not have any significant ($p > 0.05$) effect on plasma cholesterol levels and total phospholipid levels of both testes and prostate, when compared with the control.

The phospholipid profile of the testes and prostate are shown in Tables 2 and 3. Cadmium significantly ($p < 0.05$) reduced phosphatidylcholine, phosphatidylethanolamine and sphingomyeline levels in testes when compared with the control. However, when compared with the group that was treated with only cadmium, rats that were treated with Cd and 75 mg vitamin E showed a significant ($p < 0.05$) increase in phosphatidylcholine level. A significant increase in sphingomyeline was observed in all the Cd and vitamin E treated rats when compared with the group that was treated with only cadmium. In the prostate, phosphatidylcholine and sphingomyeline were significantly reduced in rats that were treated with 75 and 150 mg vitamin E kg^{-1} body wt. when compared with the group that was treated with only cadmium. However, pre-treatment with 750 mg α-tocopherol before cadmium treatment, caused a significant ($p < 0.05$) reduction in the phosphatidylethanolamine levels in the prostate when compared with the group that was treated with only cadmium. When compared with the control, the group that was treated with only 750 mg vitamin E kg^{-1} body wt. showed a significant ($p < 0.05$) reduction in phosphatidylethanolamine level in the testes.

In this study, PC/PE, SPM/PE and TPL/CHL ratios were used as indexes of membrane fluidity so as to establish whether or not cadmium alters this important membrane phenomenon. The results presented in Table 4, show that cadmium decreased the TPL/CHL and PC/PE

Table 1. Effects of cadmium, α-tocopherol and α-tocopherol plus cadmium treatments on total cholesterol, total phospholipid and total phospholipid / cholesterol ratio in testes and prostate of rat.

Parameters	Groups					
	1 (-Cd -Vit)	2 (+Cd -Vit)	3 -Cd+V750	4 (+Cd+V75)	5 (+Cd+V150)	6 (+Cd+V750)
Testicular Total Cholesterol (CHL) (mg/ g tissue)	13.87 ± 1.34	$32.36 \pm 6.06^{*}$	$47.77 \pm 5.73^{*}$	21.46 ± 2.68	9.83 ± 0.22^{a}	$37.57 \pm 5.28^{*}$
Prostate Total Cholesterol (CHL) (mg/ g tissue	42.50 ± 5.30	$93.03 \pm 9.45^{*}$	$81.66 \pm 3.60^{*}$	30.83 ± 4.43^{a}	22.19 ± 1.60^{a}	45.82 ± 4.84^{a}
Testicular Total Phospholipid (TPL) (mg /g tissue)	1.64 ± 0.22	1.41 ± 0.14	1.65 ± 0.22	1.26 ± 0.04	1.24 ± 0.12	1.45 ± 0.06
Prostate Total Phospholipid (TPL) (mg/ g tissue)	1.66 ± 0.19	1.46 ± 0.07	1.63 ± 0.11	1.25 ± 0.06	1.42 ± 0.08	1.45 ± 0.11
Plasma Total Cholesterol (PCHL) (mg / dl)	36.01 ± 3.37	37.31 ± 4.66	$45.91 \pm 2.63^{*}$	36.94 ± 3.60	37.70 ± 3.38	$40. 23 \pm 1.08$

Values are ± SD (n = 5).
*Values on the same row followed by asterisks differ significantly (p< 0.05) from control.
[a] Values on the same row followed by an alphabet differ significantly (p<0.05) from the group that was treated with only cadmium.
-Vit - Cd = group was neither given vitamin E nor cadmium and served as the control.
- Vit +Cd = group was not given vitamin E but was treated with cadmium and served as the test control.
+ V750 - Cd = group received only750mg vitamin E and served as the vitamin control.
+ V75 + Cd = group was given 75mg vitamin E and administered cadmium.
+V150 + Cd = group was given 150mg vitamin E and administered cadmium.
+ V750 + Cd = group was given 750mg vitamin E and administered cadmium

Table 2. Effects of cadmium, α-tocopherol and α-tocopherol plus cadmium treatments on testes phospholipid profile.

Parameters	Groups					
	1(-Cd-Vit)	2(+Cd-Vit)	3(-Cd+V750)	4(+Cd+V75)	5(+Cd+V150)	6(+Cd+V750)
Phosphatidylcholine (PC) (mg/ g tissue)	6.44 ± 0.01	$2.93 \pm 0.01^{*}$	5.08 ± 0.02	7.50 ± 1.50^{a}	$4.23 \pm 0.12^{*}$	$4.06 \pm 0.02^{*}$
Phosphatidylethanolamine (PE) (mg/ g tissue)	5.30 ± 0.11	$3.98 \pm 0.04^{*}$	$4.30 \pm 0.51^{*}$	$3.32 \pm 1.00^{*}$	$2.32 \pm 0.17^{*a}$	$4.19 \pm 0.31^{*}$
Sphingomyeline (SPM) (mg/g tissue)	3.31 ± 0.50	$1.47 \pm 0.42^{*}$	2.73 ± 0.27	3.98 ± 0.05^{a}	$4.15 \pm 0.16^{*a}$	3.02 ± 0.06^{a}

Values are mean ± SD (n = 5).
*Values on the same row followed by asterisks differ significantly (p < 0.05) from control.
[a]Values on the same row followed by an alphabet differ significantly (p < 0.05) from the group that was treated with only cadmium.

Table 3. The effect of 4-weeks α-tocopherol pretreatment on cadmium induced changes in prostate phospholipid profile.

Parameters	Groups					
	1(-Cd-Vit)	2(+Cd-Vit)	3(-Cd+V750)	4(+Cd+V75)	5(+Cd+V150)	6(+Cd+V750)
Phosphatidylcholine (PC) (mg/ g tissue)	0.003 ± 0.000	0.005 ± 0.001	$0.006 \pm 0.001^{*}$	0.003 ± 0.000^{a}	0.002 ± 0.000^{a}	$0.009 \pm 0.000^{*a}$
Phosphatidylethanol-amine (PE) (mg/ g tissue)	0.005 ± 0.000	0.004 ± 0.001	$0.010 \pm 0.001^{*}$	0.005 ± 0.001	0.003 ± 0.000	0.002 ± 0.000^{a}
Sphingomyeline (SPM) (mg/g tissue)	0.005 ± 0.000	0.008 ± 0.001	0.005 ± 0.001	0.004 ± 0.001^{a}	0.003 ± 0.000^{a}	0.009 ± 0.002

Values are mean ± SD (n = 5).
*Values on the same row followed by asterisks differ significantly (p< 0.05) from control.
[a] Values on the same row followed by an alphabet differ significantly (p<0.05) from the group that was treated with only cadmium.
See table 1 footnote for other interpretations.

Table 4. The Effect of cadmium, α-tocopherol and α-tocopherol plus cadmium treatments on phosphatidylcholine (PC)/Phosphatidylethanolamine (PE), Sphingomyeline(SPM)/Phosphatidylethanolamine (PE) and Total phospholipid (TPL)/ Cholesterol(CHL) molar ratios in the testes and prostate of rat.

Organs	Parameters	Groups					
		1(-Cd-Vit)	2(+Cd-Vit)	3(-Cd+V750)	4(+Cd+V75)	5(+Cd+V150)	6(+Cd+V750)
Testes	PC/PE molar ratio	1.15	0.70	1.11	2.12	1.73	0.92
	SPM/ PE molar ratio	2.04	3.66	1.02	2.51	1.14	2.19
	TPL/CHL molar ratio	0.030	0.011	0.009	0.015	0.033	0.010
Prostate	PC/PE molar ratio	0.567	1.181	0.569	0.567	0.631	4.25
	SPM/ PE molar ratio	0.55	1.01	0.20	0.68	0.44	0.92
	TPL/CHL molar ratio	0.010	0.004	0.005	0.010	0.016	0.008

molar ratios but increased SPM/PE molar ratio in the testes when compared with the control. However, treatment with graded doses of α-tocopherol ameliorated these effects in the testes, with the 150 mg/kg body wt. dose being more effective. In the prostate, cadmium increased the PC/PE and SPM/PE ratios while the TPL/CHL ratio was reduced, when compared with the control. Treatment with 150 mg α-tocopherol Kg^{-1} body wt. increased TPL/CHL and PC/PE ratio but reduced SPM/PE ratio in the prostate.

DISCUSSION

The present study examined the effects of cadmium, and pre-treatment of rats with α-tocopherol before cadmium, on the ability of the toxicant to cause changes in the pattern of lipids in the testes and prostate.

Cadmium increased total cholesterol levels in the testes and prostate of rats. If this increase was due to dietary cholesterol, it would have reached the testes and prostate via the blood, thereby leading to a significant elevation in plasma cholesterol level. However, in this study, plasma cholesterol level was not significantly altered by cadmium in any of the rat treatment groups. Again it has been established that there is a blood – testes or blood – male reproductive tract barrier for cholesterol (Shimamato and Sifikitis, 1998; Wong et al., 2004). Evidently, the high testicular cholesterol level observed in this study cannot be attributed to diet. Rather, it is attributable to the intra - gonad alteration in lipid distribution; namely increased mobilization from the membrane of the cells within the testes and / or increased prostatic secretion of cholesterol into the seminal plasma in response to the presence of Cd within the gonad and accessory glands. The later view is more probable since cholesterol is normally secreted into the seminal plasma by the prostate (Sofikitis and Miyagawa, 1991) to protect the spermatozoa against environmental shock. The mechanism by which Cd stimulates increased cholesterol level in the prostate is not known. However, this metal causes oxidative stress in a number of tissues

including the testes (Kara et al., 2007). It is therefore likely that secretion and build-up of cholesterol in the testes and prostate is a biological event that is meant to protect spermatozoa from oxidative stress and damage. The increase in cholesterol level in the testes of rats exposed to high doses of vitamin E only (Table 1, group 3) compared with the control rats is in agreement with earlier reports on increased liver (Alfin- Slater et al., 1972), brain (Dahl et al., 1974) and plasma (Mansour et al., 1992) cholesterol levels in rats and elderly men given high daily doses of α-tocopherol (Vitamin E). Pre-treat-ment with moderate dose of, 150 mg α-tocopherol kg^{-1} body wt was effective in reducing the high cholesterol levels in the testes and prostate. The presence of high level of cholesterol in the testes and prostate may be an indication of decreased androgen production by the testes. This is conceivably so because this hormone is produced by leydig cells (a group of cells that make up the testes) and the function of stimulated leydig cells are impaired by high cholesterol levels (Shimamoto and Sofikitis, 1998). The Cd-induced increase in cholesterol production as observed in this study will therefore affect negatively the leydig cell function. Optimal leydig cell function and testosterone secretion are known to be prerequisites for the normal activation of spermato-genesis (Hikim et al., 2005). Pre-treatment with low levels of vitamin E (75 and 150 mg/kg body wt) was effective in reducing cholesterol to levels close to that of the control while pre-treatment with high dose 750 mg kg^{-1} body wt. alone, or in combination with Cd enhanced cholesterol concentrations to levels higher than the control. This study reveals that the toxic effect of Cd in the testes may involve leydig cell dysfunction. Mechanistically, it could be caused indirectly by Cd when it elevates testicular and prostate cholesterol levels. However, moderate doses of vitamin E appear to be capable of obviating this effect of Cd on testicular cholesterol level.

Total phospholipids / cholesterol (TPL/CHL), phospha-tidylcholine/ phosphatidyl ethanolamine (PC/PE) and sphingomyeline / phosphatidyl ethanolamine (SPM / PE) molar ratios are known indexes of membrane fluidity (Bangur et al., 1995). Increase in the PC/PE and SPM/PE molar ratios and a decrease in the TPL/CHL molar ratio indicate decreased membrane fluidity (Bangur et al., 1995).

In this study, PC/PE, SPM/PE and TPL/CHL ratios were used as indexes of membrane fluidity so as to establish whether or not cadmium alters this important membrane phenomenon. The study shows that cadmium decreased the TPL/CHL and PC/PE molar ratios but increased SPM/PE molar ratio in the testes. Increase in both PC/PE and SPM/PE molar ratios should indicate decreased membrane fluidity but this study shows a decrease in PC/PE and an increase in SPM/PE ratios. Since the two ratios counterbalance each other, the net effect is that cell membranes in the testes will be neither completely fluid nor completely rigid in the presence of cadmium. In the prostate, the PC/PE and SPM/PE ratios were increased while the TPL/CHL ratio was reduced. These effects on prostate phospholipid ratios will bring about complete decrease in its membrane fluidity. The contrasting effects of this toxicant on the testes and prostate lend credence to the suggestion that the effect of Cd on tissue phospholipid may be organ dependent. This effect on the testes and prostate phospholipid ratios was not generally reversed in rats exposed to 75 and 750 mg vitamin E kg^{-1} bd wt., respectively, before cadmium intoxication. In terms of PC/PE ratio, pretreatment of rats with lower doses of vitamin E (75 and150 mg vit. E kg^{-1} bd wt. respectively) before Cd exposure improved membrane fluidity in the testes and prostate. However, if only SPM/PE and TPL/CHL were used to determine membrane fluidity, this membrane phenomenon will be increased in the testes and prostate when Cd − intoxication is preceded by vitamin E treatment at a dose of 150 mg kg^{-1} bd. wt. Therefore, an increase in TPL/CHL ratio and a corresponding decrease in SPM/PE ratio increase membrane fluidity in the presence of Cd rather than the decrease observed in rats exposed to Cd alone. This effect of Cd on the testes is similar to that reported by Pandya et al. (2004) that long term exposure to aluminium causes an increase in cholesterol level and a decrease in TPL/CHL ratio in the brain of rats.

In conclusion, the mechanism of cadmium toxicity of the testes and prostate may involve elevation of cholesterol levels in these organs. Evidently, moderate doses of vitamin E protect the testes and prostate from Cd − induced alteration in membrane fluidity while high doses of the vitamin, when administered alone has effect similar to Cd on the testes.

REFERENCES

Amara S, Abdelmelek H, Garrel C, Guiraud P, Douki T, Ravanat J, Favier A, Sakly M, Rhounia KB (2008). Preventive effect of Zinc against cadmium − induced oxidative stress in rat testes. J. Reprod. Dev. 54(2): 129-134.

Alfin- slater RB, Aftergood L, Kisshineff S (1972). Investigations on hypervitaminosis E in rats. Abst. Int. Congr. Nutr. 9: 191.

Bangur CS, Howland JL, Katyare SS (1995). Thyroid Hormone Treatment alters Phospholipid Composition and Membrane Fluidity of the Rat Brain Mitochondria. Biochem. J. 305: 29-32.

Benoff S, Jacob A, Hurley IR (2000). Male infertility and Environmental Exposure to Lead and Cadmium. Human Reprd. Update. 6: 107-121.

Curzner MI, Davidson AN (1967). Quantitative Thin Layer Chromatography of Lipids. J. Chromatogr. 27: 388-397.

Dahl S (1974). Vitamin E in Clin. Med. The Lancet. 1: 465

Fiske CH, Subarrow Y (1925). The Colorimetric Determination of Phosphorus. J. Biol. Chem. 66: 375-400.

Hikim AS, Swerdloff RS, Wang C (2005). The Testes. In: Endocrinology, Basic and Clinical Principles. Shlomo Melmed and Corn Michael P (eds). Humana Press, New York, pp 405-408.

Jenson B (1976). Rat Testicular Lipids and Dietary Isomeric Fatty Acids in Essential Fatty Acid Deficiency. Lipids, 11(3): 179-188.

Kara H, Cevik A, Konar V, Dayangac A, Yilmaz M (2007). Protective effects of antioxidants against Cd-induced oxidative damage in rat testes. Biol. Trace Elem. Res. 120: 205-211.

Khorasani AM, Cheung AP, Lee CG (2000). Cholesterol Inhibitory effects on Human Sperm-induced Acrosome Reaction. J. Androl., 21 (4): 586-594.

.King LM, Banks AW, George WJ (1999). Differences in Cadmium Transport to the Testis, Epididymis and Brain in Cd-sensitive and Resistant Murine Strains 129/J and A/J 289. J. Pharmacol. Exp. Ther., 2: 825-830.

.Lee IP, Dixon RL (1973). Effects of cadmium on spermatogenesis studied by velocity sedimentation cell separation and serial mating. J. Pharmacol. Exptl. Ther. 187 (2): 641-651.

.Mansour A, El–mossallamy N, Fouad S, Darkish H (1992). Biochemical Response to Chronic Cadmium Intoxication: Changes in Total Cholesterol Content of Different Brain Areas. J. Egypt. Ger. Soc. Zool. O7A: 27-34.

Pandya JD, Dave RK, Katyare SS (2004). Effect of Long-term Aluminum Feeding on Lipid / Phospholipid Profiles of Rat Brain Myelin. Lipids in Health and Disease. 3: 13-22.

Prozialeck WC, Edwards JR, Woods JM (2006). The Vascular Endothelium as a Target of Cadmium Toxicity. Life Sci. 79 (16): 1493-1506.

Shimamoto K, Sofikitis N (1998). Effect of hypercholesterolemia on testicular function and sperm physiology. Yonago Acta. Medica. 41: 23-29.

Sofikitis N, Miyagawa I (1991). Secretary dysfunction of the male accessory genital gland due to prostate infections and fertility: A selected review of the literature. Jpn. Fertil. Steril. 36: 690-699.

.Wong CH, Mruk DD, Lui WY, Cheng CY (2004). Regulation of blood − testes barrier dynamics: an in vivo study. J. Cell Sci. 117 (5): 783-798.

Zollner N, Kirsch K (1962). Total Lipid Determination Using the Phospholipid Reaction. Z. Ges. Exp. Med. 135-145.

28

Antioxidative activity and catechin content of four kinds of *Uncaria gambir* extracts from West Sumatra, Indonesia

Tuty Anggraini[1,2,3]*, Akihiro Tai[1], Tomoyuki Yoshino[1] and Tomio Itani[1]

[1]Faculty of Life and Environmental Sciences, Prefectural University of Hiroshima, 562 Nanatsuka, Shobara, Hiroshima 727-0023, Japan.
[2]Faculty of Agricultural Technology, Kampus Unand Limau Manis, Andalas University, 25163 West Sumatra, Indonesia.
[3]562 Nanatsuka, Shobara, Hiroshima 727-0023, Japan.

Gambir cubadak (GC), gambir udang (GU), gambir riau mancik (GRm) and gambir riau gadang (GRg) are popular cultivars of *Uncaria gambir* in Siguntur, West Sumatra, Indonesia. The aqueous extract of gambir has been used as traditional medicine to treat diarrhea, sore throat and some studies have attributed it to the presence of antioxidant properties. The purpose of this study was to characterize the antioxidative activity and properties of four kinds of gambir extract. The antioxidative activity and properties were determined using 1,1-diphenyl-2picrylhydrazyl (DPPH) radical scavenging activity and HPLC. Reaction times of 2 min and 30 min were used to compare the measurement of DPPH. Cell viability was determined using a cytotoxicity assay. Results indicated that the four kinds of *U. gambir* provided antioxidants that were effective and safe. Total polyphenol contents of GC, GU, GRm, and GRg were 13.86, 13.60, 13.58 and 13.90 g 100 g^{-1}, respectively. Catechin is a major component of gambir extracts. GC and GRm contain caffeic acid (0.99 and 0.98 µg ml^{-1}), while in GU and GRg, it is not detected. The catechin contents of GC, GU, GRm and GRg was 104.5, 101.2, 99.4 and 108.5, 104.5 µg ml^{-1}. In conclusion, the results indicated that GC, GU, GRm and GRg, showed similar tendencies as antioxidants. The presence of catechin influences the antioxidant properties and the reaction time of 30 min was recommended for the measurement of DPPH scavenging activity because of slow acting antioxidant material in gambir.

Key words: Antioxidant, catechin, DPPH, *Uncaria gambir*.

INTRODUCTION

Gambir (*Uncaria gambir*) is a member of the Rubiaceae family and contains an officially recognized pharmacological compound (Heitzman et al., 2005). Gambir is the aqueous extract of the leaves and young twigs of *U. gambir*. The species are widely distributed in tropical regions, which vary based on region. Gambir extract has been used for the treatment of diarrhea and as an astringent medicine in Asian countries (Taniguchi et al., 2007b). Interest in the use of complementary medicine against potent oxidants, to alleviate

inflammatory conditions and improve health conditions is increasing in developed countries (Marshall, 2000). There are four cultivars of gambir in Siguntur, West Sumatra, Indonesia, with the local names: Gambir cubadak (GC), gambir udang (GU), gambir riau mancik (GRm) and gambir riau gadang (GRg). The leaf type of GC is bigger than that of GU, GRm and GRg. GU leaves are partially red in color. GRm leaves are smaller in size than those of GRg (Figure 1).

The *Uncaria* genus has been instrumental in the discovery of natural medicinal products (Heitzman et al., 2005; Sandoval et al., 2002; Taniguchi et al., 2007a). Studies have revealed that certain *Uncaria* species contain tannins and condensed tannins with antioxidant properties, which are responsible for some of *uncaria*'s

*Corresponding author. E-mail: tuty_anggraini@yahoo.co.id.

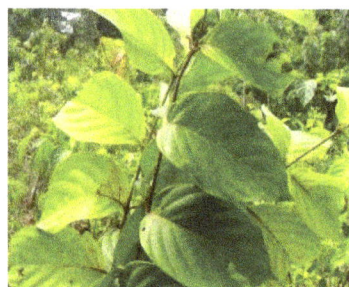

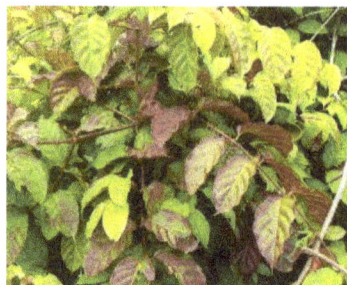

Gambir cubadak (GC)   Gambir udang (GU)

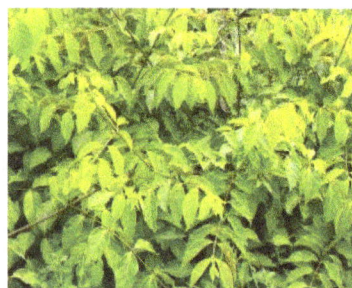

Gambir riau mancik (GRm)   Gambir riau gadang (GRg)

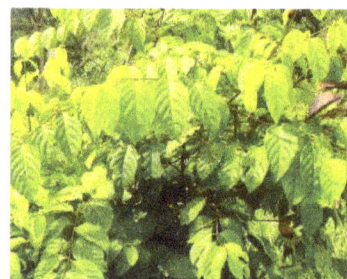

Figure 1. Photographs of GC, GU, GRm and GRg.

pharmacological effects (Desmarchelier et al., 1997). Catechin is a group that occupies an intermediary position in the tannin hierarchy as a family of catechin tannins (Bhat et al., 1998). The presence of catechin in green tea and fermented tea is associated with health protective and cancer preventive properties in animal models, due to its antioxidant activity (Sang et al., 2002). The focus of this research is to compare the antioxidative activity of four kinds of *U. gambir* from Siguntur, West Sumatra. There are four predominant species of *U. gambir*, which are used interchangeably in traditional medicine for their antioxidant properties (Laus, 2004). However, there is a lack of scientific data comparing the efficacy of the four cultivars of gambir from West Sumatra and the potential differences among them. The results of this paper are very important for the gambir farmers in West Sumatra. The determination of the highest antioxidants activity among four kinds of gambir, increase the prize and indirectly increase the farmers income. To fill this need, we have established a research program focusing on the four species of gambir, with the purpose of determining potential differences in their antioxidant activities and properties. Caffeic acid measurement could be more valuable to antioxidant property of gambir. Caffeic acid is a member of antioxidants in *Uncaria* species (Heitzman et al., 2005). For 1,1-diphenyl-2picrylhydrazyl (DPPH) measurements, the original Blois method recommended a reaction time of 30 min; shorter times have also been used. Using a modified Blois method, we compared DPPH radical scavenging activity reaction times of 2 and 30 min.

MATERIALS AND METHODS

Materials

Raw materials

Gambir extracts (GC, GU, GRm and GRg) were obtained from a gambir farmer in Siguntur, West Sumatra, Indonesia.

Chemicals and reagents

DPPH was obtained from Wako Pure Chemical Industries, Ltd, Osaka, Japan. Dulbecco's phosphate buffered saline (DPBS) was obtained from Invitrogen, California, United States. Gallic acid (for total polyphenol standard curve) was obtained from Katayama Chemical, Osaka, Japan. Sodium carbonate, ethanol and methanol were purchased from Wako Pure Chemical Industries, Ltd. Epicatechin, catechin, and caffeic acid were purchased from Wako Chemical Industries, Ltd. HPLC-grade solvents were degassed in an ultrasonic bath before use.

Preparation of gambir extract

Gambir extract was prepared using a traditional method. Gambir leaves and stems were boiled for 1.5 h and then pressed to obtain the extract. Next, the viscous extract was placed in a 'paraku' (a container specifically for the viscous gambir extract made from wood, 3 m × 30 cm × 10 cm (L×W×H)) for 24 h . The extract was then molded and sun-dried for approximately 3 days.

DPPH radical scavenging activity

DPPH radical scavenging activity was determined according to the method of Blois (1958) with a slight modification. Briefly, a 200 µM DPPH solution of DPPH radical solution in 99.5% ethanol was prepared (3.94 mg in 50 ml 99.5% ethanol), and then 300 µl of this solution was mixed with 150 µl of 200 mM MES(2-Morpholinoethanesulfonic acid, monohydrate) buffer, 150 µl distilled water, 150 µl of 50 mM MES buffer and 1 µl of gambir extracts (15 µl (concentration 0.25 mg ml^{-1}), 30 µl (0.50), 45 µl (0.75), 60 µl (1.00), 90 µl (1.50), 120 µl (2.00), 180 µl (3.00), 240 µl (4.00) and 300 µl (5.00)) with total volume, 900 µl. For control absorbance, DPPH was substituted with the 99.5% ethanol solution.

For gambir extract preparation, 10 mg of gambir extract was diluted with 99.5% ethanol up to a volume of 25 ml. Four milliliters of this extract was added to 1 ml of 200 mM MES buffer, 0.2 ml of distilled water, and 0.8 ml of 50% ethanol. The reactions were allowed to proceed for 2 and 30 min at room temperature. The absorbance of the samples was measured at 517 nm. Radical scavenging activity was expressed as the inhibition percentage of free radicals by the sample and was calculated using the following formula:

% DPPH radical scavenging activity = [(control absorbance − extract absorbance) × 100
/ control absorbance]

Total polyphenol content

100 mg of gambir sample was resuspended in 10 ml ethanol. From the solution, 0.125 ml of extract was added to 1.5 ml of distilled water and 0.123 ml of phenol and incubated for 6 min at room temperature. After incubation, 1.25 ml of sodium carbonate (7%) and 1 ml of distilled water was added. The solution was incubated for 90 min at room temperature, and absorbance was measured at 760 nm (Singleton et al., 1999; Sakanaka et al., 2005). The standard curve consisted of 6 mg of gallic acid in 10 ml distilled water.

Separation and analysis of gambir extract

The gambir extract was resuspended in ethanol. A Hitachi (Tokyo, Japan) liquid chromatographic system, consisting of a D-2500 Chromato-Integrator, an L-7100 pump, an L-7420 UV-Vis spectrophotometric detector, an L-7300 column oven, and a degasser (Gastorr-720, FLOM, Tokyo, Japan), was used. The gambir extract (5 µl) was subjected to HPLC analysis using a Develosil ODS-HG-5 column (4.6 i.d. ×150 mm, Nomura Chemical, Aichi, Japan) with a guard column (4.0 i.d. × 100 mm, Develosil ODS-HG-5) and at a flow rate of 0.7 ml/min. The elution was performed using a linear gradient system with just solvent: MeOH/H$_2$O/acetic acid (10:88:2 v/v). The gradient was achieved within 30 min. Absorbance at 280 nm was monitored. Catechin and epicatechin contents were determined from the peak area of the samples with reference to calibration of authentic samples. Absorbance at 325 nm was used for caffeic acid.

Cytotoxicity assay

IEC-6 cell (Intestinal Epithelial Cell line no. 6) was utilized for toxicity test. The cells were cultured on a 96 wells plate in which mixed standard fetal bovine serum (Thermo Fisher Scientific Inc., USA) and DMEM (Invitrogen, USA) and used for the toxicity test after 48 h cultivation. For toxicity test, the cells were washed by 100 µl of PBS (Invitrogen, USA) at room temperature and 100 µl of FBS/DMEM was cultured with sample for 24 h. Sample concentrations were 1, 10, 25, 50, 75, 100, 150 and 200 µg/ml. Cells were added with 10 µl of WST-1 (Roche, USA) and incubated

for 4 h. Absorbance of cells were measured by absorption spectrometer at 440 nm.

RESULTS AND DISCUSSION

DPPH radical scavenging activity and total polyphenol content

We measured the DPPH radical scavenging activity of gambir extract, since this method has been widely used to test the ability of compounds to act as free radical scavengers and evaluate antioxidative activity. The DPPH radical scavenging activity method gives a strong absorption at 517 nm by visible spectroscopy (purple color). Experiments were conducted to assess the capacity of GC, GU, GRm and GRg extracts to scavenge stable free radicals (DPPH). The DPPH radical scavenging activity was correlated with concentration. Although the original method recommends a reaction time of 30 min, shorter times have also been used. Therefore, we compared reaction times of 2 and 30 min.

Based on the DPPH data from the 2-min reaction time, the four kinds of gambir extract (GC, GU, GRm and GRg,) exhibited very strong antioxidant activity (Figure 2). The DPPH radical scavenging activity for 0.25 to 5.0 mg/ml GRm, GRg, GC and GU was 22.10 to 92.78, 20.38 to 93.07, 22.84 to 92.63 and 20.79 to 90.50%, indicating that values increased with increasing concentrations. Total polyphenol content of gambir ranged from 13.58 (GRm) to 13.90 (GRg) g 100 g^{-1}, while GU and GC were 13.60 and 13.86 g 100 g^{-1}, respectively (Table 1). The evaluation of gambir antioxidant activity is increasingly important, since it has been found that phenolic compounds are one of the most effective antioxidants. The high total phenolic content in gambir might be due to the presence of catechins. The antioxidative properties of catechins are manifested particularly by their ability to inhibit and scavenge free radicals (Apea-Bah et al., 2009). The concentrations of 3.00 to 5.00 mg ml^{-1} have almost the same antioxidant activity, but for 0.25 to 2.00 mg ml^{-1}, the antioxidant activity increased based on the concentration of the sample. The results showed that GC, GU, GRm and GRg antioxidant activity was concentration-dependent. With respect to DPPH radical scavenging activity, the results indicated that GC, GU, GRm and GRg, showed similar tendencies as antioxidants. The results of the 30-min reaction time differed from the 2-min reaction time (Figure 3). Among the four kinds of gambir, the DPPH radical scavenging activity rate for the 1.00, 1.50, 2.00, 3.00, 4.00 and 5.00 mg ml^{-1} samples was comparable, ranging from 92.0 to 93.1%. The DPPH radical scavenging activity values of GC GU, GRm, GRg, indicate, again, the efficiency of catechins as free radical scavengers. According to William et al. (1986) and Evelyn et al. (1960), tannins are classified into hydrolysable and condensed tannins based on their structure. Hydrolyzable tannins are characterized

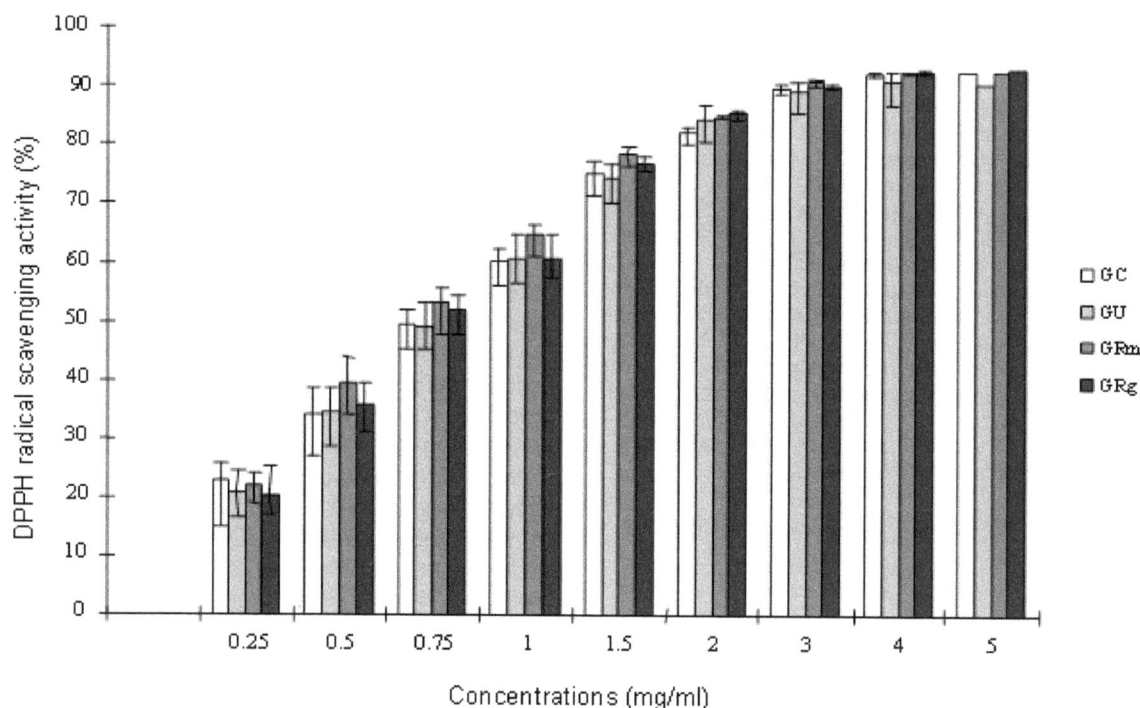

Figure 2. Gambir DPPH radical scavenging activity at a reaction time of 2 min. Gambir concentration were 0.25, 0.5, 0.75, 1, 1.5, 2, 3, 4 and 5 mg ml[-1] for GC, GU, GRm and GRg. The data are the means ± s.d of three replications. GC: Gambir Cubadak; GU: Gambir Udang; GRm: Gambir Riau mancik, and GRg: Gambir Riau gadang.

Table 1. Total polyphenol content of GC, GU, GRm and GRg.

Gambir	Polyphenol (g 100 g[-1])
Gambir Cubadak (GC)	13.86 ± 0.11
Gambir Udang (GU)	13.60 ± 0.19
Gambir Riau mancik (GRm)	13.58 ± 0.10
Gambir Riau udang (GRg)	13.90 ± 0.17

The data are the means ± s.d of three replications.

by having several gallic acid groups, or acids clearly derivable from gallic acid, united by ester linkage to a central glucose residue. Condensed tannins are polymers of flavan-3-ols (catechins) or flavan-3,4-diols or a combination of both. Catechins are a major component of condensed tannins, considered to be recalcitrant (Arunachalam et al., 2003). A reaction time of 30 min resulted in greater DPPH scavenging activity than the 2-min reaction time; this difference reflects the optimal reaction of catechins and slow acting antioxidant material in gambir. Radicals obtained from anti-oxidants with molecular structures are stable species which then stop the oxidation chain. The reaction mechanism between the antioxidants and DPPH depends on the structural conformation of the antioxidant Some compounds react very quickly with DPPH, but the majority of the compounds tested, the reactions are slower and the mechanisms seem to be more complex (Bondet et al., 1997).

Separation and analysis of gambir extract

Separation of catechin, epicatechin and caffeic acid was carried out using HPLC (Figure 4). The catechin content of gambir ranges from 99.4 to 108.5 µg ml[-1] (Table 2). The antioxidant activity was correlated directly with catechin concentration. There is another report that shows catechin content of gambir from Indonesia ranged from 0.22 to 0.76 /g and epicatechin 1.40 to 23.90 mg/g (Taniguchi et al., 2007b). Gambir was formerly cultivated extensively in Indonesia as a commercial source of tanning materials and catechins are the most abundant polyphenolic constituent in the plant (Das and Griffiths, 1967; Taniguchi et al., 2007b).

Among the four kinds of gambir, the epicatechin a caffeic acid contents were detected at very low concentrations. Therefore, catechin, as compared to epicatechin and caffeic acid, shows potential as the source

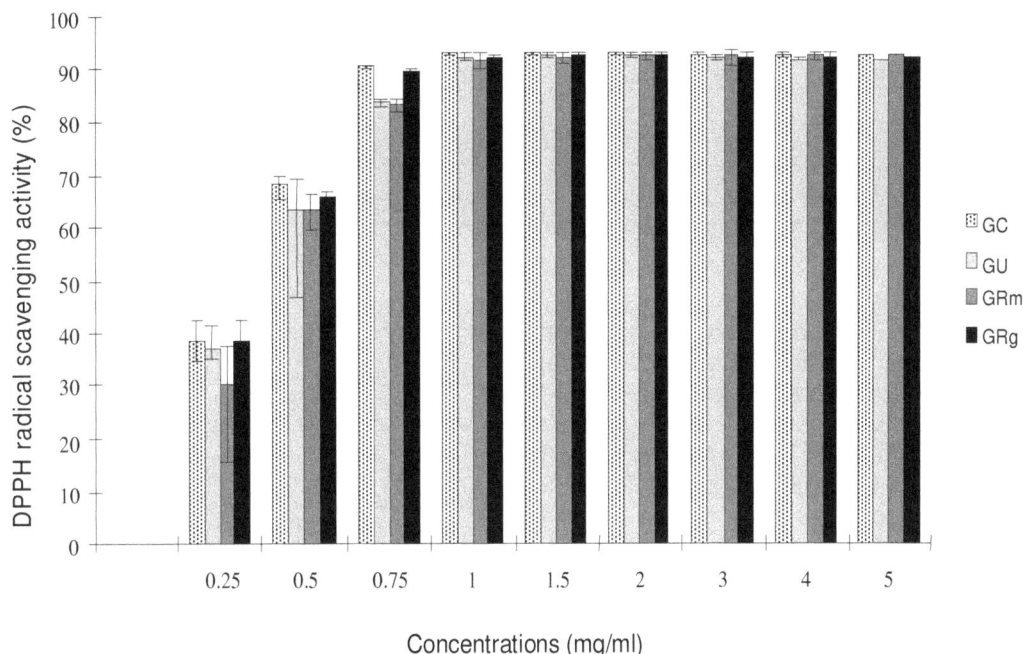

Figure 3. Gambir DPPH radical scavenging activity at a reaction time of 30 min. Gambir concentration were 0.25, 0.5, 0.75, 1, 1.5, 2, 3, 4 and 5 mg ml^{-1} for GRm, GRg, GC and GU. The data are the means ± S.D of three replications. GC: Gambir Cubadak; GU: Gambir Udang; GRm: Gambir Riau mancik; GRg: Gambir Riau gadang.

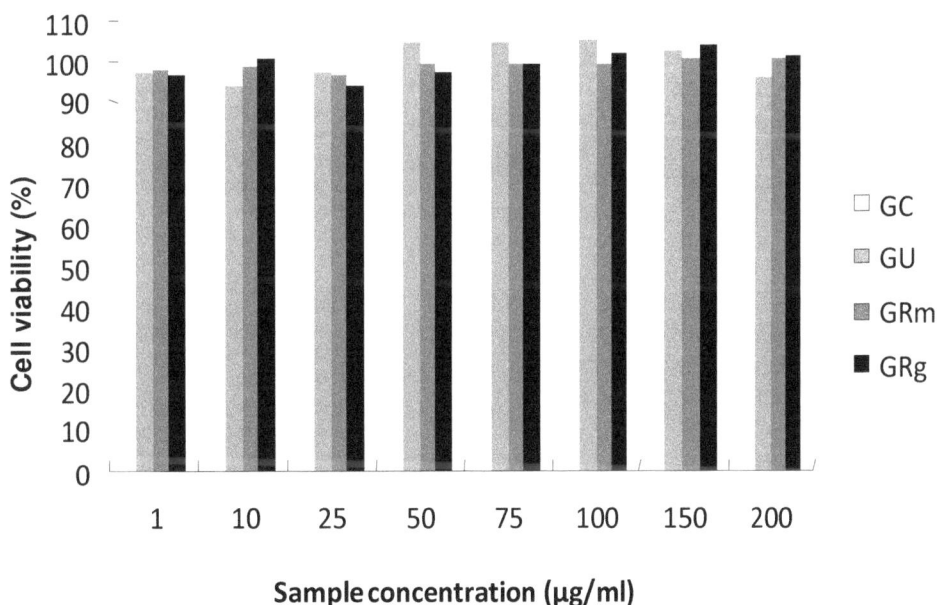

Figure 4. Cytotoxicity assay of gambir extracts. The effect of various concentrations of GC, GU, GRm and GRg on IEC6 cell viability was determined. I : Standard deviation of 3 times experiment.

of the antioxidant activity of gambir extracts in Siguntur, West Sumatra. Catechin is the only major flavonoid in *U. gambir*, and epicatechin and/or caffeic acid are/is minor flavonoids with difference among 4 kinds of gambir.

Cytotoxicity assay

Cytotoxicity is a measure of cellular viability and is used to assess whether compounds have a toxic effect.

Table 2. Concentration of catechin, epicatechin and caffeic acid in gambir extracts.

Gambir extract	Catechin (µg/ml)	Epicatechin (µg/ml)	Caffeic acid (µg/ml)
GC	104.5	0.80	0.99
GU	101.2	0.62	-
GRm	99.4	0.49	0.98
GRg	108	0.74	-

Gambir extract is used interchangeably in traditional medicine. It was revealed that in a cytotoxicity assay using IEC-6, the antioxidant in gambir was safe (Figure 4). The range of normalized gambir values ((gambir/control) × 100) were as follows: GC: 96.3 to 103.8%; GU: 94.4 to 104.6%; GRm: 96.6 to 100.3%, and GRg: 93 to 103.7%. The gambir extract showed no negative effects against IEC-6, as indicated by more than 93% live cells (for concentration 1 to 200 µg/ml). The result showed different tendency with grape seed extract (GSE), where GSE concentration from 3.9 to 15.6 µg/ml did not affect IEC-6 cell viability but higher concentrations (62.5 to 1.000 µg/ml) reduced cell viability (Cheah et al., 2009).

Conclusion

Although different in appearance, the four cultivars of *U. gambir* of Siguntur, West Sumatra, Indonesia (GC, GU, GRm and GRg) displayed similar antioxidant activities and excellent antioxidant properties, with a remarkably potent ability to scavenge free radicals. The study has shown that 30-min reaction time for DPPH measurement is recommended because gambir contain slow acting antioxidant material. The DPPH radical scavenging activity ranged from 92.0 to 93.1% and the catechin content ranged from 99.4 to 108.5 µg/ml. Total polyphenol content was as follows: 13.86 (GC), 13.60 (GU), 13.58 (GRm) and 13.90 g/100 g (GRg). Catechin was identified as the major bioactive compound in gambir. Of notable importance is that the antioxidant in gambir is safe.

ACKNOWLEDGMENTS

The authors would like to thank the Ministry of National Education of the Republic of Indonesia for the financial support programs.

REFERENCES

Apea-Bah FB, Hanafi M., Dewi RT, Fajriah S, Darmawan A, Artanti N, Lotulung P, Ngadymang P, Minarti B (2009). Assessment of the DPPH and α-glucosidase inhibitory potential of gambier and qualitative identification of major bioactive compound. J. Med. Plants Res., 3: 736-757.

Arunachalam M, Raj MM, Mohan N, Mahadevan A (2003). Biodegradation of catechin. Proc. Indian Natn. Sci. Acad., 4: 353-370.

Bhat TK, Singh B, Sharma OP (1998). Microbial degradation of tannins – a current perspective. Biodegradation, 9: 343-357.

Bondet V, Brand-Williams W, Berset C (1997). Kinetics and mechanisms of antioxidant activity using the DPPH free radical method. Lebensm.-Wiss. U.-Technol., 30, 609-615.

Blois M (1958). Antioxidant determinations by the use of a stable free radical. Nature, 26: 1199-1200.

Cheah KY, Howarth GS, Beck RY, Wright TH, Whitford EJ, Dayne C, Butter RN, Bastian SEP (2009). Grape seed extract protects IEC-6 cells from chemotherapy-induced cytotoxicity and improves parameters of small intestinal mucositis in rats with experimentally-induced mucositis. Cancer Biol. Ther., 8:4, 382-390.

Das NP, Griffiths LA (1967). Studies on flavonoid metabolism biosynthesis of (+)-[14C] catechin by the plant Uncaria gambir Roxb. Biochem. J., 105: 73-77.

Desmarchelier C, Mongelli E, Coussio J, Ciccia G (1997). Evaluation of the in vitro antioxidant activity in extracts of Uncaria tomentosa (Willd) DC. Phytother. Res., 11: 254-256.

Evelyn SR, Maohs EA, Roux DG (1960). The oxidative condensation of (+) Catechin. Biochem. J., 76: 23-27.

Heitzman M.E, Neto CC, Winiarz E, Vaisberg AJ, Hammond GB (2005). Ethnobotany, phytochemistry and pharmacology of Uncaria (Rubiaceae). Phytochem., 66: 5-29.

Laus G (2004). Advances in chemistry and bioactivity of the genus Uncaria. Phytother. Res., 18: 259-274.

Marshall E (2000). Bastions of tradition adapt to alternative medicine. Sci., 288: 1570-1572.

Sakanaka S, Tachibana Y, Okada Y (2005) Preparation and antioxidant properties of extract of Japanese persimmon leaf (kakinoha-cha). Food Chem., pp. 569-575.

Sandoval M, Okuhama NN, Zhang XJ, Condezo A, Lao J, Angeles FM, Musah RA, Bobrowski P, Miller MJ (2002). Anti-inflammatory and antioxidant activities of cat's claw (Uncaria tomentosa and Uncaria guianensis) are independent of their alkaloid content. Phytomed., 9: 325-337.

Sang S, Cheng X, Stark RE, Rosen RT, Yang CS, Ho CT (2002). Chemicals studies on antioxidant mechanism of tea catechins: Analysis of radical reaction products of catechin and epicatechin with 2,2-diphenyl-1-picrylhydrazyl. Bioorg. Med. Chem., 10: 2233-2237.

Singleton VL, Orthofer R, Lamuela-Raventos RM (1999). Analysis of total phenols and other sustrates and antioxidants by means of Folin-Ciocateu reagent. Methods in Enzymol., 299, pp. 152-178.

Taniguchi S, Kuroda K, Doi K, Tanabe M, Shibata T, Yoshida T, Hatano T (2007a). Revised Structures of gambiriins A1, A2, B1 and B2, chalcane-flavan dimers from gambir (Uncaria gambir extract). Chem. Pharm. Bull., 55: 268-272.

Taniguchi S, Kuroda K, Doi K, Yoneda Y, Tanabe M, Shibata T, Yoshida T, Hatano T (2007b). Evaluation of gambir quality based on quantitative analysis of polyphenolic constituents. Yakugaku Zasshi, 127: 1291-300.

William F, Boominathan K, Vasudevan N, Gurujeyalakshmi G, Mahadevan A (1986). Microbial degradation of lignin and tannin. J. Sci. Ind. Res., 45: 232-243.

29

In vitro biochemical investigations of the effects of *Carica papaya* and *Fagara zanthoxyloides* on antioxidant status and sickle erythrocytes

Imaga, Ngozi O. A.[1]*, Shaire Esther A.[1], Ogbeide Samson[1] and Samuel K. Akindele[2]

[1]Department of Biochemistry, College of Medicine, University of Lagos, P. M. B. 12003, Idi-Araba, Lagos State, Nigeria.
[2]Department of Biochemistry, Nigerian Institute of Medical Research, P. M. B. 2013, Yaba, Lagos State, Nigeria.

Various works have identified a number of herbal applications that have ameliorating effects on sickle cell disorders. The antisickling activities of dried *Carica papaya* leaves and roots of *Fagara zanthoxyloides* are being investigated in this study to determine the antioxidant properties of the plant extracts and their effects on homozygous sickle cell (SS) erythrocytes *in vitro*. The antisickling activity of both extracts were determined as well as analyses of hematological parameters, hemolysis of SS cells and formation of membrane associated denatured hemoglobin (MADH) used to measure the effects of plant extracts on the erythrocyte. Folin-C total phenol and beta-carotene methods of assay were used to determine antioxidant activity, while the effect of plant extracts on oxidative stress was measured by assaying for superoxide dismutase, catalase, gluthathione transferase levels and lipid peroxidation. Results confirmed the potent antisickling activity of both plants. The levels of the oxidative stress enzymes (superoxide dismutase (SOD), catalase (CAT) and glutathione (GST) and lipid peroxidation were reduced after blood samples had been incubated with the extracts. The extracts therefore protected membrane integrity resulting in a reduction of red blood cells (RBC) hemolysis without met-hemoglobin formation. Both plant extracts possess potent antioxidant activity which may be responsible for their observed antisickling action.

Key words: *Fagara*, *papaya*, oxidative stress enzymes, antioxidant activity, hemolysis.

INTRODUCTION

First-line clinical management of sickle cell anemia include use of Folic acid, amino acids (as nutritional supplements), Penicillin prophylaxis (helps prevent infection) and anti-malarial prophylaxis (helps prevent malaria attack) for example, Paludrine[R] in varying doses in childhood, adulthood and pregnancy. The faulty 'S'

gene is not eradicated in treatment, rather the condition is managed and synthesis of RBC induced to stabilize the patient's hemoglobin level. Further management and treatment of this disorder with compounds or techniques which directly affect the hemoglobin (Hb) molecule (for example, Hydroxyurea, Bone Marrow Transplantation and Blood Transfusion) are very expensive and out ofreach of the masses and besides expose the patient to mutagenicity, iron overload and other fatal risks (Brittain and Han, 2004; Steinberg, 2004; Amrolia, 2003; Saunthararajah and Maziarz, 2003; Nagel, 1998). It is acknowledged world-wide that traditional medicine can be explored and exploited to be used along-side synthetic pharmaceutical products for enhanced health manage-ment. Due to the high mortality rate of sickle cell patients, especially in children, and since chemotherapy has its adverse effects, there is need for rational drug development that must embrace not only synthetic drugs but also natural products (phytomedicines/herbal drugs),

---

*Corresponding author. Email: ngoziawaimaga@yahoo.com.

Abbreviations: SS, Sickle cell; MADH, membrane associated denatured hemoglobin; GST, glutathione; SOD, superoxide dismutase; CAT, catalase; RBC, red blood cells; Hb, hemoglobin; EDTA, ethylenediaminetetraacetic acid; FRIN, forestry research institute of Nigeria; HbAA, hemoglobin AA; HbSS, hemoglobin SS; PHBA, para-hydroxybenzoic acid; TBARS, thiobarbituric acid; MCHC, mean corpuscular hemoglobin concentration; RDW, red cell distribution width; MDA, malondiadehyde; SCD, sickle cell disease.

naturally occurring antisickling agents which can be obtained from our vast forest resources and can be used to effectively manage the sickle cell patient and treat the anemic condition accompanying this disorder.

Active constituents of medicinal plants and naturally occurring compounds, known as antisickling agents, which improve the health of sickle cell individuals are rich in aromatic amino acids, phenolic compounds and antioxidant nutrients (Abraham et al., 1991) which are thought to be responsible for their observed antisickling action. An herbal preparation of *Cajanus cajan* was found to contain phenylalanine, carjaminose and hydroxybenzoic acid as active constituents and are thought to be the reason for its antisickling effect (Ogoda et al., 2002). The antisickling activities of dried *C. papaya* leaves and roots of *F. zanthoxyloides* are being investigated in this study because some indigenes use their extracts as folk medicine therapies for sickle cell crisis and also there are recent scientific reports on the antisickling activity of dried leaves of *C. papaya* and roots of *F. zanthoxyloides* (Sofowora et al., 1975; Imaga et al., 2009). A previous study showed that unripe papaya fruit extract has antisickling activity (Oduola et al., 2006). Another study found *C. papaya* leaf extract to have an appreciable potent antisickling activity, greatly affecting the time course for sickling in a dose-dependent manner, the most effective doses being 5 and 10 mg/ml extract concentration (Imaga et al., 2009). The effect of varied concentrations of the plant extracts on erythrocyte membranes, analyzed using the osmotic fragility test, revealed appreciable membrane protective effects of the herb and an inhibitory action on hemolysis of red blood cells. The toxicity profile of the plants have also been assessed by histological and biochemical analyses and did not reveal any substantial toxicity of the plants (Sofowora et al., 1975; Oyedapo and Famurewa, 1995; Elekwa et al., 2005; Imaga et al., 2009). However, adequate biochemical studies concerning the mechanism of action of these antisickling agents are yet to be fully understood. This offers an opportunity through this work to evaluate the antioxidant properties of the plant extracts and asses their effects on homozygous SS erythrocytes.

MATERIALS AND METHODS

Chemicals

Chemicals used were of analytical grade obtained from Sigma Chemical Company and used without further purification.

Blood samples

5 ml venous blood samples were collected with full informed consent from SS individuals aged between 18 and 20 years, who came in for routine visits at the SS Out-Patients' Clinic of the Lagos University Teaching Hospital, Idi-araba, Lagos, Nigeria. The blood samples were collected in sodium Ethylenediaminetetraacetic acid (EDTA) bottles and used for the experiments.

Collection of plant material

Sun-dried *C. papaya* (fruit bearing) leaves and *F. zanthoxyloides* roots were collected during the dry season in December 2009 at the Forestry Research Institute of Nigeria (FRIN), Ibadan, Nigeria. The plants were authenticated by Mr. T. K. Odewo of FRIN and samples kept at their herbarium.

Extraction of plant material

Organic extraction

C. papaya ground leaves were extracted using the methods of Ogoda et al. (2002), as follows: 400 g of dark brown, smooth textured powdered sample was extracted with 1.5 L of petroleum ether using a Soxhlet extractor for 6 h. The petroleum ether extract obtained was further evaporated to dryness using vacuum rotary evaporator. The marc was further extracted with 1.5 L of aqueous methanol (1:3 v/v) using the soxhlet extractor for another 6 h. The obtained methanolic extract was evaporated to dryness using vacuum rotary evaporator. Both extracts were freeze dried and stored at 4°C. This process was repeated to obtain petroleum ether and methanolic extracts for *F. zanthoxyloides*. Thus the herbal extracts were obtained via soxhlet extraction (with petroleum ether 60 to 80°C and aqueous methanol (1:3, 60 to 80°C) as solvents and stored at 4°C in freeze dried form.

Aqueous extraction

Powdered *C. papaya* (400 g) was weighed into a clean bowl and 2.5 L of hot distilled water was poured in and the bowl covered. This was allowed to infuse for 3 h and then cooled at room temperature. The mixture was sieved with a clean muslin cloth. The resultant aqueous extract was freeze-dried and stored in the refrigerator at 4°C till use. This process was repeated to obtain aqueous extracts for the ground sample of *F. zanthoxyloides*.

In vitro hemoglobin studies

Antisickling activity

5 ml blood samples obtained from patients were centrifuged at 5,000 rpm for 10 min in phosphate buffered saline thrice to obtain the RBC which were then resuspended in normal saline and used for the analysis according to earlier described methods of Imaga et al. (2009). The aqueous and methanol extracts of *C. papaya* leaves and *F. zanthoxyloides* roots were used in this experiment, with para-hydroxybenzoic acid as the chemical standard. 1 ml SS blood cell suspensions were pre-incubated with 0 to 10 mg/ml concentrations of the extracts in the presence of 2% sodium metabisulphite solution and the time course of the effect of varied concentrations of extracts on the sickling of SS erythrocytes was microscopically analyzed. A plot of percentage sickling inhibition against extract concentration was analyzed for possible explanation of the observed antisickling effect.

Determination of haematological parameters, MADH

The effects of the *papaya* and *Fagara* aqueous-methanol extracts on hematological parameters, hemolysis of SS cells and formation of (MADH)/met-hemoglobin in SS blood cells were determined using the methods of Ekeke and Shode (1985), Iyamu et al. (2002) and Abdulmalik et al. (2005).

Determination of complete blood count

Blood samples were collected from hemoglobin AA (HbAA) and hemoglobin SS (HbSS) individuals. Complete blood cell count (full hematological parameters) was determined using Sysmex 21 KXN. The HbSS blood samples were incubated with papaya extract or *Fagara* extract as follows: 1 g each of methanol and aqueous extracts of papaya and *Fagara* was dissolved in 100 ml normal saline. The solution was filtered and 0.5 ml of the filtrate was added to 1 ml of HbSS blood sample. This was incubated for 30 min after which complete blood cell count was determined using Sysmex 21 KXN. HbAA blood sample served as positive control and HbSS blood sample not incubated with plant extract served as the negative control.

Hemolysis of SS cells

The time-course of hemolysis as a function of the *papaya* and *Fagara* concentrations was examined over a 4 h period at plant extract concentration of 5 mg/ml. Blood samples collected from HbSS individuals were used for this experiment. The red blood cells were washed twice in physiological saline by centrifugation at 5000 rpm for 2 min and resuspended in normal saline. Iml of the solution was incubated in 5 mg/ml extract each of *papaya* and *Fagara* in the ratio 1:1 for 4 h. I ml of the solution was also incubated in para-hydroxybenzoic acid (PHBA) in the same ratio for the same duration (as the control). At 10 min intervals, an aliquot of mixture was removed and absorbance read at 415 nm.

Formation of methemoglobin and membrane associated (denatured) hemoglobin (MADH)

Aliquots (0.5 ml) of SS blood were diluted in 1.5 ml normal saline in each of four tubes. A reagent blank was put in the first tube- contained all reagents except the HbSS blood sample. 1 ml of PHBA was added to the second tube while1ml of *Fagara* extract was added to the third tube. To the fourth tube was added 1ml of *C. papaya* extract. The tubes were incubated for 4 h. At 10 min interval, 0.5 ml of each of the mixtures was lysed with hemolysing solution (phosphate buffer pH 8) and absorbance was read at 630 nm.

Antioxidant assay

Tests for the presence of phenolic compounds (indicative of antioxidant activity) contained in the plant extracts was done according to the methods of Wilson and Walker (2001), Padma et al. (2006) and Canini et al. (2007).

Estimation of total phenolic content

0, 1, 2, 3, 5 and 10 ml of prepared garlic extract solution (the control) were pipetted into different 100 ml volumetric flasks and diluted to volume with distilled water. This was done to prepare a calibration curve with each volumetric flask having: 0, 50, 100, 150, 250 and 500 µg garlic extract stock. 7.9 ml of distilled water was pipetted into different tubes; 6 for the standards and 5 for the extracts. 0.1ml of each calibration solution sample was pipetted into the separate tubes. To the resulting solution, 0.5 ml of Folin-Ciocalteau reagent and 1.5 ml of Na_2CO_3 were added. In place of the standard (Garlic stock) solution, the individual papaya and *Fagara* aqueous and organic extracts were added into test tubes $T_7 - T_{11}$. All the test tubes were incubated in a thermostatic water-bath at 40°C for 30 min. Their absorbance readings were then taken at 765 nm using a UV-VIS GENESYS 8 spectrophotometer.

Total antioxidant activity (β–carotene assay)

β-carotene (2 mg) was dissolved in 10 ml of chloroform, after which the chloroform was removed under vacuum. From the solution, 2 ml was pipetted into a 100 ml round bottom flask. 0.5 ml of purified oleic acid, 5 ml of tween 20 emulsifier and 100 ml of distilled water were added to the mixture in the round bottom flask, then mixed vigorously. 4.8 ml of the emulsion formed was pipetted into each test tube containing different concentrations of the extracts (that is, 2, 4, 6, 8, 10 µg/ml). For comparison purposes, standard antioxidant vitamins, vitamin C (Ascorbic acid) and Vitamin E (α-tocopherol) were used. As soon as the emulsion was added to each tube, zero time absorbance was measured on a UV-VIS spectrophotometer at 470 nm. The tubes were then placed in a water bath at 50°C and the measurement of their absorbance was continued for 2 h. Graphs of absorbance against time were plotted for the different concentrations of extracts. A control devoid of the extracts but containing all other reagents used was also prepared for the assay as a standard.

Effect of the extracts on antioxidant /oxidative stress enzymes (SOD and Catalase), Lipid peroxidation (MDA) and Glutathione transferase (GST)

These give the measure of the extracts protective anti-oxidative effects on the RBC membrane. The antioxidant enzyme assays were done in 3 stages: (a) With AA blood serum alone; (b) With SS blood serum alone (c) with AA blood serum + SS blood serum + prepared extract (that is, vitamin C, *C. papaya* and *F. zanthoxyloides* extracts) where vitamin C served as a positive control, being a known antioxidant. Vitamin C solution was prepared by dissolving 1g of vitamin C in 100 ml of distilled water.

Catalase activity assay

This was determined by the method of Cohen and Dembiec (1970); by measuring the decrease in H_2O_2 concentration and reading the absorbance value at 240 nm. To 0.2 ml (200 µl) of serum or serum-extract sample (for both AA and SS blood), 1.8 ml of 30 mM H_2O_2 was added. Reagent buffer was used as the blank and their absorbance readings were taken at 240 nm, at 60 s intervals for 5 min.

Superoxide dismutase (SOD) activity

SOD enzyme activity was determined according to the method described by Sun and Zigman (1978). Here, the SOD enzyme assay determines the difference between superoxide anion decomposition and production that is, its ability to inhibit the autoxidation of epinephrine. The assay was performed in 3.0 ml of 50 mM Na_2CO_3 buffer (in 2 different test tubes) to which 0.02 ml of each serum sample was added. 0.03 ml of the epinephrine stock solution was then added to the above before taking absorbance readings at 480 nm for 3 to 5 min.

Determination of glutathione-s-transferase (GST) activity

The activity of GST was determined according to the method of Habig et al. (1974). 0.1 ml of CDNB solution was pipetted into a conical flask before adding 1ml of phosphate buffer and 1.7 ml of distilled water. Next, the mixture was incubated at 37°C for 5 min. After the incubation, 0.1 ml of the serum sample and also 0.1 ml of GSH solution (using an automatic micropipette) were added. A blank devoid of the serum was prepared for background correction.

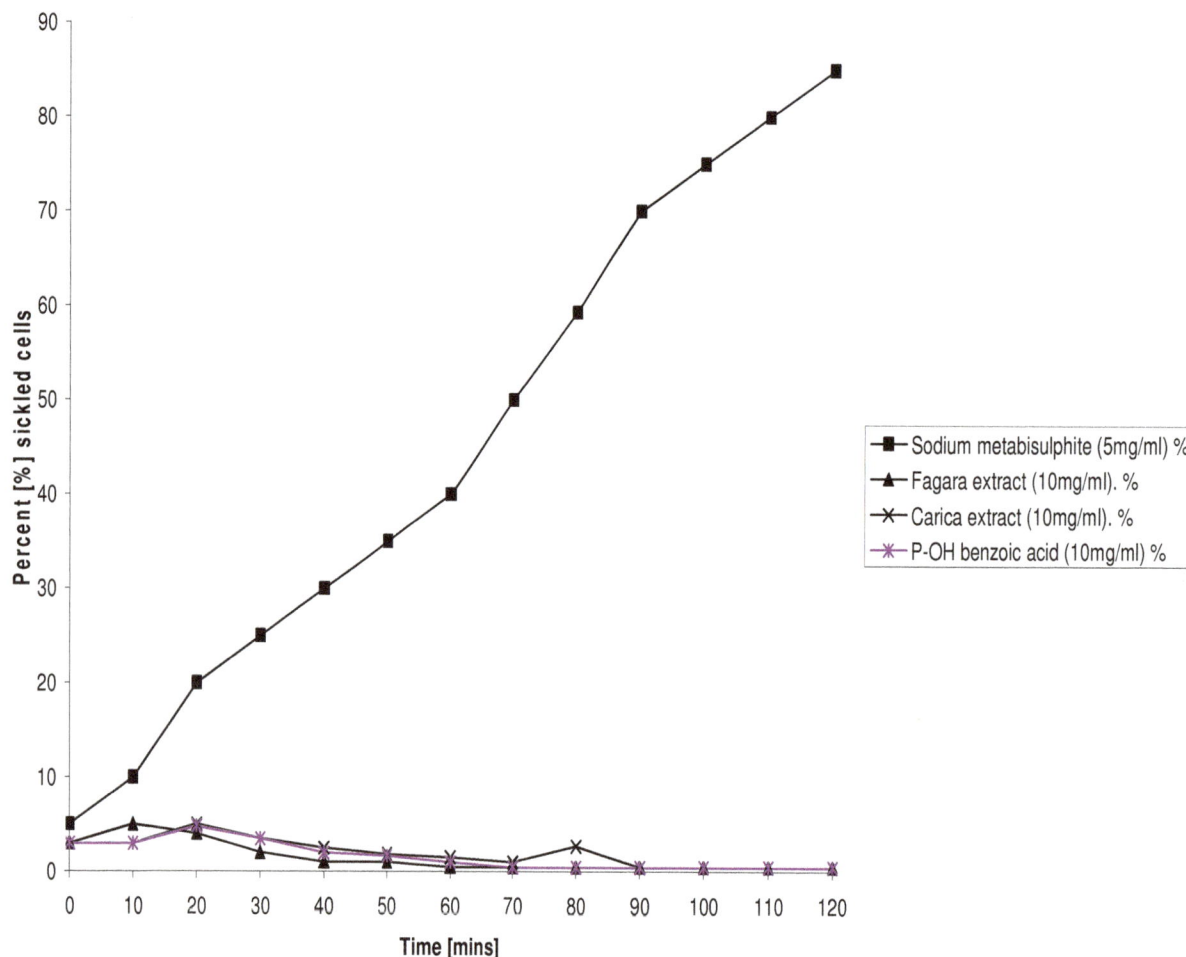

Figure 1. Timecourse of *Papaya* and *Fagara* extracts on sickling. Sickle cell suspensions pre-incubated with extracts prior to exposure to 2% sodium metabisulphite solution.

Absorbance readings at 340 nm were taken for 5 min at 60 s interval using a GENESYS 8 UV-VIS spectrophotometer.

Lipid peroxidation analysis

The Thiobarbituric acid (TBARS) assay method was used for the lipid peroxidation analysis. It is used to measure total free radical damage in a biological system; where Malondialdehyde, the end product of lipid peroxidation serves as a convenient index and can be measured spectrophotometrically at 535 nm to assay for the extent of lipid peroxidation in a sample. 1ml of serum sample was added to 2 ml of TCA-TBA-HCl reagent (1:1:1) in a test tube and mixed thoroughly. The mixture was then heated for 15 min in a boiling water bath and cooled. After cooling, the flocculent precipitate was removed by centrifugation at 1000 g for 10 min. The absorbance of the sample was then determined at 535 nm against a blank.

Statistical analyses

Data from the various studies are presented as mean ± SEM (standard error of mean). The results were analyzed for statistical significance using Microsoft Word© software systems, (2007).

Students't-test and satterwhaites' method of one way analysis of variance were used to compare mean values between groups. *p<0.05* was taken to indicate a statistical significance.

RESULTS

Antisickling activity of plant extracts

Antisickling data was obtained from a typical three independent experiments performed in duplicate using blood samples from SS individuals. Results showed that the time course for 60% sickling was 40 min for the control (SS blood without extract). *F. zanthoxyloides* showed higher antisickling activity after 40 min of incubation compared to *C. papaya* and chemical standards used (Figure 1).

Effect of extract on the blood cell components

In order to study the potential adverse effects of *C.*

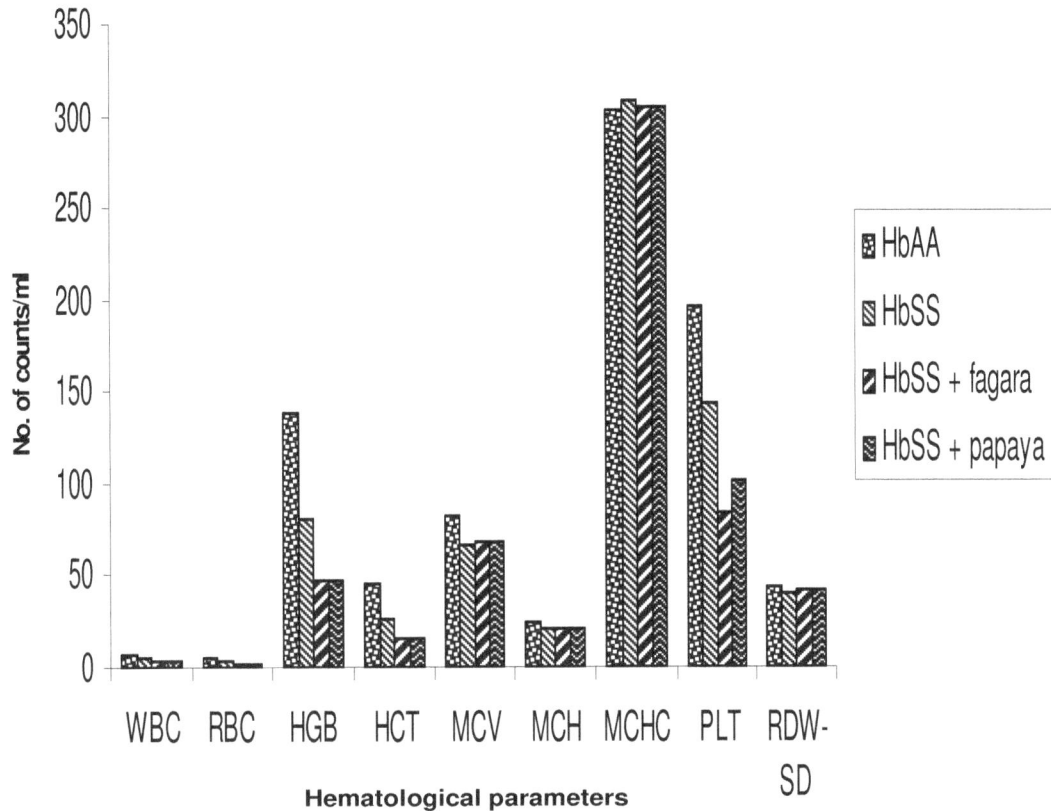

Figure 2. Effect of *Papaya* and *Fagara* extracts on some hematological parameters.

papaya on the blood cells, SS cells were incubated in the presence of 5 mg/ml concentration of extract. A full blood count, rate of hemolysis of SS cells and formation of met-hemoglobin was done. The mean corpuscular hemoglobin concentration (MCHC) and the red cell distribution width (RDW) indicated no statistically significant differences between extract-treated and control samples (Figure 2). Though there were marked differences in the Platelet count, PLT and blood volume, HCT (hematocrit/Packed Cell Volume) as shown, results obtained are not statistically significant.

Effect of extract on the rate of RBC hemolysis

The rate of hemolysis of blood samples incubated with plant extract was determined. The results indicated after 2 h incubation with the blood samples that both papaya and control PHBA lowered the incidence of RBC lysis (Figure 3), unlike the *Fagara* extract.

Effect of extract on the inhibition of met-hemoglobin formation

The rate of formation of met Hb (indirectly the level of MADH formed) was also determined. The results

indicated after 2 h incubation with the blood samples that both *C. papaya* and control PHBA decreased the formation of met-Hb better than *Fagara* extract (Figure 4).

Total phenolic compounds present in *Papaya* and *Fagara* extracts

The total phenol compounds present in the plant extracts was analyzed using the Folin-C method of assay. As shown, aqueous *C. papaya* extract had the highest total phenol (antioxidant) concentration of 540 mg/L, (Figure 5) followed by aqueous *F. zanthoxyloides* with a concentration of 500 mg/L when compared with garlic extracts (a strong phenolic compound).

Effect on total antioxidant status

The plant extracts showed high total antioxidant properties. Figure 6 shows that aqueous *C. papaya* had the highest inhibition of beta carotene bleaching activity over the methanol and petroleum ether extracts and thus the highest antioxidant property at a concentration of 4 µg/ml, when compared with vitamin A positive control. Aqueous extracts of *C. papaya* and *F. zanthoxyloides* showed high total antioxidant properties. Aqueous extract

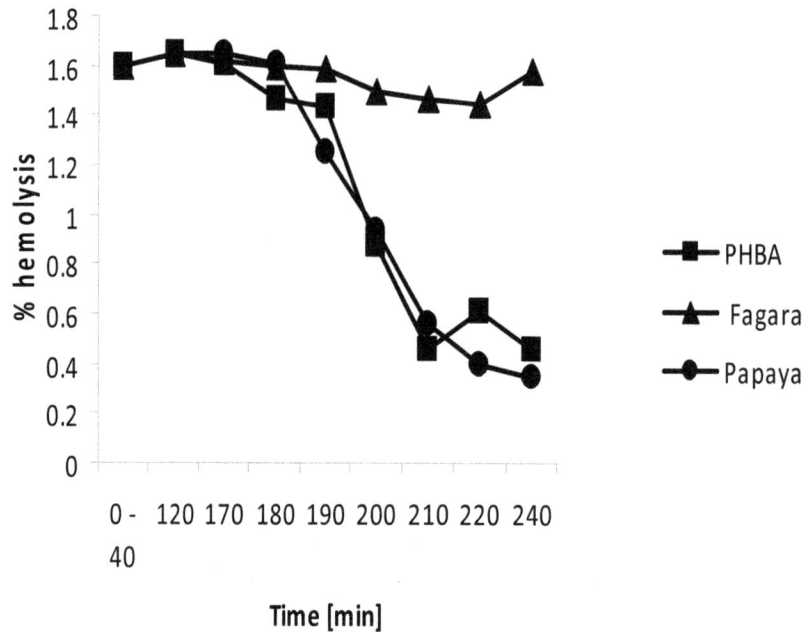

Figure 3. Effect of *Papaya* and *Fagara* extracts on RBC hemolysis.

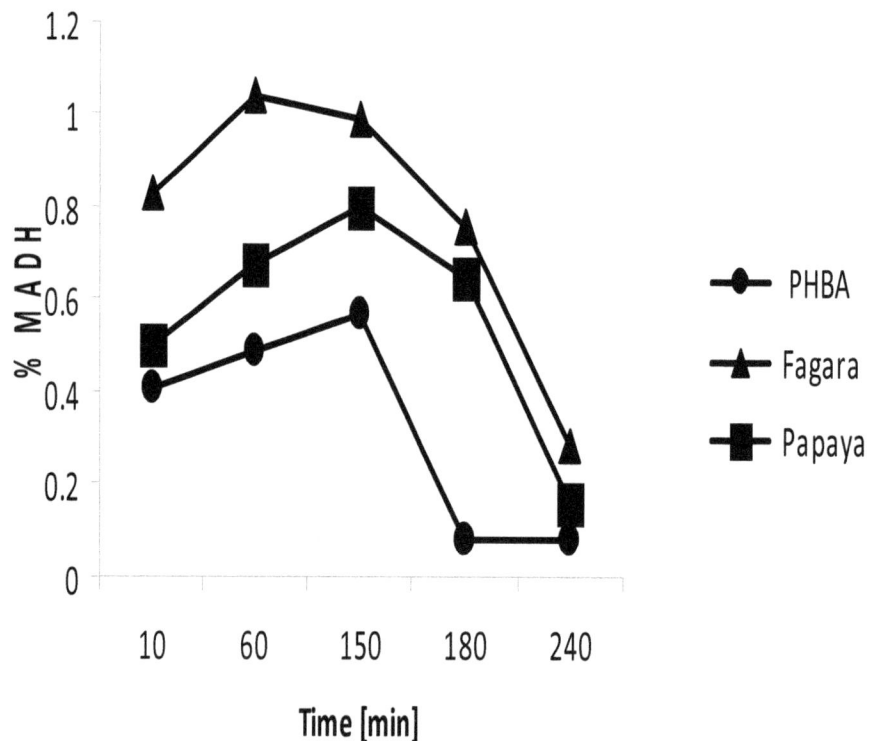

Figure 4. Effect of *Papaya* and *Fagara* extracts on Met-Hb formation (% MADH).

of papaya exhibited a higher and more stable antioxidant activity than the aqueous extract of *Fagara*, but both extracts had higher activity over vitamins A and E at 4 µg/ml concentration as shown in Figure 7. Methanol extracts of *C.papaya* and *F. zanthoxyloides* also showed high total antioxidant properties. Methanol extract of *Fagara* exhibited a higher antioxidant activity than the methanol extract of papaya. Both extracts had higher activity over vitamins A and E but gave unstable activity as shown in Figure 8.

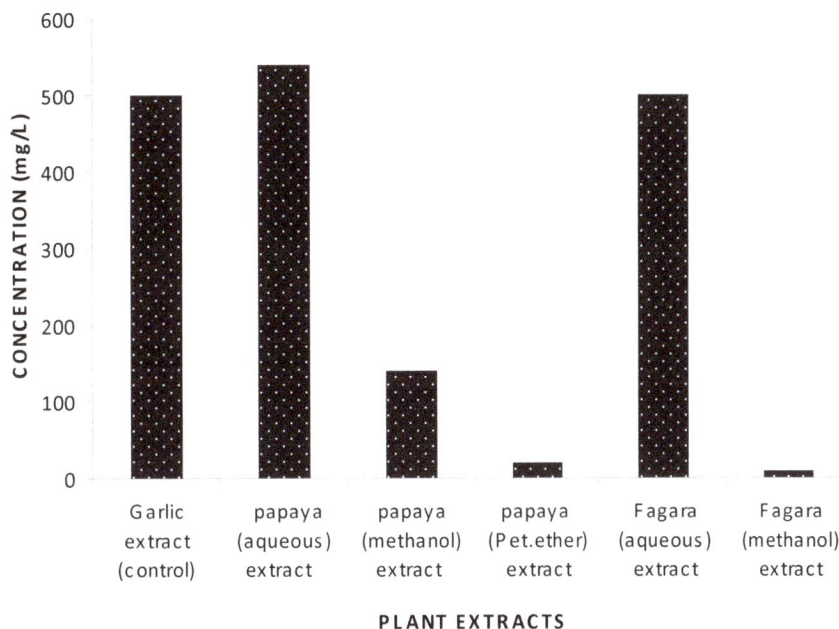

Figure 5. Total phenolic compounds present in *Papaya* and *Fagara* extracts.

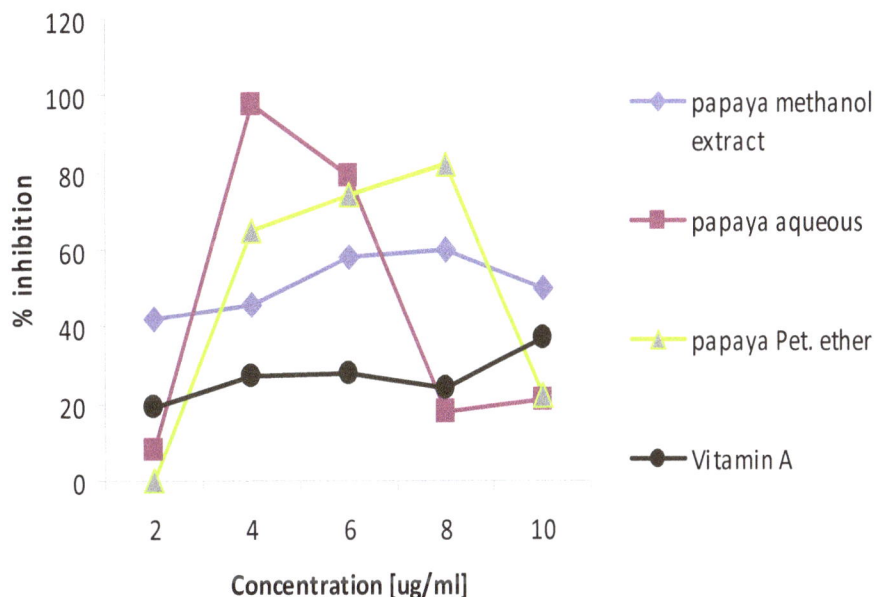

Figure 6. Antioxidant effects of *C. papaya* extracts via beta-carotene inhibition.

Antioxidant property of papaya and Fagara extract: Effect on oxidative stress and lipid peroxidation

The methanol extracts of both *C. papaya* and *F. zanthoxyloides* also showed considerably good antioxidant effects with regards to their effects on oxidative stress enzymes (SOD, CAT and GST) and lipid peroxidation in SS serum samples. From Figure 9, it can be seen that both *F. zanthoxyloides* and *C. papaya* methanol extracts inhibited oxidative stress appreciably in HbSS samples when compared with vitamin C extracts as shown by the decreased level of SOD enzymes after supplementation and in the absence of any extract. *Papaya* lowered SOD activity more than *Fagara*. The methanol extract of *F. zanthoxyloides* had stronger antioxidant activity and resisted the effect of oxidative stress as seen by CAT enzymes levels when compared with methanol extract of *C. papaya*. It was however also observed that both methanol plant extracts did not give substantial resistance to oxidative stress when compared

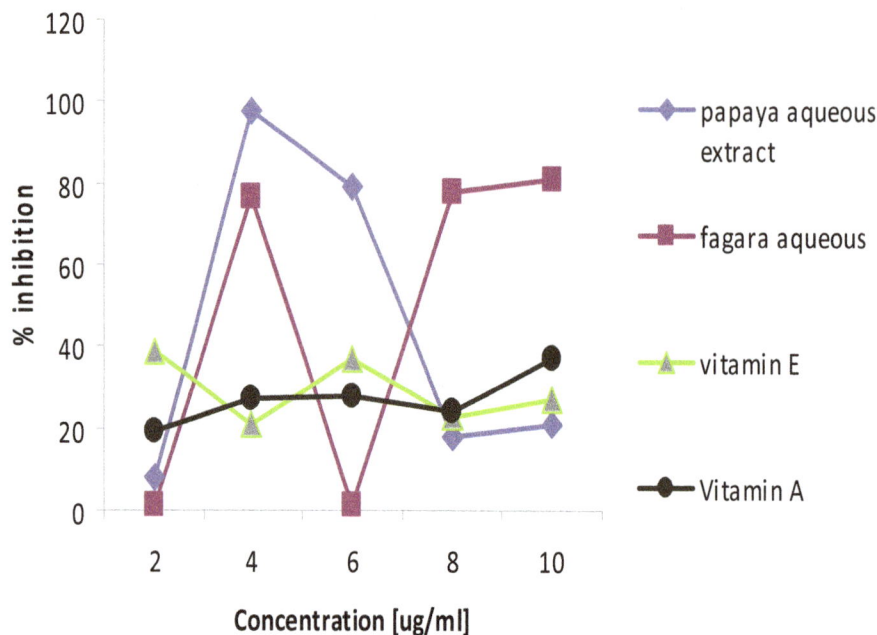

Figure 7. Antioxidant effects of aqueous extracts of *Papaya* and *Fagara* via beta-carotene inhibition.

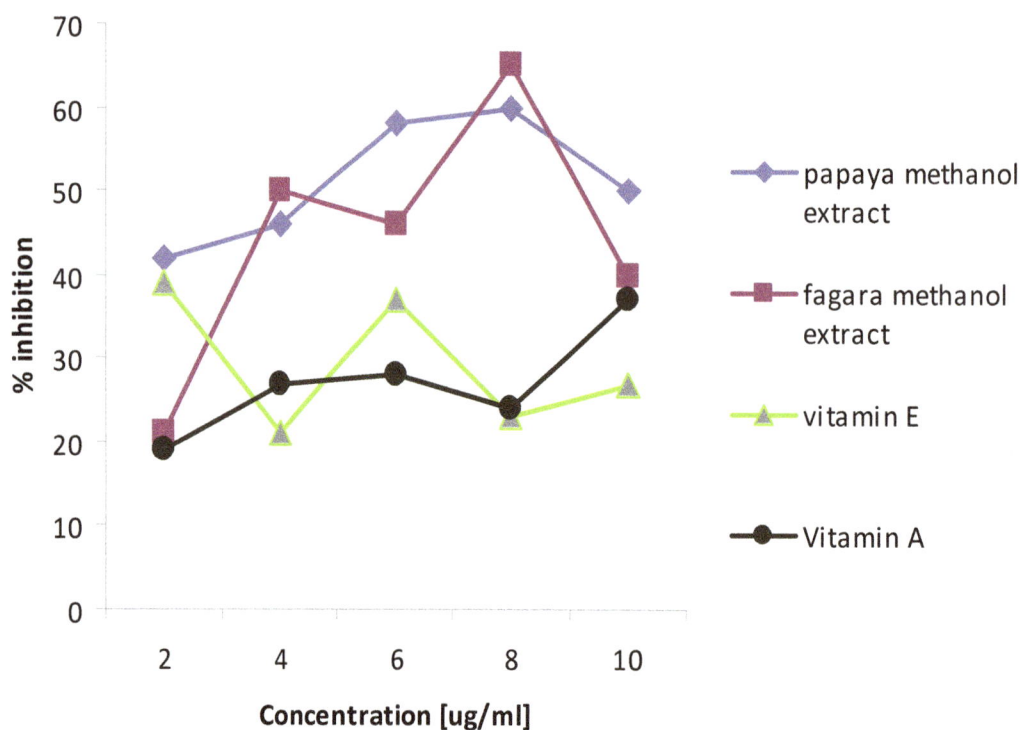

Figure 8. Antioxidant effects of methanol extracts of *Papaya* and *Fagara* via beta- carotene inhibition.

with vitamin C extract and in the absence of extracts as shown in Figures 10 and 11 shows that the methanol extract of *F. zanthoxyloides* induced higher resistance to oxidative stress in SS blood sample when compared with the papaya and vitamin C extracts. Figure 12 shows that the production of malondiadehyde (MDA) was reduced in SS serum sample incubated with *F. zanthoxyloides* and *C. papaya* methanol plant extracts (when compared with that of blood serum sample alone) hence reduction in lipid peroxidation activity.

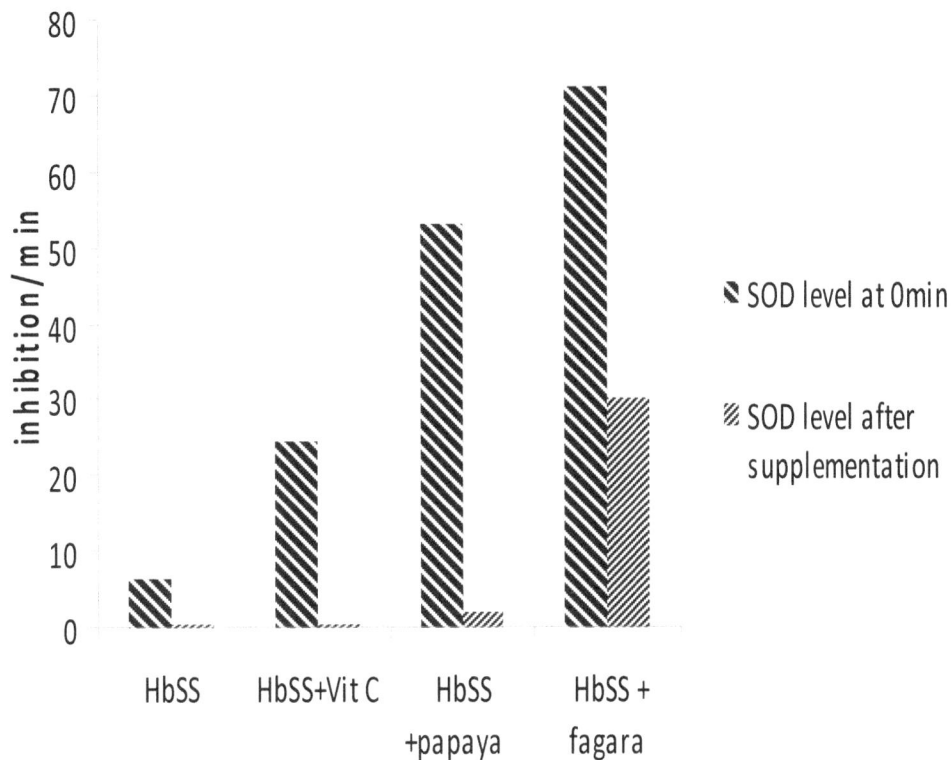

Figure 9. Effect of *Papaya* and *Fagara* extracts on SOD activity in HbSS samples.

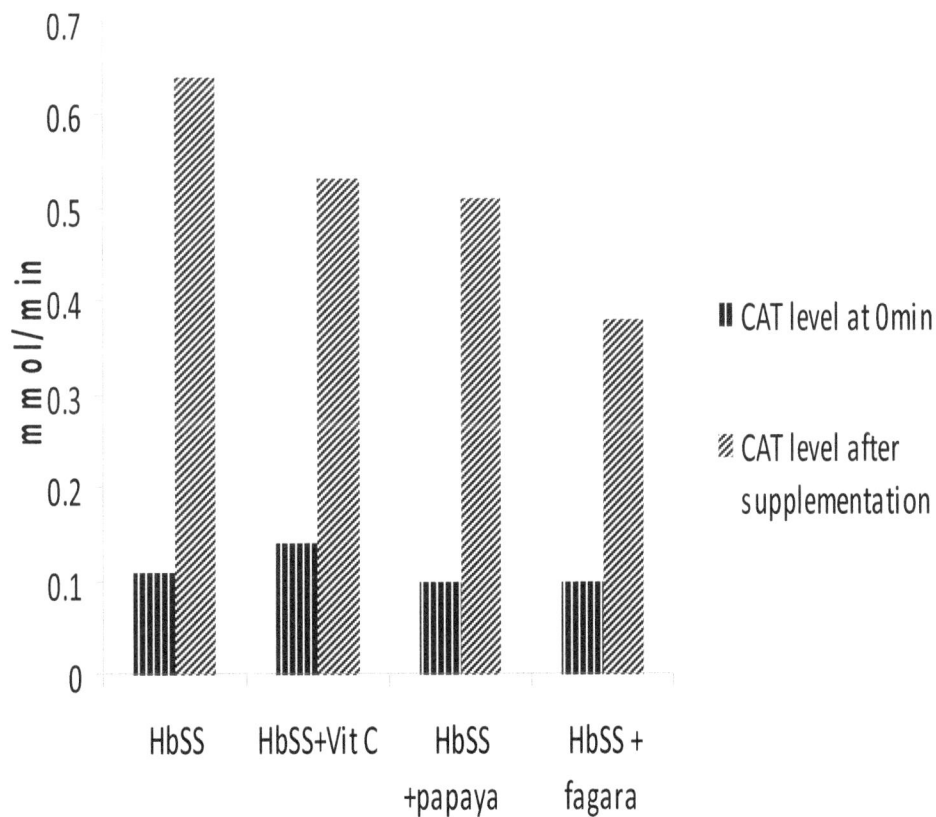

Figure 10. Effect of *Papaya* and *Fagara* extracts on catalase activity in HbSS samples.

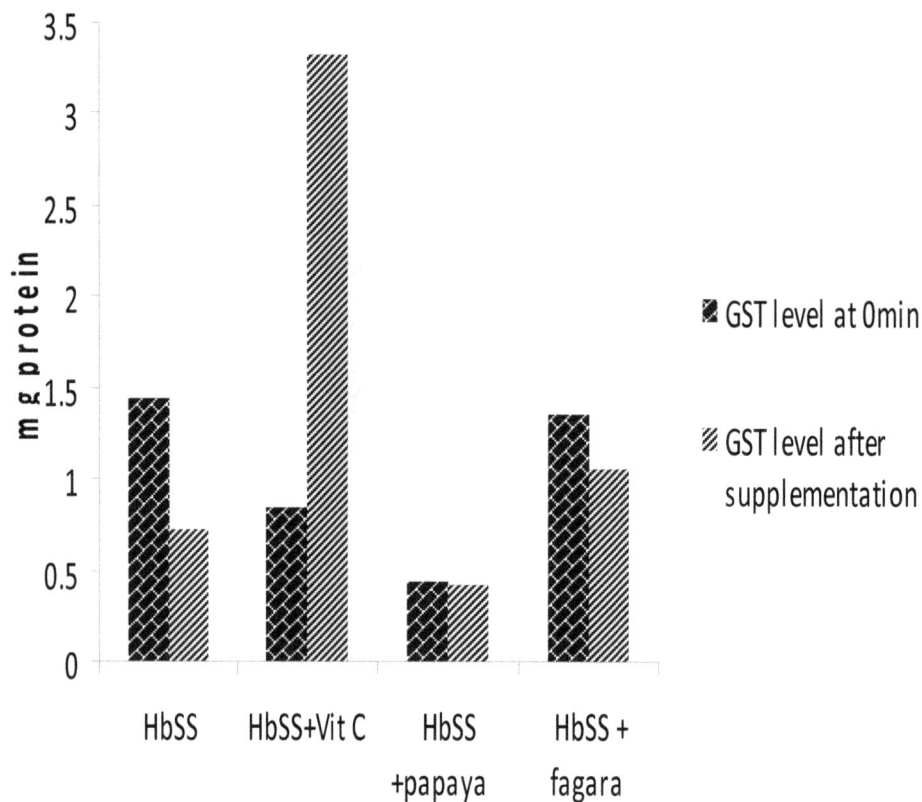

Figure 11. Effect of *Papaya* and *Fagara* extracts on glutathione activity in HbSS.

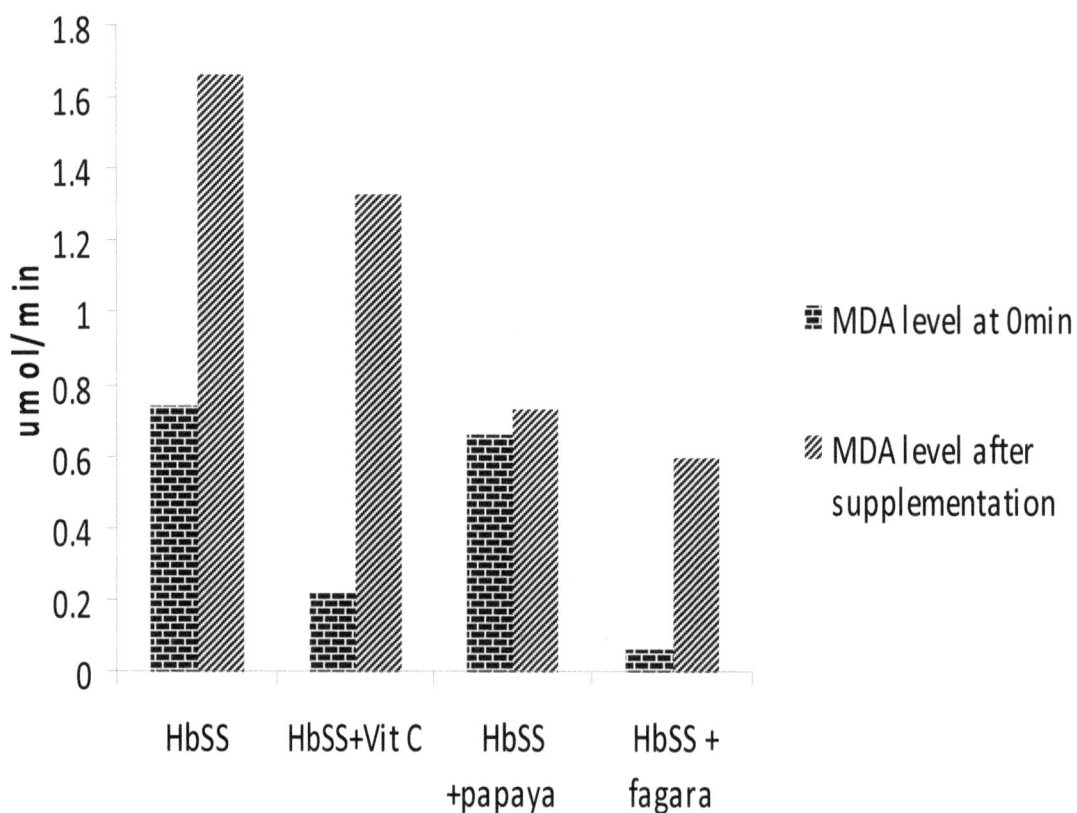

Figure 12. Effect of *Papaya* and *Fagara* extracts on lipid peroxidation [level of MDA] in HbSS.

DISCUSSION

For sickle cell disease (SCD), the study of antioxidants especially in various antisickling agents is of great importance because different antisickling agents have different degrees of effect. Antioxidants (scavengers of free radicals) are believed to be major components of these antisickling agents that add to their potential (Tatum and Chow, 1996). Thus, it is believed that the higher the antioxidant property of an antisickling agent, the higher its possible antisickling effect, as this enables it reduce oxidative stress that contributes to sickle cell crisis. In this research, the *C. papaya* leaf and *F. zanthoxyloides* root extracts induced membrane stabilization in dense sickle and normal red cells without deleterious effects on the erythrocytes. Aqueous extracts of *C. papaya* and *F. zanthoxyloides* have shown high total antioxidant properties (via β-carotene bleaching assay) and higher phenolic properties than garlic acid. This might explain why decoctions of these plants (used locally) over the years give relief to various oxidative stress associated diseases. The levels of the oxidative stress enzymes (SOD, CAT and GST) were reduced after blood samples had been incubated with the extracts. Lipid peroxidation, measured indirectly by the percentage of MDA inhibited by plant extract, was also reduced by the extracts.

These findings further confirm the antioxidant activity inherent in the plant extracts. HbSS individuals already in distress during oxidative stress-induced RBC membrane lysis do not need this situation aggravated by a plant extract that causes more oxidative stress to the erythrocyte membrane. The observed low levels of the oxidative stress enzymes show that papaya and *Fagara* extracts can quickly mop up free-radicals produced during sickle cell crisis and thus help preserve the integrity of the membrane. The extracts protected membrane integrity resulting in a reduction of RBC hemolysis during osmotic and oxidative stress without met-hemoglobin formation. This membrane stabilization effect is an additional benefit of the antisickling plants and confirms earlier reports on the membrane-stabilizing properties of the extracts on red blood cells as measured by their osmotic fragility (Imaga et al., 2009). The plant extracts' drastic antisickling effects could have been potentiated by their antioxidant activity and ability to maintain RBC membrane integrity under osmotic or oxidative stress.

Conclusion

C. papaya dried leaf extract and *F. zanthoxyloides* roots when used in 1 to 10 mg/ml concentrations *in vitro*, have no deleterious effects on erythrocytes and possess potent antioxidant activity which may be responsible for their observed antisickling action.

REFERENCES

Abdulmalik OO, Safo MK, Chen Q, Yang J, Burguara C, Ohene-Frempong K, Abraham DJ, Asakura T (2005). 5-hydroxylmethyl – 2-furfural modifies intracellular sickle hemoglobin and inhibits sickling of red blood cells. British J. Hematol., 128: 552-561.

Amrolia PJ (2003). Therapeutic Challenges in Childhood Sickle Cell Disease Part 2: A Problem-oriented approach. Br. J. Hematol., 120: 737-743.

Brittain JE, Han J (2004). Mechanism of CD47-induced $α_4β_1$ Integrin Activation and Adhesion in Sickle Reticulocytes. J. Biol. Chem., 279(41): 42393-42402.

Canini A, Daniela A, Giuseppe D, Tagliatesta P (2007). Gas chromatography-mass spectrometry analysis of phenolic compounds from *Carica papaya* L. leaf. J. Food Comp. Anal., 20(7): 584-590

Cohen GD, Dembiec JM (1970). Measurement of catalase activity in tissue extracts. Anal. Biochem., 34: 30-38.

Ekeke GI, Shode FO (1985). The Reversion of Sickled cells by *Cajanus cajan*. Planta medica, 6: 504-507.

Elekwa I, Monanu MO, Anosike EO (2005). Effects of aqueous extracts of *Zanthoxylum macrophylla* roots on membrane stability of human erythrocytes of different genotypes. Biokemistri, 17(1): 7-12.

Habig WH, Pabst MS, Jekpoly WB (1974). Glutathione transferase: a first enzymatic step in mercaptuiric acid formation. J. Biol. Chem., 249: 7130-7139.

Imaga NOA, Gbenle GO, Okochi VI, Akanbi SO, Edeoghon SO, Oigbochie V, Kehinde MO, Bamiro SB (2009). Antisickling Property of *Carica papaya* leaf extract. Afr. J. Biochem. Res., 3(4): 102-106.

Iyamu EW, Turner EA, Asakura T (2002). *In vitro* effects of Niprisan (Nix – 0699): a naturally occurring, potent antisickling agent. Br. J. Hematol., 118: 337-343.

Nagel RL (1998). A Knockout of a Transgenic Mouse – Animal Models of Sickle Cell Anemia. New Eng. J. Med., 339: 194-195.

Oduola T, Adeniyi FAA, Ogunyemi EO, Bello IS, Idowu TO (2006). Antisickling agent in an extract of unripe pawpaw (*Carica papaya*): Is it real? Afr. J. Biotech., 5(20): 1947-1949.

Ogoda OJ, Akubue PI, Okide GB (2002). The Kinetics of Reversal of Pre-sickled Erythrocytes by the Aqueous Extract of *Cajanus cajan* seeds. Phytother. Res., 16: 1-3.

Oyedapo OO, Famurewa AJ (1995). Antiprotease and membrane stabilizing activities of extracts of fagara zanthoxyloides, Olax subscorpioides and Tetrapleura Tetraptera. Int. J. Pharmacognosy, 33(1): 65-69.

Padma SV, Vandna TL, Warjeet S, Ningomban S (2006). Antioxidant properties of some exclusive species of Zingiberacea family of Manipur Elect. J. Environ. Agric. Food Chem., 5(2): 1318-1324.

Sauntharsarajah E, Maziarz RT (2003). Drug holds Promise as an Alternative for Sickle Cell Patients Unable to tolerate Standard Treatment. Blood, 12: 786-790.

Sofowora EA, Issacs-Sodeye NA, Ogunkoya LO (1975). Antisickling properties of Fagara. Lloydia, 38: 169-171.

Steinberg MH (2004). Sickle Cell Disease. Hematology, 1: 35.

Sun M, Zigman S (1978). An improved spectrophotometric assay for Superoxide Dismutase based on Epinephrine autoxidation. Anal. Biochem., 90: 81-89.

Tatum VL, Chow CL (1996). Antioxidant status and susceptibility of sickle erythrocytes to oxidative and osmotic stress. Free Radical Res., 25(2): 133-139.

Wilson K, Walker J (2001). Principles and Techniques of Practical Biochemistry, 5th edition, pp. 485-680.

30

In vitro anthelmintic potentials of *Xylopia aethiopica* and *Monodora myristica* from Nigeria

Ekeanyanwu R. C.[1]* and Etienajirhevwe O. F.[2]

[1]Department of Biochemistry, Imo State University, P.M.B 2000, Owerri, Imo State, Nigeria.
[2]Department of Science Laboratory Technology, Delta State Polytechnic, Otefe, Nigeria.

Monodora myristica and *Xylopia aethiopica* are two spices that have been traditionally used as a vermifuge in Ayurveda. The main aim of the research work was to investigate the phytochemical constituents of the aqueous, ethanol and methanol extracts of the two spices and the anthelmintic activity of the extracts of their seeds against *Eudrilus eugeniae*. The four concentrations (10, 20, 50 and 100 mg/ml) of each of the extracts from the two spices were studied in the bioassay which involved the determination of time of paralysis and time of death of the worm. Albendazole (15 mg/ml) was used as a standard reference drug in the assay. At the concentration of 100 mg/ml, the aqueous, ethanol and methanol extracts of the two spices showed very significant activities as compared to the standard drug Albendazole (15 mg/ml). The seed extracts of *M. myristica* and *X. aethiopica* produced a significant anthelmintic activity.

Key words: *Monodora myristica*, *Xylopia aethiopica*, phytochemicals, anthelmintics, *Eudrilus eugeniae*.

INTRODUCTION

Spices are a group of exoteric food adjunct that have been in use for thousands of years to enhance the sensory qualities of foods. The quality and variety consumed in tropical countries is particularly extensive. These spice ingredients imparts characteristics flavour, aroma or piquancy and colour to foods. Some spices can also modify the texture of foods. Spices are used in wines, beverages, foods, cosmetics, tooth pastes, and in medicines as adjuvant. Some have antimicrobial and soothing properties (Srinivasan, 2005). A spice being a vegetable substance of indigenous or exotic origin, being aromatic, is used to enhance the flavour of food. They are derived from rhizomes, bark of fruits, seeds, leaves, fruits, and other parts of plants (Kochlar, 1986). The inhibitory effect of spices oils could be attributed to the presence of aromatic nucleus containing a polar functional group.

Monodora myristica commonly called African nutmeg is

a perennial edible plant that grows wild in evergreen West Africa forests (Burubai et al., 2009). Its seeds usually embedded in a white sweet smelling pulp, was reported to possess valuable economic and medicinal value (Okafor, 1987; Okigbo, 1977). In Nigeria and other African countries, the kernel obtained from the seeds is a popular spicing agent as well as an aromatic stimulating addition to medicine and snuff (Ekeanyanwu et al., 2010). Also, the seeds when ground into powder and taken acts as stimulant, relieving constipation and can as well be sprinkled on sore especially those caused by guinea worm (Burkill, 1985).

Xylopia aethiopica has been reported in literature to possess medicinal and nutritional values (Nwachukwu, 2000). Chemical constituents include essential oils, resins, annonacin, reberoside, avicien, rebersole, alkaloids, tannins, oxalate, and flavonoids. The fruits are used as spices and aqueous decoction is used especially after child birth probably for its antiseptic properties and to arrest bleeding. This plant has a wide spectrum of biological activities and has played a crucial role in traditional medicines because of their valuable physiological and pharmaceutical properties (Ogbonnia

*Corresponding author. E-mail: ekeanyanwuraphael@yahoo.com.

et al., 2008). The fruits have been found to contain volatile aromatic oil, fixed oil and rutin (Burkhill, 1985). It is used in the treatment of digestive system motility, bronchitis, stomach aches, febrile pains, and rheumatism. This fruit of *X. aethiopica* has been reported to act as antioxidant, hypolipidaemia and hypoglycaemic agents, hence, confirming its use as an antidiabetic agent (Ameyaw and Owusu-Ansah, 1998).

The helminth which infect the intestine are Cestodes example tape worms (*Taenia solium*), nematodes example hookworm (*Ancyclostoma duodenate*), round worm (*Ascaris lumbricoides*) and trematodes or flukes (*Shistosoma mansoni* and *Schistosoma hematobolium*). The disease originated from parasite infection causing severe morbidity includes lymphatic filariasis, ochocerciasis, and schistosomiasis (Mali and Mahta, 2008). Traditional medicines hold a great promise as a source of easily available effective anthelmintic agents to the people, particularly in tropical countries including Nigeria. It is in this context that the people consume plants or plant derived preparations to cure helminth infections (Satyavati, 1990). Ideally an anthelmintic agent should have broad spectrum of action, high percentage cure with a single therapeutic dose, free from toxicity to the host and should be cost effective. None of the synthetic drugs available meets the requirement (Mali and Mahta, 2008). Resistance of these parasites to existing drugs (Walter and Prichard, 1985) and their high cost warrants search for newer anthelmintic agents.

Therefore, the present study was carried out to determine the phytochemicals composition of the aqueous, ethanol and methanol extracts of *M. myristica* and *X. aethiopica* and to estimate their anthelmintic activity.

MATERIALS AND METHODS

Plant materials

The dry fruits of *M. myristica* and *X. aethiopica* were collected between the month of June and November, 2011. They were identified and authenticated at the department of Botany, University of Nigeria Nsukka through comparison with a voucher specimen present in the herbarium.

Extract from the plant materials

The *M. myristica* and *X. aethiopica* fruits were sorted cleaned and milled using a laboratory mill (Retsch, 5657, GmbH, Germany). A quantity, about 300 g each of the dried and ground *M. myristica* and *X. aethiopica* fruits were defatted by shaking them with a volume, 2 L of n-hexane for 1 h, 3 times to extract the oil respectively. The defatted fruit flours of *M. myristica* and *X. aethiopica* were then dried separately in desiccators under vacuum until all traces of the n-hexane is removed. The aqueous, ethanol, and methanol extracts of *M. myristica* and *X. aethiopica* were obtained by stirring each of 100 g of the dry defatted flour of both spices with 300 ml of distilled hot water, ethanol and methanol for each of the extracts respectively at room temperature (27±1°C) for 24 h. The mixtures were then filtered using a clean muslin cloth and then whatman No.1 and evaporated to dryness. The extracts were then stored at 4°C for further use.

Standard drug used

For the present study, Albendazole was used as the standard drug (Wang, 2010). The concentration of the standard drug was prepared in normal saline to give 15 mg/ml concentration.

Worm collection and authentication

Adult African worms of the genius and species *Eudrilius eugeniae* (Family: Eudrildae) were used to study the anthelmintic activity. The earthworms were obtained from nearby areas of faculty of Biological sciences, University of Nigeria, Nsukka in the month of November, 2011 and authenticated at the department of Zoology. They were washed with normal saline to remove all the traces of faecal matter and waste surrounding their body. The African earthworm (*E. eugeniae*) 3 to 7 cm in length and 0.1 to 0.3 cm in width weighing 0.6 to 5.01 g were used for all experiment protocols. The earthworms resembled the intestinal roundworm both anatomically and physiologically and hence used to study the anthelmintic activity (Lakshananam et al., 2011). Ethical approval was obtained from the animal ethics committee of the Department of Veterinary Medicine, University of Nigeria Nsukka. Procedures were performed in accordance with current guidelines for the care of laboratory animals and ethical guidelines for investigation of experimental animals (Anonymous, 2004).

Phytochemical analysis of the extracts

The phytochemical study for the presence or absence of phytochemicals in the extracts was carried out according to the method described by Harborne (1984).

Alkaloids

A quantity, 0.2 g of each of the extracts was added to 5 ml of 2% hydrochloric acid and heated on boiling water for 10 min. They were then allowed to cool and then filtered. To 1 ml of the filtrate in a test tube was tested with alkaloids reagent, Wagner's and Mayer's reagent and results compared to blank. Turbidity or precipitation indicated the presence of alkaloids.

Tannins

A quantity, 0.2 g of each of the extracts was boiled with 5 ml of 45% ethanol for 5 min. The mixture was filtered hot using a filter paper and filtrate collected in a beaker. 2 ml of the filtrate was mixed with 10 ml of distilled water and then a drop of Iron Chloride solution was added. A blue-black or blue-green precipitate indicates the presence of tannins.

Saponin

A quantity, 0.1 g of each of the extracts was measured into a beaker and 20 ml of distilled water was added, the beaker was heated in a water bath for over 5 min. The mixtures were filtered using a filter paper into another beaker to obtain a filtrate. 2 ml of each of the filtrate was measured to another test tube and 10 ml of distilled water was added, it was shaken vigorously for over a minute. Frothing which persist on warming indicated the presence of Saponin.

Resins

A weighed quantity, 0.2 g of each of the extracts was poured into 20 ml of distilled water in a beaker. A precipitate occurring indicates the presence of resins.

Steroids

A quantity, 0.1 g of each of the extracts were added a mixture of 10 ml of lead acetate solution (90% w/v) and 20 ml of 50% aqueous ethanol in a 200 ml conical flask. The mixtures were placed on boiling water for 2 min, cooled and filtered. The filtrate was extracted twice with 15 ml chloroform. Then 5 ml of the chloroform extract was evaporated to dryness on a water bath. To the residue, 2 ml of 3, 5 - dinitrobenzoic acid solution (2% in ethanol) and 1 ml of 1 N sodium hydroxide solution were added. A reddish brown interphase shows the presence of steroids.

Glycosides

A quantity, 0.2 g of each of the extracts was mixed with 30 ml of water and heated on a water bath for 5 min and filtered. 5 ml of a mixture of equal parts of Fehling's solutions A and B were added to 5 ml of the filtrate until it turned alkaline (with litmus) and then boiled on a water bath for 5 min. A brick red precipitate indicated the presence of Glycosides.

Cyanogenic glycosides

A quantity, 0.1 g of each of the extracts in a conical flask was added 10 ml of water and 1.0 ml dilute HCl. Picrate papers were suspended above the mixtures and contents of the flask were warmed at 45°C for 1 h. A control without the extracts was set up. A colour change from yellow to reddish purple of the picrate paper was indicative of a positive test.

Flavonoids

A quantity, 0.1 g of each of the extracts was added a mixture of 10 ml of lead acetate solution (90% w/v) and 20 ml of 50% aqueous ethanol in a 200 ml conical flask. The mixtures were placed on boiling water for 2 min, cooled and filtered. A volume, 5 ml of dilute ammonia was added to a portion of the aqueous filtrate followed by the addition of concentrated sulphuric acid 1 to 2 ml of potassium hydroxide solution and allowed to mix. Then into acid base mixture a small quantity of aqueous filtrate of the sample was added and observed for colour change.

Anthelmintic activity study

Twenty six groups of approximately equal sized earthworms consisting of six earthworms in each group were released into 50 ml of desired formulation. The extract was suspended in 1% Dimethyl sulphoxide (DMSO) in normal saline at 10, 20, 50, and 100 mg/ml concentrations. Each group was treated with one of the following; control (1% DMSO in normal saline), Albendazole (15 mg/ml), M. myristica extracts (10, 20, 50, and 100 mg/ml) and X. aethiopica extracts (10, 20, 50, and 100 mg/ml). Observations were made for the time taken to paralyze and / or death of individual worms.

Paralysis was said to occur when the worms do not revive even in normal saline. Death was concluded when the worms lose their motility followed with fading away of their body colour.

Statistical analysis

Numerical data were presented as mean±standard deviation and analysed using simple students' T-test. Values of $P < 0.05$ were considered as significant. All analysis was done using Statistical Package for Social Science (SPSS) software, version 17.0 by International Business Machine (IBM), USA.

RESULTS

The percentage yield of the aqueous, ethanol and methanol extracts of M. myristica seed flour after solvent evaporation were approximately 6.16, 1.17 and 3.01% respectively, while the percentage yield of the aqueous, ethanol and methanol extracts of X. aethiopica seed flour after solvent evaporation were approximately 5.0, 17.0 and 16.0% respectively (Table 1).

Preliminary phytochemical screening of the extract of M. myristica showed that the aqueous extracts contained alkaloids, tannins, saponins, resins, steroids, glycosides, flavonoids, cyanogenic glycosides, oxalates, and phytates. The alcohol extract revealed the presence of alkaloids, tannins, saponins, resins, glycosides, flavonoids, cyanogenic glycosides, oxalates and phytates, while the methanol extract also contained phytochemicals such as alkaloids, tannins, saponins, resins, glycosides, flavonoids, cyanogenic glycosides, oxalates and phytates (Table 2). The preliminary phytochemical screening of the X. aethiopica extracts showed that the aqueous extract contained alkaloids, tannins, saponins, resins, cyanogenic glycosides, glycosides and flavonoids. The ethanol extract revealed the presence of alkaloids, tannins, saponins, resins, cyanogenic glycosides, glycosides and flavonoids while the methanol extract also contained alkaloids, tannins, saponins, resins, cyanogenic glycosides, glycosides and flavonoids (Table 2).

Anthelmintic drugs like Albendazole are reported to cause paralysis of the worms so that they are expelled in the faeces of man and animals (Tiwari, 2011). The extracts not only demonstrated this property, but caused the death of the worms. The anthelmintic activities of the aqueous extract of M. myristica and X. aethiopica were more potent than the ethanol extracts of M. myristica and X. aethiopica, which were more potent than the methanol extracts. The various extracts were more potent than the standard drug Albendazole at 15 mg/ml (Table 3). At the concentration of 100 mg/ml, the ethanol, methanol and aqueous extracts of M. myristica showed very significant activities as compared to the standard drug Albendazole (15 mg/ml), the time of paralysis and death being 1.98±0.67 and 7.23±0.19 as in the case of aqueous extract, 2.30±0.28 and 8.30±0.34 in the case of ethanol extract and 4.06±0.60 and 6.30±0.88 as in the case of

Table 1. The colour, consistency and yield of the different extracts of the seeds of *M. myristica* and *X. aethiopica.*

Solvent extracts	Colour	Consistency	Yield (%)
Xylopia aethiopica extracts			
Aqueous extracts	Brown	Dry	5.0
Ethanol extracts	Brown	Sticky	17.0
Methanol extracts	Brown	Sticky	16.0
Monodora myristica extracts			
Aqueous extract	Reddish brown	Dry	6.16
Ethanol extract	Reddish brown	Dry	1.17
Methanol extract	Reddish brown	Sticky	3.01

Table 2. Qualitative phytochemical analysis of the different extracts of *M. myristica* and *X. aethiopica.*

Phytochemical composition	Aqueous extract	Ethanol extract	Methanol extract	Aqueous extract	Ethanol extract	Methanol extract
	Monodora myristica extracts			*Xylopia aethiopica* extracts		
Alkaloids	+++	++	+	+++	++	++
Tannins	++	++	++	+++	+++	+++
Saponins	+++	+++	+++	+++	+++	+++
Resins	++	+	+	+++	++	++
Steroids	-	-	-	-	-	-
Glycosides	+	+	+	+	+	+
Flavonoids	+++	+++	+++	+	+	+
Cyanogenic glycosides	+	+	+	++	++	++
Oxalates	+	+	+	+++	++	++
Phytates	+	+	+	+++	+++	+++

Key: +++ = present in high amount, ++ = present in moderately high amount, + =   = absent.

methanol extract respectively. The same trend was observed in *X. aethiopica* extracts where the anthelmintic activity of the aqueous extract of *X. aethiopica* was found to be more potent than the ethanol extract of *X. aethiopica*, which was more potent than the methanol extract. At the concentration of 100 mg/ml, the aqueous, ethanol and methanol extracts showed very significant activities as compared to the standard drug Albendazole (15 mg/ml), the time of paralysis and death being 1.63±0.36 and 6.77±0.11 in the case of the aqueous extract, 2.91±0.10 and 8.86±0.66 in the case of ethanol extract, 3.19±0.56 and 6.44±0.83 in the case of the methanol extract and 32.00±0.87 and 38.87±0.65 as in the case of the standard drug Albendazole respectively. The seed extracts of *M. myristica* and *X. aethiopica* produced a significant anthelmintic activity in dose dependent manner.

DISCUSSION

Parasitic helminths affect animals and man, causing considerable hardship, malnutrition and stunted growth.

For a drug to be considered a good anthelmintic drug, it must be able to penetrate the cuticle of the worm or gain access to the alimentary tract. Anthelmintic drugs are known to act by causing paralysis of the worm, or damaging cuticle, leading to partial digestion or to rejection by immune mechanism. Anthelmintic drugs also interfere with the metabolism of worm, and since the metabolic requirement of these parasites vary greatly from one species to another (Aisawarya et al., 2010).

Albendazole has been known to affect worms by destroying the cytoskeletal structure of the worm thereby causing paralysis (Nikesh et al., 2011). The cytoskeletal structure of the helminth includes microfilaments, microtubules and β-tubulins. Under normal conditions, microtubule assembly is dependent on β-tubulin function where the β-tubulin dimmers are continually being polymerised from one end and then depolymerised at the other end of the microtubule (Tiwari, 2011). Albendazole is known to bind to the β-tubulin, preventing their assembly. This results to depletion of parasites glycogen stores, reducing the formation of ATP, disrupting the metabolic pathways and ultimately leading to the parasites death.

Table 3. The Anthelmintic activities of *M. myristica* and *X. aethiopica* extracts.

Treatment	Groups	Concentration (mg/ml)	Time of paralysis (min) (Mean±SD)	Time of death (min) (Mean±SD)
Control	1	-	-	-
Albendazole	2	15	32±0.87	38.87±0.65
Monodora myristica extracts				
	3	10	6.39±0.66*	12.86±0.11*
Aqueous extract	4	20	5.01±0.91*	11.77±0.83*
	5	50	3.66±0.23*	10.68±0.14*
	6	100	1.98±0.67*	7.23±0.19*
	7	10	8.48±0.18*	13.78±0.26*
Ethanol extract	8	20	6.39±0.30*	12.39±0.02*
	9	50	4.59±0.02*	12.15±0.33*
	10	100	2.30±0.28*	8.30±0.34*
	11	10	10.47±0.36*	13.41±0.47*
Methanol extract	12	20	8.46±0.86*	11.26±0.31*
	13	50	6.07±0.77*	11.26±0.31*
	14	100	4.06±0.60*	6.30±0.88*
Xylopia aethiopica extracts				
	15	10	5.44±0.76*	11.04±0.22*
Aqueous extract	16	20	4.63±0.01*	10.61±0.67*
	17	50	2.44±0.89*	8.76±0.44*
	18	100	1.63±0.36*	6.77±0.11*
	19	10	10.84±0.36*	16.81±0.13*
Ethanol extract	20	20	7.22±0.44*	15.88±0.90*
	21	50	4.03±0.56*	12.61±0.17*
	22	100	2.91±0.10*	8.86±0.66*
	23	10	10.44±0.70*	14.46±0.12*
Methanol extract	24	20	8.67±0.83*	13.06±0.30*
	25	50	6.11±0.50*	12.01±0.14*
	26	100	3.19±0.56*	6.44±0.83*

Values are Mean ± SD for each group of five rats. *Means significantly different at P<0.05 compared with the Albendazole treated group.

Preliminary phytochemical tests of the crude extracts of *M. myristica* and *X. aethiopica* revealed the presence of tannins, flavonoids and alkaloids, among other constituents contained within them. Phytochemicals such as tannins, alkaloids, flavonoids and saponins have been demonstrated to possess anthelmintic activities. Chemically, Tannins are polyphenolic compounds (Bate-smith, 1962). Some synthetic phenolic anthelmintics example niclosamide, oxyclozanide and bithionol are known to interfere with energy generation in helminth parasites by uncoupling parasite specific fumarate reductase mediated oxidative phosphorylation reaction. It could be possible that tannins contained in our extracts produced similar effects. From the result of our analysis, there is moderately high amount of tannin in our aqueous, ethanol and methanol extracts. Another feasible anthelmintic effect of tannins is that they can bind to free proteins in the gastrointestinal tract of the host animal (Athanasiadou et al., 2001) as glycoprotein on the cuticle of the parasite (Thompson and Geary, 1995) and cause death to it.

Alkaloids may have acted on the central nervous system of the earth worms causing paralysis (Roy, 2010). This study suggests that the effect could be due to presence of the steroidal alkaloids oligosaccharides which have been reported to suppress the transfer of sucrose from the stomach to the small intestine which could diminish the availability of glucose to helminths together with its antioxidant effect which is capable of reducing the nitrate generation. The extracts may have also induced possible inflammatory effect in the gastric and intestinal mucosal which could have interfered in local homeostasis, essential in the development of helminths.

The main biologic activity ascribed to saponins based on recent research is their membrane permeability property. The main possible actions of saponins are changes in membrane permeability and pore formation, similar with two conventional anthelmintic drugs such as praziquantel and toltrazuril. The anthelmintic drug affects the permeability of the cell membrane of earth worm, causing vacuolisation and disintegration of the teguments (Wang, 2010).

Conclusions

The traditional claim that the seeds of *M. myristica* and *X. aethiopica* possess vermicidal property has been confirmed as our various extracts from the two spices displayed activity against the worm used in the study. Further studies to isolate and reveal the active compounds contained in the organic extracts of *M. myristica* and *X. aethiopica* seeds and to establish the mechanism of action are required to be done in future.

REFERENCES

Ameyaw Y, Owusu-Ansah E (1998). Morphological studies of two plants species used in Ethno medicine. J. Herbs Spices Med. Plants, 5(4): 60–85.

Aisawarya G, Reza KH, Radhika G, Rahul V (2010). Study for anthelmintic activity of Cashew apple (*Anarcadium occidentais*) extract. Int. J. Pharm. Sci. Rev. Res., 6(1): 44–47.

Anonymous (2004). Australian Code of Practice for the Care and Use of Animal for Scientific Purposes. 7th edition, http://www.nhmrc.gov.au/publications/synopses/ea16syn.htm.

Athanasiadou S, Kyriazakis I, Jackson F, Coop RL (2001). Direct anthelmintic effects of condensed tannins towards different gastrointestinal nematodes of sheep: *In vitro* and *in vivo* studies. Vet. Parasitol., 99: 205–219.

Bate-Smith EC (1962). The phenolic constituent of plants and their taxonomic significance, dicotyledons. J. Linn. Soc. Bot., 58: 95–103.

Burkill H (1985). The useful plants of West Tropical Africa. Kew: Royal Botanical Gardens, 2: 25.

Burubai W, Amulla E, Daworiye P, Suowari T, Nimame P (2009). Proximate composition and some technological properties of African Nutmeg (*Monodora myristica*) seeds. Electron. J. Environ. Agric. Food Chem., 8: 396–402.

Ekeanyanwu RC, Ogu GI, Nwachukwu UP (2010). Biochemical characteristics of the African Nutmeg, *Monodora Myristica*. Agric. J., 5(5): 303–308.

Harborne JB (1984). Phytochemical methods, 2 ed. London-New York: Chapman and Hall, p. 279.

Kochlar SL (1986). Spices. Macmillian publication Publication London, pp. 50–65.

Lakshananam B, Mazumber MP, Sasmal D, Ganguly S, Jena SS (2011). *In vitro* anthelmintic activity of some 1- substituted imidazole derivatives. Acta Parasitol. Globalis, 2(1): 1–5.

Mali GR, Mehta AA (2008). A review of anthelmintic plants- Natural Product Radiance, 7(5): 466–475.

Nikesh M, Binitha G, Rekha S, Ravindra N, Anto Sharing M (2011). Comparative *In vitro* Anthelmintic Activity of Chloroform and Acetone Extracts of *Mentha piperita*. Int. J. Pharm. Biol. Arch., 2(3): 945–948.

Nwachukwu N (2000). Nutritional and antinutritional substances in some selected Indigenous spices, PhD thesis, FUTO, Nigeria.

Ogbonnia S, Adekunle AA, Bosa MK, Enwuru VN (2008). Evaluation of acute and subacute toxicity of *Alstonnia congensis* Engler bark and *Xylopia aethiopica* (Dunal) A. Rich (Annonaceae) fruits mixtures used in treatment of diabetes. Afr. J. Biotechnol., 7(6): 701–705.

Okafor JC (1987). Development of forest tree crops for food supplies in Nigeria. For. Ecol. Man, 1: 235–247.

Okigbo BN (1977). Neglected plants of horticultural importance in traditional farming systems of tropical Africa. Acta Horticult., 53: 131–150.

Roy H (2010). Preliminary phytochemical investigation and anthelmintic activity of *Acanthospermum hispidum* D.C. J. Pharm. Sci. Technol., 2(5): 217–221.

Satyavati GV (1990). Use of plant drugs in Indian traditional systems of medicine and their relevance to primary healthcare, In: Farnsworth NR and Wagner H(eds.), Economic and medicinal plant research, 4, plant and traditional medicine, Academic press Ltd., London.

Srinivasan K (2005). Role of spices beyond food flavouring: Neutraceuticals with multiple health effects. Food Rev. Int., 21: 167–188.

Thompson DP, Geary TG (1995). The structure and function of helminth surfaces. In: Marr J.J. (eds). Biochemistry and Molecular Biology of Parasites. 1st ed. New York: Academic Press, pp. 203–232.

Tiwari P, Kumar B, Kumar M, Kaur M, Debnath J, Sharma P (2011). Comparative anthelmintic activity of aqueous and ethanolic stem extract of *Tinospora cordifola*. Int. J. Drug Dev. Res., 3(1): 70–83.

Walter PJ, Prichard KK (1985). Chemotherapy of parasitic infections, W.C. Campbell and L.S. Rew (Eds), Plenum, New York, pp. 278–539.

Wang GX (2010). *In vivo* anthelmintic activity of five alkaloids from macleaya microcarpa (maxim) fedde against *Dactylogyrus intermedius* in *Carassius auratus*. Vet. Parasitol., 171: 305–313.

31

Antioxidant capacity of bioactive compounds extracted from selected wild and domesticated cereals of Zimbabwe

Kudakwashe Chitindingu[1,2]*, Jill J. F. Chitindingu[1], Mudadi A. N. Benhura[1], Amos Marume[3], Isaac Mutingwende[3], Michael Bhebhe[1] and Maud Muchuweti[1]

[1]Department of Biochemistry, University of Zimbabwe, M. P. 167, Mount Pleasant, Harare, Zimbabwe.
[2]Department of Biotechnology, Chinhoyi University of Technology, Chinhoyi, Zimbabwe.
[3]School of Pharmacy, College of Health Sciences, University of Zimbabwe, M. P. 167, Mount Pleasant, Harare, Zimbabwe.

Bioactive compounds were extracted from 6 wild and 4 domesticated cereal grains of Zimbabwe, using 50% methanol with the aim of testing their capability to prevent phospholipid peroxidation and β-carotene bleaching. The highest yield of phenolic compounds was obtained from *Eleusine indica* (a wild cereal) with 7.16 mg GA/100 mg sample, while the least yield was obtained from *Amaranthus hybridus* with 1.13 mg GA/100 mg sample. Antioxidant activities of the cereal extracts were studied using the β-carotene-linoleic acid and the inhibition of phospholipid peroxidation assays. It was shown that *Sorghum arundinaceum* had the greatest (77%) increase in inhibition of phospholipid when its concentration was increased from 20 to 80 mg/ml, while *Eleusine corocana*, a domestic cereal grain had the least. Relative to a standard BHA (an artificial antioxidant), *E. indica* was found to have the highest ability (67%) to prevent bleaching of β-carotene, while *Pennisetum* spp with 17.3% inhibition, had the least ability. Owing to the ability of the cereal grain extracts to act as antioxidants, the studies can be further extended to exploit the phenolic extracts as replacements of artificial antioxidants like butylated hydroxyl anisole (BHA) in food and health supplements and nutraceuticals.

Key words: Wild cereal grains, antioxidants, phospholipid peroxidation, health supplements.

INTRODUCTION

Natural plants have received attention as sources of biologically active substances including antioxidants, antimutagens and anticarcinogens (Singh et al., 2004). Antioxidants play a crucial role in preventing diseases because of their ability to capture, deactivate or repair the damage caused by a group of molecules or atoms called free radicals that are implicated in many diseases (Wang et al., 1997). Free radicals, such as superoxide ($O_2^{\bullet-}$, $OOH^{\bullet}$), hydroxyl ($OH^{\bullet}$) and peroxyl ($ROOH^{\bullet}$) radicals play an important role in oxidative stress related to the pathogenesis of various important diseases (Slater,

1984). In addition, these molecules are considered to induce lipid peroxidation causing the deterioration of foods. In healthy individuals, the production of free radicals is balanced by the antioxidative defense system. Oxidative stress is generated when the balance is in favor of the free radicals as a result of an increased production or depletion of antioxidant levels. It is common knowledge that oxidative stress, particularly due to aging, may be a contributory factor in neurodegenerative disorders, such as Alzheimer's and Parkinson's diseases.

There is therefore, a marked interest in determining the role of phytonutrients in promoting improved health and in reducing cancer, cardiovascular disease, and the effects of aging. Antioxidant phytonutrients can inhibit the propagation of free radical reactions that may ultimately lead to the development of diseases, especially those

*Corresponding author. E-mail: kchitindingu@gmail.com.

which are aging related. Many cereal grains have strong antioxidant capacities, and this capacity is due primarily to non-vitamin C phytochemicals (Prior et al., 1998). The presence of a wide range of phytochemicals such as phenolics, thiols, carotenoids, anthocyanins and tocopherol, have been suggested to exert chemo-preventive (Dragsted et al., 1993), cardioprotective (Vita, 2005) effects, and protect the human body against oxidative damage by free radicals (Halliwell and Gutteridge, 1999). The health benefits of cereal grains have notable implications for the improvement of food quality, particularly through applications in functional foods and nutraceuticals (Abdul-Hamid and Luan, 2000; Truswell, 2003). Phytochemicals in plants can function as natural antioxidants and thereby retard or even prevent rancidity of food lipids, improve sensory scores and offer greater consumer acceptance of food products (Nakatani, 1997). As a group, these naturally occurring compounds have been found to be strong antioxidants against free radicals and other reactive oxygen species (ROS), the major cause of many chronic human diseases such as cancer and cardiovascular diseases (Andreasen et al., 2001a; Yu et al., 2002, 2003).

A number of synthetic antioxidants, such as butylated hydroxyanisole (BHA), butylated hydroxytoluene (BHT) and tert-butylhydroquinone (TBHQ) have been added to foodstuffs but, because of toxicity issues, their use is being questioned (Valentaõ et al., 2002). Attention has therefore been directed toward the isolation of natural antioxidants from plant sources, especially edible plants, with the hope of finding non-toxic replacements to the synthetic antioxidants. The use of natural antioxidants in foods is limited, however, on account of the lack of knowledge concerning their molecular composition, the content of active compounds in the raw material and the availability of relevant toxicological data.

In this study, we sought to investigate inhibitory effects of phenolic extracts from selected wild and domesticated cereal grains found in Zimbabwe, against oxidation of phospholipids and fatty acids. The cereal grains we chose for the study are usually consumed in times of drought and famine by poor families in Zimbabwe. These cereal grain extracts can potentially be used as replacements of artificial antioxidants in the food industry.

MATERIALS AND METHODS

Chemicals

The chemicals were all of high purity grade and were all from Sigma – Aldrich Chemie (Steinheim, Germany).

Collection of samples

Mature cereal grains were randomly collected from areas in and around Harare in Zimbabwe. Samples were sundried and stored in brown bottles away from direct sunlight until needed for use in assays. The samples collected were *Eleusine indica* (Crowfoot grass), *Sorghum arundinaceum* (common wild sorghum), *Rottiboellia cochinchinensis* (itchgrass), *Brachiaria brizantha* (upright brachiaria), *Panicum maximum* (Guinea grass), *Amaranthus hybridus* (smooth pigweed or slim amaranth), *Eleusine corocana* (finger millet), *Sorghum bicolor (Red)* (sorghum), *Sorghum bicolor (White)* (sorghum) and *Pennisetum americanum* (bulrush millet).

Extraction method for total phenolic compounds

Total phenolic compounds were extracted from the fruit samples as described by Makkar (1999). The finely ground sample (2 g) was extracted twice with cold 50% aqueous methanol (10 ml, 1:1 v/v) in a 50 ml test tube suspended in ice subject to ultrasonication for 20 min. The two extracts were combined, made up to 20 ml with 50% aqueous methanol, centrifuged at 3000 rpm for 10 min and supernatant transferred into small sample bottles ready for analysis. Analyses were done on freshly extracted samples.

Folin Ciocalteau assay for total phenolics

The Folin Ciocalteau method for determination of total phenolic compounds was carried out following the method described by Singleton and Rossi (1965). A sample (50 µl), distilled water (950 µl) was added to make up to 1 ml, then 1 N Folin reagent (500 µl) was added followed by sodium carbonate (2.5 ml). At the end of 40 min absorbencies at 725 nm were read using a spectronic 20® genesys™ spectrophotometer against a blank which contained methanol instead of sample. Gallic acid (0.5 mg/ml) was used as the standard and concentration of sample was expressed as mg GA/100 mg.

Ability to prevent oxidation of β-carotene

The β-carotene-linoleic acid assay was done following the method by Shon et al. (2003). β - carotene (2 mg) was dissolved in chloroform (10 ml). An aliquot (1 ml) of the solution was taken and chloroform was removed by vacuum on a rotary evaporator. Linoleic acid (40 mg) was added to the almost dry material followed by Tween 80 (400 mg) and distilled water (100 ml) with rigorous shaking. Aliquots (3 ml) of the mixture were combined with samples (100 µl, at a concentration of 80 mg/ml). The reaction mixture was shaken until an emulsion was formed and the absorbance at zero time was measured at 470 nm using a Shimadzu UV-1601 UV-visible spectrophotometer. Measurement of absorbance was continued at 5 min intervals for 2 h. A blank without β-carotene was used as a negative control. Butylated hydroxyl anisol (BHA) (0.5%) was used as a standard and its extent of protection of β-carotene was treated as 100% protection.

Ability to inhibit phospholipid peroxidation

Female Sprague Dawley rats (*Rattus norvegicus*) were obtained from the Animal House, University of Zimbabwe and dissected to obtain the brain. The rat brain was stored at -85℃ until it was used. Homogenization of rat brain (2 g) was done in chloroform: methanol mixture (2:1, v/v) followed by centrifugation at 3000 x g for 5 min. The supernatant obtained was used as the source of phospholipids. The test run contained the phospholipids solution (50 µl), the sample extract (0.5 ml), 50% methanol (0.2 ml) and $FeSO_4$ (0.5 ml). The blank contained the phospholipid solution (50 µl) mixed with distilled water (0.5 ml) instead of the phenolic compound containing sample and methanol (0.2 ml, 50%). Ascorbic acid (0.5%) was used as the control. Incubation of the reaction mixture at 37℃ for 1 h

Table 1. Total phenolic content expressed as gallic acid equivalence as determined by Folin Ciocalteau assay for wild and domesticated cereal grains on dry weight basis. The results are presented as mean ± standard deviation of three independent measurements.

Extract	Total phenolic compounds (mg GA/100 mg sample)
Amaranthus hybridus	1.13 ± 0.01
Brachiaria brizantha	3.18 ± 0.07
Eleusine corocana	6.31 ± 0.03
Eleusine indica	7.16 ± 0.10
Panicum maximum	2.58 ± 0.02
Pennisettum spp	3.09 ± 0.02
Rottiboellea cochinchinensis	3.31 ± 0.04
Sorghum arundinaceum	6.18 ± 0.03
Sorghum bicolor (Red type)	3.98 ± 0.02
Sorghum bicolor (White type)	2.10 ± 0.03

was followed by the addition of thiobarbituric acid (TBA) (0.5 ml) and trichloroacetic acid (TCA) (4 ml) and the solution was then heated in a boiling water bath for 15 min. After cooling the sample on ice, absorbance was read at 532 nm on a spectronic 20® genesys™ spectrophotometer.

Statistical analysis

Results are expressed as the means ± standard deviation (vertical error bars) of three replicates. One way analysis of variance (ANOVA) and the Student's *t* test were used to determine the statistical difference. Statistical significance was $p < 0.05$, unless otherwise stated.

RESULTS AND DISCUSSION

Total phenolics

In Table 1, variations in total phenolic content of wild cereal samples expressed as gallic acid equivalence, are shown. The total phenolic content varied considerably ($p < 0.05$) between cereal samples, with the highest total phenolic content being exhibited by *E. indica* (a wild cereal) with 7.16 mg GA/100 mg sample, while the least amount was found in *A. hybridus* 1.13 ± 0.01 mg GA/100 mg sample). There was also variation within cereals of the same family. *S. arundinaceum*, *S. bicolor* (Red) and *S. bicolor* (White) belong to the same family and their phenolic contents were found to be 6.18, 3.98 and 2.05 mg GA/100 mg sample respectively. This wide variation may be due to the different environmental conditions the three cereal grains are exposed to and their genetic makeup (Singh et al., 2004). The wild cereal, *S. arundinaceum*, had a higher phenolic compound concentration compared to both the domestic varieties that is the red and the white varieties.

Of the domestic sorghum samples, the red variety also exhibited a larger concentration than the white variety. This may be due to their differences in colour, where the red variety may contain more anthocyanidins than the

white variety (He and Giusti, 2010; Janero, 1990). The total phenolic content follows the order: *E. indica* > *E. corocana* > *S. arundinaceum* > *S. bicolor* (Red) > *R. cochinchinensis* > *B. brizantha* > *Pennisetum* spp > *P. maximum* > *S. bicolor* (White) > *A. hybridus*. The previous results were obtained using the Folin-Ciocalteu method. Characteristics of the phenolic extracts were investigated further using the phospholipid peroxidation and β-carotene-linoleic acid model system assays to measure antioxidant activity.

Inhibition of phospholipid peroxidation assay

Lipid peroxidation is an oxidative alteration of polyunsaturated fatty acid in the cell membranes that generates a number of degradation products. Malonyldialdehyde (MDA), one of the major products of lipid peroxidation, has been studied widely as an index of lipid peroxidation and as a marker of oxidative stress (He and Giusti, 2010; Janero, 1990). In this study, the ability of cereal extracts to prevent lipid peroxidation was followed using a system that contained rat brain homogenates whereas peroxidation was induced by addition of $FeCl_2$-H_2O_2. From Figure 1, it is evident that methanolic extracts from *S. arundinaceum*, *E. indica*, *E. corocana*, *S. bicolor* (White), and *S. bicolor* (Red) caused protection of phospholipid as shown by the decrease in absorbance as sample concentration was increased. *A. hybridus*, *P. maximum*, *B. brizantha*, *R. cochinchinensis* and *Pennisetum* spp caused protection of phospholipid from peroxidation as indicated in Figure 2.

Addition of cereal grain extracts to the Fe^{2+}-H_2O_2 system resulted in a decrease in the formation of tissue MDA levels, suggesting that the cereal extracts were scavengers of ·OH. Therefore, the ·OH-scavenging activity observed in this study indicates a possible application for the cereal extracts in the management of diseases involving free radicals and oxidative damage, such as lipid peroxidation. Comparatively, the order of

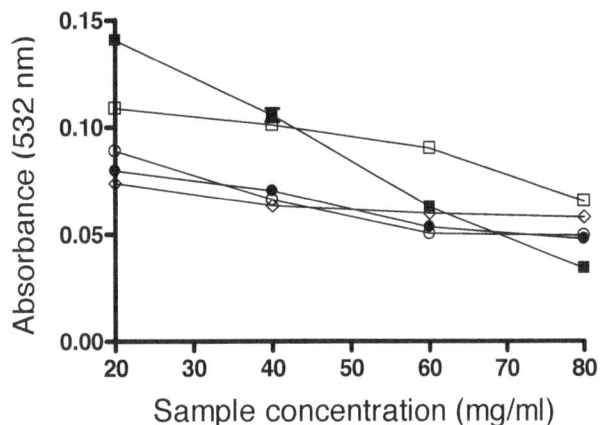

Figure 1. Inhibition of phospholipid peroxidation by the methanolic extracts of *Sorghum arundinaceum* (■), *Eleusine indica* (○), *Eleusine corocana* (◊), *Sorghum bicolor (White)* (●) *Sorghum bicolor (Red)* (□). The lower the absorbance reading, the lower the amount of MDA that was formed which in turn was an indication of the extract's ability to inhibit phospholipid peroxidation. The results are presented as mean ± standard deviation of three independent measurements.

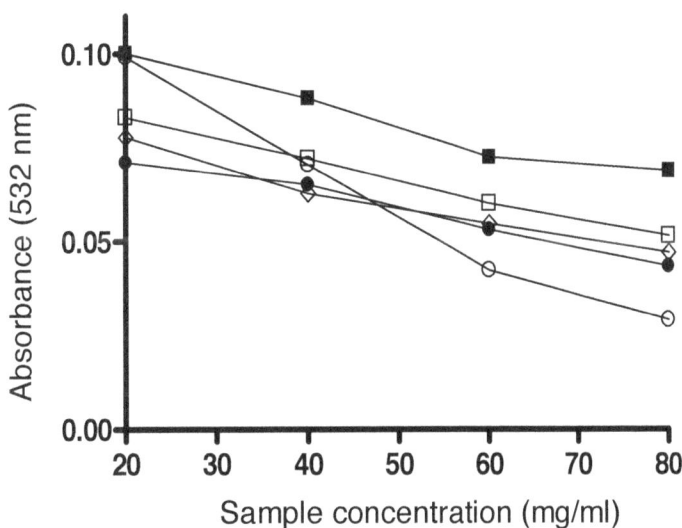

Figure 2. Inhibition of phospholipid peroxidation by the methanolic extracts of *Amaranthus hybridus* (□), *Panicum maximum* (●), *Brachiaria brizantha* (■), *Rottiboellia cochinchinensis* (○) and *Pennisetum* spp (◊). The lower the absorbance reading, the lower the amount of MDA that was formed which, in turn, was an indication of the extract's ability to inhibit phospholipid peroxidation. The results are presented as mean ± standard deviation of three independent measurements.

inhibition of lipid peroxidation follows the order: *S. arundinaceum* > *E. indica* > *S. bicolor* (White) = *S. bicolor* (Red) = *P. maximum* > *Pennisetum* spp > *A. hybridus* > *B. brizantha* > *R. cochinchinensis* > *E. corocana* as shown in Figures 1 and 2. This order was obtained by calculating the absorbance of each sample at a concentration of 80 mg/ml as a percentage of its absorbance at 20 mg/ml.

S. arundinaceum showed the greatest (77%) increase in inhibition of phospholipid when its concentration was increased from 20 to 80 mg/ml. The inhibition was dose dependant for all samples and the increase in inhibition as concentration of sample increased was significant (P>0.05) for all cereal grain antioxidant extracts.

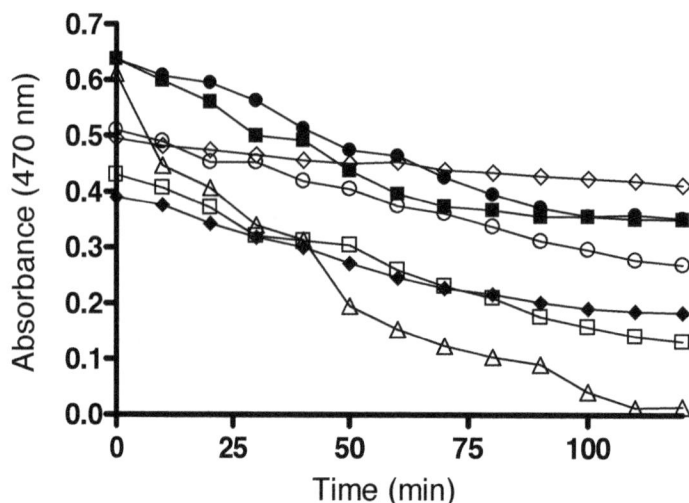

Figure 3. Antioxidant activity of extracts of *Sorghum arundinaceum* (■), *Eleusine indica* (●), *Eleusine corocana* (♦), *Sorghum bicolor (White)* (□) *Sorghum bicolor (Red)* (○) in β-carotene/linoleic acid system. BHA (◊) was used as the positive control and in the negative control (Δ), no sample was added. Slow decrease in absorbance signifies protection of β-carotene. Results are presented as the mean ± Standard deviation of three independent measurements.

S. bicolor (White), *S. bicolor* (Red) and *P. maximum* inhibited phospholipid peroxidation to the same extent when dosage of sample was increased. This may be because the cereal grains contain similar phenolic compounds that are responsible for preventing phospholipid peroxidation. Cetojević-Simin et al. (2010) also reported that plants contain phytochemicals that had protective effects against lipid peroxidation. However, there is need to characterize the phytochemicals by HPLC-MS method to positively identify the constituent phenolic compounds. *S. arundinaceum* is a wild cereal, whereas *S. bicolor* (White) and *S. bicolor* (Red) have been domesticated.

The wild cereal grains exhibited greater potential to prevent lipid peroxidation than its domestic counterparts and the protective capability may be due to the fact that the *S. arundinaceum* has a deeper red colour which is usually indicative of a lot of phenolic compounds, mainly anthocyanidins (Cetojević-Simin et al., 2010; He and Giusti, 2010). The same trend that the sorghums show exists between *E. indica* (45%) and *E. corocana* (23%). *E. indica* is the wild cereal grain which exhibited greater response to increase in dose than *E. corocana*.

Antioxidant activity in the β-carotene bleaching assay

Oxidation of carotenoids, which is induced by light, heat or peroxyl radicals (Ursini et al., 1998) results, in bleaching (Huang et al., 2005). Antioxidants that can donate hydrogen atoms to quench radicals can prevent or reduce decolorisation of carotenoids (Burda and

Oleszek, 2001). All the cereal extracts had the ability to delay the bleaching of β-carotene. For the negative control, no sample was added to prevent bleaching of β-carotene, so rate of discolouration was rapid. Butylated Hydroxy-toluene (BHT) was used as the positive control. In Figures 3 and 4, the extent of protection of β-carotene over 2 h is shown. Relative to BHA, the order of protection of β-carotene can be shown from Table 2 and it is as follows: *E. indica* > *S. bicolor* (Red)> *E. corocana*> *S. arundinaceum* > *A. hybridus* > *S. bicolor* (White) > *P. maximum* > *B. brizantha* > *R. cochinchinensis*> *Pennisetum* spp. There was no notable trend between the wild and the domestic cereal grains in this assay but all cereal grains showed ability to protect β-carotene over time. *E. indica*, a wild cereal grain had 67.5% of the β-carotene remaining unbleached after 2 h, which was the highest percentage of all the cereal grains under study. *Pennisetum* spp, a domestic cereal had the least amount of β-carotene remaining after 2 h. Different extracts of various cereal grains have also been reported to have potential inhibiting activity against the oxidation of β-carotene molecules (Cardador-Martìnez et al., 2002).

The differences in ability to protect against bleaching may depend on the phenolic compound constituents in the individual grains. Environmental factors also affect the amount of potential antioxidant in the sample (Osier and Lindroth, 2001). To be able to determine which phenolic compounds were effective as antioxidants in both assays, the active compounds can be isolated by fractionation and then the structures elucidated by mass spectroscopy. All the cereal grains, wild and domesticated contain phenolic compounds. *E. indica* was shown

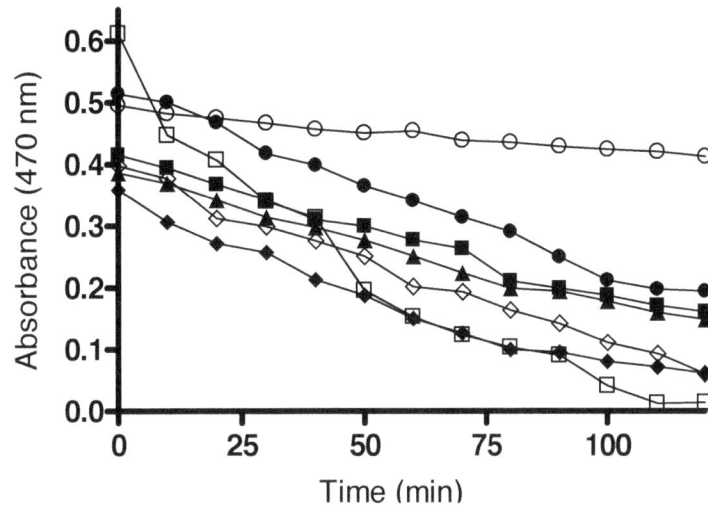

Figure 4. Antioxidant activity of extracts of *Amaranthus hybridus* (■), *Panicum maximum* (▲), *Brachiaria brizantha* (●), *Rottiboellia Cochinchinensis* (◊) and *Pennisetum spp* (♦) in β -carotene/linoleic acid system. BHA (○) was used as the positive control and in the negative control (□), no sample was added. Slow decrease in absorbance signifies protection of β-carotene. Results are presented as the mean ± Standard deviation of three independent measurements.

Table 2. Antioxidant activity of extracts of wild and domestic cereal grains expressed as a percentage relative to a BHA standard. Assumption is that, after 2 h BHA inhibited bleaching of β-carotene by 100%.

Sample	Relative β-carotene remaining after 2 h, expressed as a percentage with 100% meaning that bleaching of β-carotene was completely prevented
BHA	100
No sample	0
Amaranthus hybridus	46.9
Brachiaria brizantha	38.7
Eleusine corocana	62.3
Eleusine indica	67.8
Panicum maximum	40.7
Pennisetum spp	17.3
Rottiboellia cochinchinensis	20.1
Sorghum arundinaceum	59.7
Sorghum bicolor (Red)	65.5
Sorghum bicolor (White)	43.7

to have the highest total phenolic content, while *A. hybridus* had the least among the cereals under studied. Only *E. indica* was shown to have a strong positive correlation between total phenolics and antioxidant activity (r^2 = 0.934). In the rest of the remaining cereal grains, there was no correlation, suggesting that ability to inhibit phospholipid peroxidation and β-carotene bleaching depended more on the quality than quantity of the constituent phenolic compounds. The highest ability (P>0.05) to prevent phospolipid peroxidation is given by *S. arundinaceum*, while *E. corocana* displayed the least activity. The ability of the wild and domesticated cereal

grains to prevent lipid peroxidation was found to be dose dependant. There was positive correlation between dose of cereal and level of prevention of lipid peroxidation (r^2 = 0.967). All cereal grains had the ability to prevent bleaching of β-carotene. The cereal grains may be used as potential sources of natural antioxidants.

ACKNOWLEDGEMENTS

We wish to thank the WF Kellog's Foundation, UNU-INRA and the University of Zimbabwe research board for funding the project.

REFERENCES

Abdul-Hamid A, Luan YS (2000). Functional properties of dietary fibre prepared from defatted rice bran. Food Chem., 68: 15-19.

Andreasen MF, Kroon PA, Williamson G, Garcia-Conesa MT (2001a). Intestinal release and uptake of phenolic antioxidant di-ferulic acids. Free Radic. Biol. Med., 31: 304-314.

Burda S, Oleszek W (2001). Antioxidant and antiradical activities of flavonoids. J. Agric. Food Chem., 49: 2774-2779.

Cardador-Martı̀nez A, Loarca-Pina GL, Oomah BD (2002). Antioxidant activity in common beans (Phaseolus vulgaris L.). J. Agric. Food Chem., 50: 6975-6980.

Cetojević-Simin DD, Canadanović-Brunet JM, Bogdanović GM, Djilas SM, Cetković GS, Tumbas VT, Stojiljković BT (2010). Antioxidative and antiproliferative activities of different horsetail (Equisetum arvense L.) extracts. J. Med. Food, 13(2): 452-459.

Dragsted LO, Strube M, Larsen JC (1993). Cancer-protective factors in fruits and vegetables: biochemical and biological background. Pharmacol. Toxicol., 72: 116-135.

Halliwell B, Gutteridge JMC (1999). Free Rad. Biol. Med. 3rd ed. Oxford University Press: Oxford, U.K. pp. 60-67.

He J, Giusti MM (2010) Anthocyanins: natural colorants with health-promoting properties. Annu. Rev. Food Sci. Technol., 1: 163-87.

Huang D, Ou B, Prior RL (2005). The chemistry behind antioxidant capacity assays. J. Agric. Food Chem., 53: 1841-1856.

Janero DR (1990). Malondiadehyde and thiobarbituric acid reactivity as diagnostic indices of lipid peroxidation and peroxidative tissue injury. Free Radic. Biol. Med., 9: 515-540.

Makkar HPS (1999). Quantification of Tannins in Tree Foliage: A laboratory manual for the FAO/IAEA Co-ordinated Research project on 'Use of nuclear and Related Techniques to Develop Simple Tannin Assay for Predicting and Improving the Safety and Efficiency of Feeding Ruminants on the Tanniniferous Tree Foliage. Joint FAO/IAEA Division of Nuclear Techniques in Food and Agriculture, Vienna, Austria. pp. 1-29

Nakatani N (1997). Antioxidants from spices and herbs. In F. Shahidi (Ed.), Natural antioxidants. Chemistry, health effects, and applications. Champaign: AOCS Press, pp. 64-75.

Osier TL, Lindroth RL (2001). Effects of genotype, nutrient availability, and defoliation on aspen phytochemistry and insect performance. Oecologia, 148: 293-303.

Prior RL, Cao G, Martin A, Sofic E, McEwen J, O'Brien C, Lischner N, Ehlenfeldt M, Kalt W, Krewer G, Mainland CM (1998). Antioxidant capacity as influenced by total phenolic and anthocyanin content, maturity, and variety of Vaccinium species. J. Agric. Food Chem., 46: 2686-2693.

Shon MY, Kim TH, Sung NJ (2003). Antioxidant and free radical scavenging activity of Phillinus baumii (Phellinus of Hymenochaetaceae) extracts. Food Chem., 82: 593-597.

Singh SK, Hawkins C, Clarke ID, Squire JA, Bayani J, Hide T, Henkelman RM, Cusimano MD, Dirks PB (2004). Identification of human brain tumour initiating cells. Nature, 432(7015): 281-282.

Singleton VL Rossi JA (1965). Colorimetry of Total Phenolics with Phosphomolybdic-phosphotungstic acid Reagent. Am. J. Enol. Viticulture, 16:144-158.

Slater TF (1984). Free radical mechanisms in tissue injury. Biochem. J., 222: 1-15.

Truswell AS (2003). Cereal grains and coronary heart disease. Eur. J. Clin. Nutr., 56: 1-14.

Ursini F, Zamburlini A, Cazzolato G, Maiorino M, Bon GB, Sevanian A (1998). Postprandial plasma lipid hydroperoxides: A possible link between diet and atherosclerosis. Free Radic. Biol Med., 25: 250-252.

Valentaõ P, Fernandes E, Carvalho F, Andrade PB, Seabra RM, Bastos ML (2002). Antioxidative properties of cardoon (Cynara cardunculus L.) infusion against superoxide radical, hydroxyl radical, and hypochlorous acid. J. Agric. Food Chem., 50: 4989-4993.

Vita JA (2005). Polyphenols and cardiovascular disease: effects on endothelial and platelet function. Am. J. Clin. Nutr., 81: 292S-297S.

Wang H, Cao G, Prior RL (1997). Oxygen radical absorbing capacity of anthocyanins. J. Agric. Food Chem., 45: 304-309.

Yu L, Haley S, Perret J, Harris M, Wilson J, Qian M (2002). Free radical scavenging properties of wheat extracts. J. Agric. Food Chem., 50: 1619-1624.

Yu L, Perret J, Harris M, Wilson J, Haley S (2003). Antioxidant properties of bran extracts from "Akron" wheat grown at different locations. J. Agric. Food Chem., 51: 1566-1570.

32

The role of ascorbic acid in the treatment of *Plasmodium Berghei* infected mice

H. O. T. Iyawe* and A. O. Onigbinde

Department of Biochemistry Ambrose Alli University, P. M. B. 14, Ekpoma Nigeria.

This work aimed at examining the effect of malaria parasites and ascorbic treatments in mice. The relevance of this research derives from the desire to understand the role of ascorbic acid in malaria infection. In this study design, three groups of ten mice each categorized as non-parasitized-non-treated (control), parasitized-non-treated (PnT) and parasitized ascorbic acid treated (P+asT) were used. Results collected and analyzed using adequate statistical software revealed that parasitism in mice had significant (p < 0.05) increases in erythrocyte fragility, total and indirect bilirubin, total protein and globulin but decreased (p < 0.05) mice packed cell volume (PCV). Plasma malondialdehyde (MDA) significantly (p < 0.05) increased while superoxide dismutase (SOD) and catalase (CAT) decreased (p < 0.05). Liver SOD and CAT as well as kidney MDA of parasitized non treated mice were observed to increase (p < 0.05) following *Plasmodium berghei* infection. Ascorbic acid treatment of parasitized mice was observed to reverse the effects of *P. berghei* in mice. The findings suggest ascorbic acid to be critical in the management of malaria parasite infection.

Key words: *Plasmodium berghei*, ascorbic acid, antioxidants, erythrocyte fragility, oxidative stress.

INTRODUCTION

In the tropics and subtropical regions of the world, the endemic nature of malaria as well as the mortality associated with the infection particularly among children under the ages of five years have been reported (WHO, 2000; Nmorsi et al., 2007).

It is also documented that malaria parasites inside erythrocytes exert oxidative stress within the parasitized red blood cells (Hunt and Stocker, 1990; Potter et al., 2005). The parasites are suggested to generate reactive oxygen species (ROS) from which they are protected (Potter et al., 2005), through one or more of the named pathways: Electron transport chain (Deslauriers et al., 1987), haemoglobin and cytosolic proteins degradation (Atamma and Ginsburg, 1993), or redox reactions of hemin (Har-El et al., 1993). The formation of ROS by malaria parasites if not checked by the host cytoprotective enzymes and antioxidants could led to oxidative damage and there are increasing evidence that injuries contribute to pathophysiology of many diseases (Gora et al., 2006).

The potential toxicity of free radical generated by malaria parasites are counteracted by a large number of cytoprotective enzymes and antioxidants. One of such antioxidant is ascorbic acid (Behrman et al., 2001), a water soluble vitamin that reacts with radicals and effectively protects cell against lipid peroxidation (Frei et al., 1990). For cell protection ascorbic acid has been reported to act as scavenger for superoxide radicals, sulphur-centred radical, singlet oxygen and hydroxyl radical (Gutteridge and Halliwell, 1994). Though the effect of ascorbic acid combination treatment with chloroquine in malaria infection has been reported (Iyawe et al., 2006), the specific role of ascorbic acid in the management of oxidative stress occasioned by malaria parasites is not clear. Therefore, this study is an attempt to elucidate the possible specific role of ascorbic acid in oxidative stress occasioned by malaria parasites.

MATERIALS AND METHODS

Animals and parasites

Thirty albino male mice of 8 weeks were used in the study and the animals were handled in a very humane manner. Observation protocols and method used for maintaining ANKA strains of *Plasmodium berghei* in our laboratory has been previously described (Iyawe and Onigbinde, 2009).

---

*Corresponding author. E-mail: iyawehanson@yahoo.com.

Procedures

Three groups of animals respectively categorized as control (None parasitized non–treated), parasitized non–treated (PnT) and parasitized but ascorbic acid-treated (P+asT) were used. The animals were allowed free access to feed on Grower's mash (from Bendel feeds and flourmills Ltd. Ewu Edo State Nigeria) and water. At the end of the experiment, the mice were anaesthetized with chloroform and blood collected by cardiac puncture into sample tubes from where plasma used for assay was harvested.

Drug preparation and administration

Three milliliters of ascorbic acid containing 100 mg/5 ml w/v (NAFDAC REG NO. 04 – 0262) manufactured by Emzor Pharmaceutical Industries Ltd., Lagos Nigeria was made up to 60 ml with sterile distilled water. The preparation brought the active component of each drug to 3 mg/ml. The drug was administered (25 mg/Kg BW) intraperitoneally for three days.

Tissue extracts preparation and assays

Kidney, liver and heart tissues of subjects were obtained as previously described (Iyawe and Onigbinde, 2009). Lipid peroxidation, superoxide dismutase activity, catalase activity, assay of glutathione levels, glucose–6–phosphate dehydrogenase activity (G6PD), gamma glutamyltransferase activity (GGT), Alanine aminotransferase (ALT) and aspartate aminotransferase (AST) assay, serum bilirubin (total, conjugated and unconjugated),Total serum albumin and proteins, Globulin concentration and Erythrocyte fragility were respectively determined as previously described (Iyawe and Onigbinde, 2009).

STATISTICAL ANALYSIS

Data collected from this study were subjected to one factor analysis of variance (ANOVA) using computer software (InStat, Graphpad Software, SanDiego, CA). P < 0.05 was considered significant. LSD was used to determined differences in means at 95% confidence interval.

RESULTS

Parasitized mice had their erythrocyte fragility, total and direct bilirubin increased significantly (p < 0.05) but reduced (p < 0.05) mice packed cell volume (PCV). Ascorbic acid treatment significantly (p < 0.05) reduced erythrocyte fragility, significantly (p < 0.05) increased PCV in mice compared to PnT animals (Table 1). *P. berghei* infected mice had their total protein and globulin significantly (p < 0.05) increased. Ascorbic acid treatment also reduced (p < 0.05) Plasma total protein and globulin levels compared to PnT (Table 2). Parasitized mice plasma MDA increased (p < 0.05) while SOD and CAT activities reduced (p < 0.05). Treatment of parasitized mice with ascorbic acid reduced (p < 0.05) plasma MDA while SOD and CAT enzymes increased significantly (p < 0.05) compared to PnT (Table 3). Parasitemia increased liver tissue SOD and CAT, including kidney MDA (p < 0.05). Ascorbic acid treatment of parasitized mice liver and kidney reduced kidney MDA compared to PnT and

reduced (p < 0.05) liver SOD and CAT compared to PnT (Table 4).

DISCUSSION AND CONCLUSION

The reductions in total serum protein and globulin observed in ascorbic acid treated mice as compared to PnT mice group may perhaps indicate the contribution of the organic molecule to erythropoesis. It is most likely that ascorbic acid may perform useful function in bone marrow to enhance blood cells formation, as indicated in this study by the recorded increased packed cell volume (PCV). This may imply that the iron released as a result of parasite degradation of haemoglobin may probably be recycled for blood cells production.

Ascorbic acid and reduced glutathione are important chain breaking antioxidants responsible for scavenging free radicals and suppression of peroxidation in aqueous and lipid region of the cell (Gora et al., 2006). It is reported to exist in blood as oxidised dihydroascorbic acid (DHAA) and reduced ascorbic acid forms (RAA) and its transportation across cell membranes is in the form of DHAA, which is less ionized at physiological pH and therefore, more permeable to membrane (Mann and Newton, 1975). The decrease in oxidative stress in ascorbic acid treated group compared to PnT mice group may be that the most potent membrane antioxidant α-tocopherol has probably become more effective as ascorbic acid can supply required reducing equivalents to tocopheroxyl radical (Sies, 1991), a product of α-tocopherol reaction with membrane free radical. As a result, the ascorbic acid is oxidized to dehydroascorbic acid (DHAA) which is reconverted to ascorbic acid by plasma reduced glutathione. This reaction may account for the observed reductions in plasma MDA and GSH.

It could be hypothesized that the observed reduction in G6PD activity under parasitized condition may be due to G6PD enzyme inhibition by ascorbic acid. There is evidence that malarial parasites inside the erythrocytes exert oxidative stress within the parasitized red blood cell from which they are protected by a number of parasite encoded enzymes, by ascorbic acid, vitamin E, by glutathione and that parasite antioxidant defence is believed to include export of oxidized glutathione to the erythrocyte cytosol (Postma et al., 1996; Potter et al., 2005). Apart from the parasite induced ROS, phagocytic leucocytes are able to engulf infectious agents within the phagocytic food vacuole leading to the formation of the enzyme NADPH-oxidase involved in the formation of superoxide anion that is involved in the killing of the pathogen (Karupiah et al., 2000). It is therefore not unlikely that in other to control the superoxide anion and its derivatives such as hydrogen peroxide, cellular synthesis of SOD and CAT may have occurred under increased oxidative stress condition to cause an increase in the plasma levels of these enzymes and hence their observed increased activities.

Table 1. Effect of *P. berghei* and ascorbic acid treatments on some biochemical indices in parasitized mice.

Parameters	Control	PnT	P+asT
Erythrocyte fragility (%)	0.00 ± 0.00^a	37.15 ± 0.77^b	25.35 ± 3.27^c
Packed Cell Volume (%)	42.71 ± 2.17^a	26.83 ± 2.33^b	35.17 ± 2.65^c
Total Bilirubin (mg/dL)	0.16 ± 0.02^a	0.76 ± 0.12^b	0.35 ± 0.07^c
Direct Bilirubin (mg/dL)	0.10 ± 0.03^a	0.68 ± 0.12^b	0.28 ± 0.04^c
Indirect Bilirubin (mg/dL)	0.06 ± 0.02^a	0.08 ± 0.01^a	0.06 ± 0.03^a

Mean $\pm$ SD triplicate determinations (n = 10). Values in same row with different alphabet are significantly different (p < 0.05).

Table 2. Effect of *P. berghei* and ascorbic acid treatments on parasitized mice plasma proteins and some liver function enzymes.

Parameters	Control	PnT	P+asT
Total Protein (g/L)	67.72 ± 4.17^a	89.43 ± 6.24^b	70.36 ± 2.70^a
Albumin (g/L)	36.63 ± 2.15^a	39.14 ± 3.50^a	38.62 ± 1.60^a
Globulin (g/L)	31.09 ± 2.65^a	50.29 ± 6.18^b	31.75 ± 3.67^a
AST Activity (U/L)	32.07 ± 5.41^a	36.55 ± 4.93^a	35.61 ± 3.64^a
ALT Activity (U/L)	28.17 ± 4.93^a	30.67 ± 2.86^a	28.74 ± 3.45^a
GGT Activity (U/L)	12.22 ± 2.34^a	14.27 ± 2.43^a	13.07 ± 2.52^a

Mean $\pm$ SD triplicate determinations (n = 10). Values in same row with different alphabet are significantly different (p < 0.05).

Table 3. Effect of *P. berghei* and ascorbic acid treatments on MDA, glutathione and some antioxidant enzymes of parasitized mice.

Parameters	Control	PnT	P+asT
Malondialdehyde (nmole/mL)	3.36 ± 0.71^a	6.54 ± 0.44^b	4.76 ± 0.54^c
Superoxide Dismutase (U/L)	148.72 ± 10.81^a	58.18 ± 18.78^b	85.21 ± 4.27^c
Catalase (U/L)	199.70 ± 0.14^a	166.27 ± 5.92^b	186.33 ± 9.16^c
Glu-6-P Dehydrogenase (U/L)	29.97 ± 0.78^a	33.55 ± 1.68^a	31.88 ± 1.78^a
Reduced Glutathione (ug/mL)	3.83 ± 0.19^a	3.48 ± 0.19^a	3.49 ± 0.26^a

Mean $\pm$ SD triplicate determinations (n = 10). Values in same row with different alphabet are significantly different (p < 0.05).

The significant reductions in total serum protein and globulin levels observed in parasitized and ascorbic acid treated mice may be linked with the formation of blood cells in the bone marrow as synthesis of blood cells may reduce the stress on the surviving T-cells and its complements in producing and secreting antibody molecules in an attempt to ameliorate the effects of the infecting parasites. Kidney cells appear to be very amenable to ascorbic acid treatment under parasitized condition as treatment is observed to significantly reduce oxidative stress observed in PnT and brought values near that of control group. The reductions in liver GSH level SOD and CAT enzyme activities observed in this study are pointers to the fact that the ascorbic acid may have reacted with other molecule to inhibit these enzymes causing the reduction in their activities, therefore resulting in the utilization of cellular reduced glutathione.

From these observations a conclusion can be drawn, that under parasitized condition in mice, ascorbic acid treatment may affect erythrocytes fragility by possibly in-

Table 4. Effects of parasites and ascorbic acid treatments on MDA, glutathione and antioxidant enzymes of parasitized mice organs.

Parameters	HERAT			LIVER			KIDNEY		
	Control	PnT	P+asT	Control	PnT	P+asT	Control	PnT	P+asT
MDA(nmole/g)	0.54 ± 0.17 [a]	0.59 ± 0.09 [a]	0.58 ± 0.11 [a]	0.74 ± 0.14 [a]	0.79 ± 0.12 [a]	0.67 ± 0.15 [a]	0.66 ± 0.10 [a]	0.71 ± 0.12 [b]	0.61 ± 0.08 [a]
SOD (U/mg)	41.51 ± 8.22 [a]	41.34 ± 7.63 [a]	41.34 ± 7.63 [a]	57.32 ± 12.53 [a]	66.67 ± 8.26 [b]	41.64 ± 7.31 [c]	41.51 ± 9.70 [a]	40.91 ± 3.16 [a]	41.34 ± 7.23 [a]
CAT (U/L)	24.89 ± 0.75 [a]	24.63 ± 0.50 [a]	24.63 ± 0.35 [a]	38.57 ± 4.71 [a]	44.16 ± 3.06 [b]	34.32 ± 5.33 [c]	24.66 ± 1.80 [a]	23.89 ± 2.47 [a]	24.31 ± 2.04 [a]
G6PD (U/mg)	0.04 ± 0.11 [a]	0.03 ± 0.08 [a]	0.03 ± 0.10 [a]	0.07 ± 0.01 [a]	0.05 ± 0.01 [b]	0.05 ± 0.01 [c]	0.04 ± 0.10 [a]	0.03 ± 0.08 [a]	0.03 ± 0.04 [a]
GSH (ug/mg)	0.37 ± 0.02 [a]	0.37 ± 0.02 [a]	0.36 ± 0.03 [a]	0.69 ± 0.10 [a]	0.58 ± 0.10 [b]	0.56 ± 0.20 [c]	0.37 ± 0.02 [a]	0.37 ± 0.02 [a]	0.37 ± 0.02 [a]

Mean ± SD triplicate determinations (n = 10). Values in same row with different alphabet are significantly different (p < 0.05).

ducing erythropoesis in bone marrow and may reduce MDA formation by supplying electrons to membrane tocopherol radicals to reduce lipid peroxidation.

REFERENCES

Atamna H, Ginsburg H (1997). The malaria parasite supplies glutathione to its host cell-investigation of glutathione transport and metabolism in human erythrocytes infected with Plasmodium falciparum. Mol. Biochem. Parasitol. 61:231-242.

Behrman HR, Kodaman HR, Preston SL, Goa S (2001). Oxidative stress and the ovary. J. Soc. Gynaecol. Invest. 8: S40-S42.

Deslauriers R, Butler K, Smith IC (1987). Oxidative stress in Malaria as probed by stable nitroxide radicals in erythrocytes infected with Plasmodium berghei: The effects of Primaquine and chloroquine. Biochim. Biophys. Acta. 931: 267-275.

Frei B, Stocker R, England L, Ames BN (1990). Ascorbate: the most effective antioxidant in human blood plasma. Adv. Exp. Med. and Biol. 264: 155-163.

Gora D, Sandhya M, Shiv G, Praveen S (2006). Oxidative stress, α-Tocopherol, Ascorbic acid and Reduced Glutathione Status in Schzophrnics. Ind. J. Clin. Biochem. 21(2): 34-38.

Gutteridge JMC, Halliwell B (1994). Antioxidants in nutrition, health and disease. Oxford University Press, Oxford pp. 45-120

Har-El R, Marva E, Chevion M, Golenser J (1993). Is hemin responsible for the susceptibility of plasmodia to oxidative stress?. Free Radic. Res. 17: 249- 262.

Hunt NH, Stocker R (1990). Oxidative stress and the redox status of malaria infected erythrocytes. Blood Cells. 16: 499 –526.

Iyawe HOT, Onigbinde AO (2009). Impact of Plasmodium berghei and Chloroquine on Haematological and Antioxidant Indices in Mice. Asian. J. Biochem. 4 (1): 30 -35.

Iyawe HOT, Onigbinde AO Aina OO (2006). Effect of chloroquine and ascorbic acid interaction on the oxidative stress of Plasmodium berghei infected mice. Int. J. Pharmacol. 2(1): 1-4.

Karupiah G, Hunt NG, King NJ Chaudhri G (2000). NADPH oxidase, Nrampl and nitric oxide synthase 2 in the host antimalarial response. Rev. Immunogent. 2: 387-415

Mann GV, Newton P (1975). The membrane transport of ascorbic acid. Ann. N. Y. Acad. Sci. 258: 243-252.

Nmorsi OPG, Ukwandu CD, Oladokun IAA, Elozino SE (2007). Severe Plasmodium falciparum malaria in some Nigerian children. J. Pediat. Infect. Dis. 2: 205-210.

Postma NS, Mommers EC, Eling WM, Zuidema J (1996). Oxidative stress in Malaria; Implication for prevention and therapy. Pham. World Sci. 18 (4): 121 – 129.

Potter SM, Mitchell AJ, Cowden WB, Sanni LA, Dinauer M, De Haan JB, Hunt NH (2005). Phagocyte-derived reactive oxygen species do not influence the progression of murine blood-stage malaria infections. Infect. Immun. 73(8): 4941-4947.

Sies H (1991). Glutathione and its role in cellular functions. Free Radic. Biol. Med. 27: 916 – 921.

World Health Organization (2000). Severe falciparum malaria. Trans R. Soc. Trop. Med. Hyg. 94(Suppl. 1): S1- S90.

Permissions

All chapters in this book were first published in AJBR, by Academic Journals; hereby published with permission under the Creative Commons Attribution License or equivalent. Every chapter published in this book has been scrutinized by our experts. Their significance has been extensively debated. The topics covered herein carry significant findings which will fuel the growth of the discipline. They may even be implemented as practical applications or may be referred to as a beginning point for another development.

The contributors of this book come from diverse backgrounds, making this book a truly international effort. This book will bring forth new frontiers with its revolutionizing research information and detailed analysis of the nascent developments around the world.

We would like to thank all the contributing authors for lending their expertise to make the book truly unique. They have played a crucial role in the development of this book. Without their invaluable contributions this book wouldn't have been possible. They have made vital efforts to compile up to date information on the varied aspects of this subject to make this book a valuable addition to the collection of many professionals and students.

This book was conceptualized with the vision of imparting up-to-date information and advanced data in this field. To ensure the same, a matchless editorial board was set up. Every individual on the board went through rigorous rounds of assessment to prove their worth. After which they invested a large part of their time researching and compiling the most relevant data for our readers.

The editorial board has been involved in producing this book since its inception. They have spent rigorous hours researching and exploring the diverse topics which have resulted in the successful publishing of this book. They have passed on their knowledge of decades through this book. To expedite this challenging task, the publisher supported the team at every step. A small team of assistant editors was also appointed to further simplify the editing procedure and attain best results for the readers.

Apart from the editorial board, the designing team has also invested a significant amount of their time in understanding the subject and creating the most relevant covers. They scrutinized every image to scout for the most suitable representation of the subject and create an appropriate cover for the book.

The publishing team has been an ardent support to the editorial, designing and production team. Their endless efforts to recruit the best for this project, has resulted in the accomplishment of this book. They are a veteran in the field of academics and their pool of knowledge is as vast as their experience in printing. Their expertise and guidance has proved useful at every step. Their uncompromising quality standards have made this book an exceptional effort. Their encouragement from time to time has been an inspiration for everyone.

The publisher and the editorial board hope that this book will prove to be a valuable piece of knowledge for researchers, students, practitioners and scholars across the globe.

List of Contributors

Abdullahi Mann
Department of Science Laboratory Technology, Federal Polytechnic Bida, P. M. B. 55, Bida, Niger State, Nigeria

Evans C. Egwim
Department of Biochemistry, Federal University of Technology Minna, P. M. B. 65, Minna Niger State Nigeria

Barnabas Banji
Department of Science Laboratory Technology, Federal Polytechnic Bida, P. M. B. 55, Bida, Niger State, Nigeria

Nda-Umar Abdukadir
Department of Science Laboratory Technology, Federal Polytechnic Bida, P. M. B. 55, Bida, Niger State, Nigeria

Mohammed Gbate
Department of Science Laboratory Technology, Federal Polytechnic Bida, P. M. B. 55, Bida, Niger State, Nigeria

J. T. Ekanem
Department of Biochemistry, University of Ilorin, P. M. B. 1515, Ilorin, Kwara State Nigeria

SP Songca
Faculty of Science, Engineering and Technology, P.O. Box 19712, Tecoma, 5247, East London, South Africa

C Sebothoma
Department of Chemistry and Biochemistry, Faculty of Science, University of Limpopo, Private Bag X 235, Medunsa, 0204, South Africa

BB Samuel
Department of Paraclinical Science, Faculty of Veterinary Science, University of Pretoria, Onderstepoort, 0110, Pretoria, South Africa

JN Eloff
Department of Paraclinical Science, Faculty of Veterinary Science, University of Pretoria, Onderstepoort, 0110, Pretoria, South Africa

P. Praveen Kumar
Food Testing Laboratory, Indian Institute of Crop Processing Technology, Pudukkottai Road, Thanjavur-613 005. Tamil Nadu, India

S. Kumaravel
Food Testing Laboratory, Indian Institute of Crop Processing Technology, Pudukkottai Road, Thanjavur-613 005. Tamil Nadu, India

C. Lalitha
Department of Biochemistry, Dhanalkshmi Srinivasan Arts and Science College for Women, Perambalur-621212, Tamil Nadu, India

C. O. Jayeola
Crop Processing and Utilization Division, Cocoa Research Institute of Nigeria, P. M. B., 5244, Ibadan, Oyo State, Nigeria

A. Oluwadun
Department of Medical Microbiology and Parasitology, Obafemi Awolowo College of Health Science, Olabisi Onabanjo University Sagamu, Ogun State, Nigeria

O. Olubamiwa
Crop Processing and Utilization Division, Cocoa Research Institute of Nigeria, P. M. B., 5244, Ibadan, Oyo State, Nigeria

H. I. Effedua
Department of Medical Microbiology and Parasitology, Obafemi Awolowo College of Health Science, Olabisi Onabanjo University Sagamu, Ogun State, Nigeria

O. E Kale
Department of Pharmacology, Obafemi Awolowo College of Health Science, Olabisi Onabanjo University Sagamu, Ogun State, Nigeria

S. Ramakrishnan
Department of Biotechnology, Sri Paramakalyani College, Alwarkurichi – 627 412, Tirunelveli District, Tamil Nadu, India

R. Venkataraman
Post graduate and Research Department of Chemistry, Sri Paramakalyani College, Alwarkurichi – 627 412, Tirunelveli District, Tamil Nadu, India

A. J. Mahadesh Prasad
Department of Biochemistry Manasagangotri, University of Mysore, Mysore-570006, India

K. Kemparaju
Department of Biochemistry Manasagangotri, University of Mysore, Mysore-570006, India

Elizabeth A. Frank
Department of Biochemistry Manasagangotri, University of Mysore, Mysore-570006, India

Cletus J. M. D'Souza
Department of Biochemistry Manasagangotri, University of Mysore, Mysore-570006, India

Chioma A. Anosike
Department of Biochemistry, University of Nigeria, Nsukka. Enugu State, Nigeria

Onyechi Obidoa
Department of Biochemistry, University of Nigeria, Nsukka. Enugu State, Nigeria

Lawrence U. S. Ezeanyika
Department of Biochemistry, University of Nigeria, Nsukka. Enugu State, Nigeria

Meshach M. Nwuba
Department of Biochemistry, University of Nigeria, Nsukka. Enugu State, Nigeria

S. Adekunle Adeniran
Department of Biochemistry, Ladoke Akintola University of Technology, Ogbomoso, Oyo State, Nigeria

L. Adedeji Adebayo
Department of Biochemistry, Ladoke Akintola University of Technology, Ogbomoso, Oyo State, Nigeria

B. Krishna Reddy
Department of Genetics, Osmania University, Hyderabad, A.P, India

M. Balaji
Department of Biotechnology, University of Kashmir, Srinagar, 190006, India

P. Uma Reddy
Department of Genetics, Osmania University, Hyderabad, A.P, India

G. Sailaja
Department of Biotechnology, University of Kashmir, Srinagar, 190006, India

K. Vaidyanath
Department of Genetics, Osmania University, Hyderabad, A.P, India

G. Narasimha
Department of Virology, Sri Venkateswara University, Tirupati, A.P, 517502, India

Showkat Ahmad Ganie
Department of Biochemistry University of Kashmir, Srinagar, 190006, India

Mohmmad Afzal Zargar
Department of Biochemistry University of Kashmir, Srinagar, 190006, India

Akbar Masood
Department of Biochemistry University of Kashmir, Srinagar, 190006, India

Ehtishamul Haq
Department of Biotechnology, University of Kashmir, Srinagar, 190006, India

Hanaa H. Abd El-Baky
Plant Biochemistry Department, National Research Centre, Dokki, Cairo, Egypt

O. C. Adumanya
Department of Nutrition and Dietetics, Imo State Polytechnic, Umuagwo, Imo State, Nigeria

A. A. Uwakwe
Department of Biochemistry, University of Port Harcourt, Rivers State, Nigeria

O. B. Odeghe
Department of Biochemistry, University of Port Harcourt, Rivers State, Nigeria

E. B. Essien
Department of Biochemistry, University of Port Harcourt, Rivers State, Nigeria

T. O. Okere
Department of Nutrition and Dietetics, Imo State Polytechnic, Umuagwo, Imo State, Nigeria

Mushafau A. Akinsanya
Department of Medical Biochemistry, Faculty of Basic Medical Sciences, Lagos State University College of Medicine (LASUCOM), PMB 21266, Ikeja, Lagos, Nigeria

Taiwo T. Adeniyi
Department of Biochemistry, College of Natural Sciences, University of Agriculture, PMB 2240, Abeokuta, Ogun State, Nigeria

Gabriel O Ajayi
Department of Medical Biochemistry, Faculty of Basic Medical Sciences, Lagos State University College of Medicine (LASUCOM), PMB 21266, Ikeja, Lagos, Nigeria

Musbau A. Oyedele
Department of Biochemistry, College of Natural Sciences, University of Agriculture, PMB 2240, Abeokuta, Ogun State, Nigeria

Chavan Atish
Department of Biotechnology, School of Bioengineering, SRM University, Kattankulathur, Tamil Nadu, India-603203, India

Suman Diggi Prasad
Department of Biotechnology, School of Bioengineering, SRM University, Kattankulathur, Tamil Nadu, India-603203, India

Rawal Mukesh
Department of Biotechnology, School of Bioengineering, SRM University, Kattankulathur, Tamil Nadu, India-603203, India

Kandasamy Surendran
Central Laboratory, Department of Biochemistry, SRM Medical College Hospital and Research Centre, SRM University, Kattankulathur, Tamil Nadu, India- 603203, India

Sivapatham Sundaresan
Department of Medical Research, SRM Medical College Hospital and Research Centre, SRM University, Kattankulathur, Tamil Nadu, India- 603203, India

Thangarajan Thangapannerselvem
Department of Biochemistry, SRM Medical College Hospital and Research Centre, SRM University, Kattankulathur, Tamil Nadu, India- 603203, India

Kelechukwu Clarence Obimba
Department of Biochemistry, College of Natural and Applied Sciences, Michael Okpara University of Agriculture Umudike. Abia State, Nigeria

G. S. El-Baroty
Department of Biochemistry, Faculty of Agriculture, Cairo University, Cairo, Egypt

H. H. Abd El-Baky
Department of Biochemistry, Faculty of Agriculture, Cairo University, Cairo, Egypt

R. S. Farag
Department of Plant Biochemistry, National Research Centre, Dokki, Cairo, Egypt

M. A. Saleh
Department of Chemistry, Texas Southern University, Houston, Texas, USA

Adenike Kuku
Department of Biochemistry, Obafemi Awolowo University, Ile-Ife, Nigeria

Oludele Odekanyin
Department of Biochemistry, Obafemi Awolowo University, Ile-Ife, Nigeria

Kemi Adeniran
Department of Biochemistry, Obafemi Awolowo University, Ile-Ife, Nigeria

Mary Adewusi
Department of Biochemistry, Obafemi Awolowo University, Ile-Ife, Nigeria

Toyin Olonade
Department of Biochemistry, Obafemi Awolowo University, Ile-Ife, Nigeria

R. Vennila
Center of Advanced Study in Marine Biology, Annamalai University, Portonovo, Tamil Nadu, India

R. K. Rajesh kumar
Center of Advanced Study in Marine Biology, Annamalai University, Portonovo, Tamil Nadu, India

S. Kanchana
Center of Advanced Study in Marine Biology, Annamalai University, Portonovo, Tamil Nadu, India

M. Arumugam
Center of Advanced Study in Marine Biology, Annamalai University, Portonovo, Tamil Nadu, India

T. Balasubramanian
Center of Advanced Study in Marine Biology, Annamalai University, Portonovo, Tamil Nadu, India

L. A. Alli
Department of Medical Biochemistry, College of Health Sciences, University of Abuja, Nigeria

A. A. Adesokan
Department of Biochemistry, Faculty of Sciences, University of Ilorin, Nigeria

O. A. Salawu
Department of Pharmacology and Toxicology, National Institute for Pharmaceutical Research and Development (NIPRD), Abuja, Nigeria

M. A. Akanji
Department of Biochemistry, Faculty of Sciences, University of Ilorin, Nigeria

A. Y. Tijani
Department of Pharmacology and Toxicology, National Institute for Pharmaceutical Research and Development (NIPRD), Abuja, Nigeria

P. Dzomba
Chemistry Department, Faculty of Science Education, P. Bag 1020, Bindura, Zimbabwe

E. Togarepi
Chemistry Department, Faculty of Science Education, P. Bag 1020, Bindura, Zimbabwe

C. Mahamadi
Chemistry Department, Faculty of Science Education, P. Bag 1020, Bindura, Zimbabwe

Sudeshna Bhattacharya
BOSE INSTITUTE, Division of Plant Biology, MC, 93/1 APC Road, Kolkata – 700 009, India

Swati Sen-Mandi
BOSE INSTITUTE, Division of Plant Biology, MC, 93/1 APC Road, Kolkata – 700 009, India

B. Sadeghi-Nejad
Department of Mycoparasitology, Medical School, Joundi-Shapour University of Medical Sciences, Ahwaz, Iran

S. S Deokule
Department of Botany, University of Pune Ganeshkhind, Pune- 411007, India

Stuart .J. Semple
Department of Biokinetics and Sport Science, University of Zululand, KwaDlangezwa, South Africa

Andrew .J. McKune
School of Physiotherapy, Optometry and Sports Science, University of KwaZulu-Natal, South Africa

Rubina Majid
Department of Biochemistry University of Kashmir J&K India

Latief Ahmad
Division of Agronomy SKUAST-Kashmir J&K India

M. A. Zargar
Department of Biochemistry University of Kashmir J&K India

Salwa H. N. Al-Rubae'i
Chemistry Department, College of Science, Al-Mustansiriya University, Baghdad, Iraq

Abass K. Al-Musawi
Chemistry Department, College of Science, Al-Mustansiriya University, Baghdad, Iraq

I. Onyesom
Department of Medical Biochemistry, Delta State University, Abraka, Nigeria

R. C. Ekeanyanwu
Department of Chemical Science, Novena University, Ogume, Delta State, Nigeria

N. Achuka
Department of Chemical Science, Novena University, Ogume, Delta State, Nigeria

M. A. Adaikpoh
Department of Biochemistry, Faculty of Life Sciences, University of Benin, P. M. B 1154, Benin City, Nigeria

F. O. Obi
Department of Biochemistry, Faculty of Life Sciences, University of Benin, P. M. B 1154, Benin City, Nigeria

Tuty Anggraini
Faculty of Life and Environmental Sciences, Prefectural University of Hiroshima, 562 Nanatsuka, Shobara, Hiroshima 727-0023, Japan
Faculty of Agricultural Technology, Kampus Unand Limau Manis, Andalas University, 25163 West Sumatra, Indonesia
562 Nanatsuka, Shobara, Hiroshima 727-0023, Japan

Akihiro Tai
Faculty of Life and Environmental Sciences, Prefectural University of Hiroshima, 562 Nanatsuka, Shobara, Hiroshima 727-0023, Japan

Tomoyuki Yoshino
Faculty of Life and Environmental Sciences, Prefectural University of Hiroshima, 562 Nanatsuka, Shobara, Hiroshima 727-0023, Japan

Tomio Itani
Faculty of Life and Environmental Sciences, Prefectural University of Hiroshima, 562 Nanatsuka, Shobara, Hiroshima 727-0023, Japan

Ngozi O. A. Imaga
Department of Biochemistry, College of Medicine, University of Lagos, P. M. B. 12003, Idi-Araba, Lagos State, Nigeria

A. Shaire Esther
Department of Biochemistry, College of Medicine, University of Lagos, P. M. B. 12003, Idi-Araba, Lagos State, Nigeria

Ogbeide Samson
Department of Biochemistry, College of Medicine, University of Lagos, P. M. B. 12003, Idi-Araba, Lagos State, Nigeria

Samuel K. Akindele
Department of Biochemistry, Nigerian Institute of Medical Research, P. M. B. 2013, Yaba, Lagos State, Nigeria

R. C. Ekeanyanwu
Department of Biochemistry, Imo State University, P.M.B 2000, Owerri, Imo State, Nigeria

O. F. Etienajirhevwe
Department of Science Laboratory Technology, Delta State Polytechnic, Otefe, Nigeria

Kudakwashe Chitindingu
Department of Biochemistry, University of Zimbabwe, M. P. 167, Mount Pleasant, Harare, Zimbabwe
Department of Biotechnology, Chinhoyi University of Technology, Chinhoyi, Zimbabwe

Jill J. F. Chitindingu
Department of Biochemistry, University of Zimbabwe, M. P. 167, Mount Pleasant, Harare, Zimbabwe

Mudadi A. N. Benhura
Department of Biochemistry, University of Zimbabwe, M. P. 167, Mount Pleasant, Harare, Zimbabwe

Amos Marume
School of Pharmacy, College of Health Sciences, University of Zimbabwe, M. P. 167, Mount Pleasant, Harare, Zimbabwe

Isaac Mutingwende
School of Pharmacy, College of Health Sciences, University of Zimbabwe, M. P. 167, Mount Pleasant, Harare, Zimbabwe

Michael Bhebhe
Department of Biochemistry, University of Zimbabwe, M. P. 167, Mount Pleasant, Harare, Zimbabwe

Maud Muchuweti
Department of Biochemistry, University of Zimbabwe, M. P. 167, Mount Pleasant, Harare, Zimbabwe

H. O. T. Iyawe
Department of Biochemistry Ambrose Alli University, P. M. B. 14, Ekpoma Nigeria

A. O. Onigbinde
Department of Biochemistry Ambrose Alli University, P. M. B. 14, Ekpoma Nigeria

www.ingramcontent.com/pod-product-compliance
Lightning Source LLC
Chambersburg PA
CBHW080652200326
41458CB00013B/4822